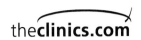

IMMUNOLOGY AND ALLERGY CLINICS OF NORTH AMERICA

Hypereosinophilic Syndromes

GUEST EDITOR
Amy D. Klion, MD

CONSULTING EDITOR
Rafeul Alam, MD, PhD

August 2007 • Volume 27 • Number 3

SAUNDERS

An Imprint of Elsevier, Inc.
PHILADELPHIA   LONDON   TORONTO   MONTREAL   SYDNEY   TOKYO

W.B. SAUNDERS COMPANY
A Division of Elsevier Inc.

Elsevier, Inc., 1600 John F. Kennedy Blvd., Suite 1800, Philadelphia, PA 19103-2899

http://www.theclinics.com

IMMUNOLOGY AND ALLERGY CLINICS	Volume 27, Number 3
OF NORTH AMERICA	ISSN 0889-8561
August 2007	ISBN-13: 978-1-4160-5083-4
Editor: Patrick Manley	ISBN-10: 1-4160-5083-3

The ideas and opinions expressed in *Immunology and Allergy Clinics of North America* do not necessarily reflect those of the Publisher. The Publisher does not assume any responsibility for any injury and/or damage to persons or property arising out of or related to any use of the material contained in this periodical. The reader is advised to check the appropriate medical literature and the product information currently provided by the manufacturer of each drug to be administered to verify the dosage, the method and duration of administration, or contraindications. It is the responsibility of the treating physician or other health care professional, relying on independent experience and knowledge of the patient, to determine drug dosages and the best treatment for the patient. Mention of any product in this issue should not be construed as endorsement by the contributors, editors, or the Publisher of the product or manufacturers' claims.

Immunology and Allergy Clinics of North America (ISSN 0889-8561) is published quarterly by Elsevier Inc., 360 Park Avenue South, New York, NY 10010-1710. Months of issue are February, May, August, and November. Business and Editorial offices: 1600 John F. Kennedy Blvd., Suite 1800, Philadelphia, PA 19103-2899. Customer Service office: 6277 Sea Harbor Drive, Orlando, FL 32887-4800. Periodicals postage paid at New York, NY and additional mailing offices. Subscription prices are $193.00 per year for US individuals, $308.00 per year for US institutions, $94.00 per year for US students and residents, $237.00 per year for Canadian individuals, 127.00 per year for Canadian students, $374.00 per year for Canadian institutions, $253.00 per year for international individuals, $374.00 per year for international institutions, $127.00 per year for international students. To receive student/resident rate, orders must be accompanied by name of affiliated institution, date of term, and the *signature* of program/residency coordinator on institution letterhead. Orders will be billed at individual rate until proof of status is received. Foreign air speed delivery is included in all *Clinics* subscription prices. All prices are subject to change without notice. POSTMASTER: Send address changes to *Immunology and Allergy Clinics of North America*, Elsevier Periodicals Customer Service, 6277 Sea Harbor Drive, Orlando, FL 32887-4800. **Customer Service: 1-800-654-2452 (US). From outside of the US, call 1-407-345-4000. E-mail: hhspcs@wbsaunders.com.**

Reprints. For copies of 100 or more, of articles in this publication, please contact the Commercial Reprints Department, Elsevier Inc., 360 Park Avenue South, New York, New York 10010-1710. Tel. (212) 633-3813 Fax: (212) 462-1935 e-mail: reprints@elsevier.com.

Immunology and Allergy Clinics of North America is covered in Index Medicus, Current Contents/Life Sciences, Science Citation Index, ISI/BIOMED, Chemical Abstracts, and EMBASE/Excerpta Medica.

Printed in the United States of America.

CONSULTING EDITOR

RAFEUL ALAM, MD, PhD, Veda and Chauncey Ritter Chair in Immunology; Professor and Director, Division of Allergy and Immunology, National Jewish Medical and Research Center, Denver, Colorado

GUEST EDITOR

AMY D. KLION, MD, Staff Physician, Laboratory of Parasitic Diseases, National Institutes of Health, Bethesda, Maryland

CONTRIBUTORS

STEVEN J. ACKERMAN, PhD, Professor of Biochemistry, Molecular Genetics, and Medicine, Department of Biochemistry and Molecular Genetics, The University of Illinois at Chicago School of Medicine, Chicago, Illinois

BARBARA J. BAIN, MBBS, FRACP, FRCPath, Professor of Diagnostic Haemotology and Honorary Consultant Haemologist, Department of Haemotology, St. Mary's Hospital Campus of Imperial College Faculty of Medicine, St. Mary's Hospital, London, United Kingdom

BRUCE S. BOCHNER, MD, Professor of Medicine, Department of Medicine, Division of Allergy and Clinical Immunology, Johns Hopkins University School of Medicine, Johns Hopkins Asthma and Allergy Center, Baltimore, Maryland

JOSPEH H. BUTTERFIELD, MD, Professor of Medicine, Division of Allergic Diseases, Mayo Clinic; and Mayo Clinic College of Medicine, Rochester, Minnesota

ELIE COGAN, MD, PhD, Professor and Dean of the Faculty of Medicine, Université Libre de Bruxelles; and Head, Department of Internal Medicine, Erasme Hospital, Université Libre de Bruxelles, Brussels, Belgium

JAN COOLS, PhD, Department of Molecular and Developmental Genetics, L.U. Leuven, Leuven, Belgium

SARAH H. FLETCHER, MBBChir, MRCP, Specialist Registrar in Haemotology, Department of Haemotology, St. Mary's Hospital Campus of Imperial College Faculty of Medicine, St. Mary's Hospital, London, United Kingdom

GERALD J. GLEICH, MD, Professor of Dermatology and Medicine, Departments of Dermatology and Medicine, University of Utah Health Sciences Center, University of Utah, Salt Lake City, Utah

MICHAEL GOLDMAN, MD, PhD, Professor of Immunology, Université Libre de Bruxelles, Brussels; and Director, Institute for Medical Immunology, Université Libre de Bruxelles, Gosselies, Belgium

McDONALD K. HORNE III, MD, Senior Clinical Investigator, Hematology Service, Department of Laboratory Medicine, W.G. Magnuson Clinical Center, National Institutes of Health, Bethesda, Maryland

AMY D. KLION, MD, Staff Physician, Laboratory of Parasitic Diseases, National Institutes of Health, Bethesda, Maryland

KRISTIN M. LEIFERMAN, MD, Professor of Dermatology, Department of Dermatology, University of Utah Health Sciences Center, University of Utah, Salt Lake City, Utah

THOMAS B. NUTMAN, MD, Head, Helminth Immunology Section; and Head, Clinical Parasitology Unit, Laboratory of Parasitic Diseases, National Institute of Allergy and Infectious Diseases, National Institutes of Health, Bethesda, Maryland

PRINCESS U. OGBOGU, MD, Clinical Fellow, Allergy and Immunology, National Institute of Allergy and Infectious Diseases, National Institutes of Health, Bethesda, Maryland

MARGOT S. PETERS, MD, Rochester, Minnesota

DOUGLAS R. ROSING, MD, Head, Cardiology Consultation Service, Cardiology Branch, National Heart, Lung, and Blood Institute, National Institutes of Health, Bethesda, Maryland

MARC E. ROTHENBERG, MD, PhD, Professor of Pediatrics and Director, Division of Immunology and Allergy, Department of Pediatrics, Cincinnati Children's Hospital Medical Center, University of Cincinnati, College of Medicine, Cincinnati, Ohio

FLORENCE ROUFOSSE, MD PhD, Associate Professor of Medicine, Department of Internal Medicine, Erasme Hospital, Université Libre de Bruxelles, Brussels; and Clinical Research Associate (Belgian National Fund for Scientific Research), Institute for Medical Immunology, Université Libre de Bruxelles, Gosselies, Belgium

JAVED SHEIKH, MD, Assistant Professor of Medicine, Division of Allergy and Inflammation, Beth Israel Deaconess Medical Center, Harvard Medical School, Boston, Massachusetts

HANS-UWE SIMON, MD, PhD, Department of Pharmacology, University of Bern, Bern, Switzerland

MICHAEL E. WECHSLER, MD, MMSc, Associate Director, BWH Asthma Research Center, Pulmonary and Critical Care Division, Brigham and Women's Hospital; and Assistant Professor, Harvard Medical School, Boston, Massachusetts

PETER F. WELLER, MD, Professor of Medicine, Division of Allergy and Inflammation; and Division of Infectious Diseases, Beth Deaconess Medical Center, Harvard Medical School, Boston, Massachusetts

LI ZUO, MD, Clinical Fellow, Division of Immunology and Allergy, Department of Pediatrics, Cincinnati Children's Hospital Medical Center, University of Cincinnati, College of Medicine, Cincinnati, Ohio

CONTENTS

Hypereosinophilic syndrome (HES) or syndromes are disorders characterized by chronic peripheral blood hypereosinophilia with damage to various organs due toeosinophilic infiltration and release of mediators. HES is most accurately described as a collection of heterogeneous disorders, with some similarities in clinical features, but many differences. Based on recent advances in molecular and genetic diagnostic techniques and increasing experience with differences in clinical features and prognosis, some subtypes of HES have been defined, such as myeloproliferative variants, including chronic eosinophilic leukemia, and lymphocytic variants, but other subtypes remain undefined. Recent evidence suggests that, in addition to differences in clinical features, the range of complications, treatment options, and prognoses differs significantly among the myeloproliferative, lymphocytic, and undefined variants of HES.

The increased numbers of activated eosinophils in the blood and tissues that typically accompany hypereosinophilic disorders result from a variety of mechanisms. Exciting advances in translating discoveries achieved from mouse models and molecular strategies to the clinic have led to a flurry of new therapeutics specifically designed to target eosinophil-associated diseases. So far, this form of hypothesis testing in humans in vivo through pharmacology generally has supported the paradigms generated in vitro and in animal models, raising hopes that a spectrum of novel therapies soon may become available to help those who have eosinophil-associated diseases.

disease identities. These diseases include primary eosinophil associated gastrointestinal diseases, gastrointestinal eosinophilia in hypereosinophilic syndrome, and all gastrointestinal eosinophilic states associated with known causes. Each of these diseases has its unique features but there is no absolute boundary between them. All three groups of gastrointestinal eosinophila are described in this article, although the focus is on primary gastrointestinal eosinophilia.

The hypereosinophilic syndromes (HESs) are characterized by persistent marked eosinophilia (>1500 eosinophils/mm^3), the absence of a primary cause of eosinophilia (such as parasitic or allergic disease), and evidence of eosinophil-mediated end organ damage. Cardiovascular complications of HES are a major source of morbidity and mortality in these disorders. The most characteristic cardiovascular abnormality in HES is endomyocardial fibrosis. Patients who have an HES also may develop thrombosis, particularly in the cardiac ventricles, but also occasionally in deep veins. Because of the rarity of these disorders, specific guidelines for the management of the cardiac and thrombotic complications of HES are lacking. This article reviews the diagnosis and management of the cardiovascular manifestations of HES.

Acute eosinophilic pneumonia, chronic eosinophilia, Churg-Strauss syndrome, and the hypereosinophilic syndrome are pulmonary eosinophilic syndromes characterized by an increased number of eosinophils in peripheral blood, in lung tissue, in sputum, in bronchoalveolar lavage fluid, or in all of these. These pulmonary eosinophilic syndromes generally are characterized by increased respiratory symptoms, abnormal radiographic appearance, and the potential for systemic manifestations. It is critical to exclude other causes of eosinophilia in patients who have lung disease, to make a quick diagnosis, and to treat aggressively with corticosteroids and other therapies to prevent long-term sequelae.

The hypereosinophilic syndromes continue to challenge our clinical acumen and skills. Prednisone, hydroxyurea, and interferon alpha 2b are three of the oldest agents that allow control of eosinophilia and its devastating clinical consequences. They still work. As our experience with them has grown, it has become evident that use of these agents in combination will control eosinophilia in most patients. Moreover, with time, the doses can frequently be reduced. Even with the advent of newer agents for treatment of hypereosinophilic syndromes, these three medications still afford an excellent, cost-effective avenue for disease management.

There has been recent progress in the understanding of the pathogenesis of the hypereosinophilic syndromes (HES). This led to the distinction of subgroups, in which the underlying cause has been identified. Consequently, new treatment options became available, such as imatinib and mepolizumab, which proved to be promising. This article summarizes these new pharmacologic approaches to the therapy of HES.

Hyperosinophilic syndromes (HES) are a group of heterogeneous disorders many of which remain ill-defined. By definition, the HES must be distinguishedfrom other disorders with persistently elevated eosinophilia with a defined cause. Although marked eosinophilia worldwide is most commonly caused by helminth (worm) infections, the diagnostic approach must include noninfectious (nonparasitic) causes of marked eosinophilia as well.

With the introduction of new diagnostic methods and treatment modalities, it has become increasingly clear that hypereosinophilic syndromes (HES) are a heterogeneous group of disorders for which a single approach to treatment is insufficient. This article discusses current treatment modalities for myeloproliferative HES, idiopathic HES, and lymphocytic-variant HES.

FORTHCOMING ISSUES

VISIT THESE RELATED WEB SITES

Access your subscription at:
www.theclinics.com

ELSEVIER
SAUNDERS

Immunol Allergy Clin N Am
27 (2007) xi–xii

IMMUNOLOGY
AND ALLERGY
CLINICS
OF NORTH AMERICA

Foreword

The Recent Progress in Hypereosinophilic Syndrome

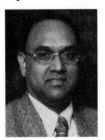

Rafeul Alam, MD, PhD
Consulting Editor

Although the physiologic function of eosinophils remains an enigma, the pathologic consequences of increased eosinophil number and eosinophil activation are well known. Hypereosinophilic syndrome (HES) is one of these eosinophilic conditions that can present with devastating and progressive multiorgan dysfunction. As the name suggests, this disorder is a syndrome, not a single disease entity. Tremendous progress has been made toward understanding the molecular basis of the myeloid variant of HES. The identification of a chromosomal deletion that leads to the expression of a spontaneously active kinase was a landmark discovery. More importantly, the expression of the fusion kinase *FIP1L1-PDGFRA* in a patient who has HES makes imatinib the treatment of choice. This is very important because imatinib is a relatively specific inhibitor for PDGFR (platelet-derived growth factor receptor), Abl family kinases (Abl1 and Abl2/Arg), and c-kit. Because of this narrow specificity, this agent has minimal side effects compared with other chemotherapeutic agents. Newer chemically related agents are now being tested clinically that are able to inhibit imatinib-resistant mutants of the tyrosine kinases. A clinical test to detect the fusion protein is now commercially available, which is of tremendous help to many practitioners.

FIP1L1-PDGFRA is expressed only in a subset of patients who have the myeloid form of HES. The exact mechanism of eosinophilia in other forms of HES is unclear. In some cases, proliferation of an aberrant CD3⁻CD4⁺

IL5-producing T cell population leads to eosinophilia. Chromosomal studies have detected persistent 6p deletion with progression to T cell lymphoma
in a few patients who have HES. Further, an impaired expression of the
CD3 gamma subunit of the T cell receptor complex has been detected.
Because IL-5 is at the root of eosinophilia in this form of the disease, an
anti–IL-5 antibody-based approach has proven to be of significant value
in controlling eosinophilia and clinical symptoms in these patients. Despite
this progress, major challenges remain ahead of us. What triggers the transition of myeloid as well as lymphoid HES to malignancy is unknown. It is
also unclear whether the current therapeutic approaches could prevent or
delay the malignant transformation of HES. To update the reader on the
state of the art, Dr. Amy Klion has brought together the leaders in the field,
who address the pathogenesis, disease variants, clinical diversity, organ-specific manifestation of HES, and the recent therapeutic advances. This is
a timely and important topic. The issue will benefit practitioners as well
as researchers, who deal with this rare but serious illness.

Rafeul Alam, MD, PhD
Head, Division of Allergy and Immunology
National Jewish Medical and Research Center
1400 Jackson Street
Denver, CO 80206, USA

E-mail address: alamr@njc.org

ELSEVIER
SAUNDERS

Immunol Allergy Clin N Am
27 (2007) xiii–xiv

IMMUNOLOGY
AND ALLERGY
CLINICS
OF NORTH AMERICA

Preface

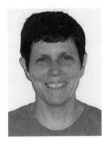

Amy D. Klion, MD
Guest Editor

Eosinophilia is a prominent feature of a wide variety of disorders, including allergic and atopic diseases, neoplasms, and helminth infections. However, the role of eosinophils in the pathogenesis of these disorders remains controversial. In contrast, hypereosinophilic syndromes (HES) are defined by the presence of marked eosinophilia (eosinophils $> 1500/\text{mm}^3$) and eosinophil-related end organ dysfunction. Consequently, HES provide a unique opportunity to study the relationship between eosinophil function, activation, and disease.

Whereas it was clear from the time of Chusid's classic definition in 1975 that HES are a heterogeneous group of disorders ranging from an aggressive myeloproliferative disease, reminiscent of leukemia, to a more benign form characterized by non life-threatening, but often times disabling, symptoms, it was not until recently that molecular and immunologic tests became available to identify specific etiologic subtypes of HES. These subtypes include a myeloproliferative variant associated with an interstitial deletion leading to a fusion tyrosine kinase (*FIP1L1/PDGFRA*-positive chronic eosinophilic leukemia) and a lymphocytic variant characterized by the presence of a clonal lymphocyte population secreting eosinophilopoietic cytokines. The identification of these subtypes has led to a reexamination of the definition, clinical manifestations, and treatment of HES. Nevertheless, despite our present diagnostic tools, as many as 50% of patients who have HES remain unclassified.

doi:10.1016/j.iac.2007.08.002   *immunology.theclinics.com*

In this issue of *Immunology and Allergy Clinics of North America*, international experts in the field of eosinophilia provide in-depth reviews of the approach to diagnosis, clinical spectrum and end organ manifestations, and options for treatment of HES, taking into account the recently described HES subtypes. The information in this issue is intended not only to provide a guide for clinicians taking care of patients who have HES, but also to highlight the recent research advances and gaps in our understanding of these rare disorders.

I would like to thank all of the authors who contributed their time and expertise; Dr. Rafeul Alam, who gave us the opportunity to publish this issue on HES; and Carla Holloway and Patrick Manley at Elsevier for their patience and editorial support.

Amy D. Klion, MD
Laboratory of Parasitic Diseases
National Institutes of Health
Building 4, Room 126
4 Center Drive
Bethesda, MD 20892, USA

E-mail address: aklion@nih.gov

ELSEVIER
SAUNDERS

Immunol Allergy Clin N Am
27 (2007) 333–355

IMMUNOLOGY
AND ALLERGY
CLINICS
OF NORTH AMERICA

Clinical Overview of Hypereosinophilic Syndromes

Javed Sheikh, MD[a],*, Peter F. Weller, MD[a,b]

[a]*Division of Allergy and Inflammation, Beth Israel Deaconess Medical Center,
Harvard Medical School, 330 Brookline Avenue, DA-617, Boston, MA 02215, USA*
[b]*Division of Infectious Diseases, Beth Israel Deaconess Medical Center,
Harvard Medical School, 330 Brookline Avenue, DA-617, Boston, MA 02215, USA*

History of hypereosinophilic syndromes

Elevated peripheral blood eosinophil counts are usually seen with helminthic parasitic infections (in countries where these parasites are common), atopic disease, and drug hypersensitivity [1,2]. In chronic cases of eosinophilia that are not secondary to these common diseases or other diseases such as malignancy and connective tissue disorders, one of the eosinophilic diseases must be considered [3]. Eosinophilic diseases include various relatively uncommon conditions characterized by tissue-associated eosinophilic inflammation and, in some cases, peripheral blood eosinophilia, such as the eosinophilic gastrointestinal diseases (EGIDs), Churg-Strauss syndrome, and what is known as the hypereosinophilic syndrome (HES) or hypereosinophilic syndromes (HESs) [4]. For a period of time, HES was referred to as the idiopathic hypereosinophilic syndrome [3], but with recent advances in knowledge of the underlying pathophysiology in a proportion of affected individuals, the use of the label "idiopathic" to describe the syndrome is no longer appropriate, and the term HES can now be used to encompass a range of types of HESs [5].

Cases of unexplained hypereosinophilia have been reported for more than a century [3,6], using terms such as Loffler's syndrome, Loeffler's fibroplastic endocarditis with eosinophilia, eosinophilic leukemia, and disseminated eosinophilic collagen disease; the terms vary, based on the clinical presentation and organs involved [7,8]. Hardy and Anderson [7] were the first to refer to these diseases collectively as "hypereosinophilic syndromes," in a 1968 review article describing three patients they compared to

---

* Corresponding author.
E-mail address: jsheikh@bidmc.harvard.edu (J. Sheikh).

0889-8561/07/$ - see front matter © 2007 Elsevier Inc. All rights reserved.
doi:10.1016/j.iac.2007.07.007   *immunology.theclinics.com*

previously reported cases. They used the plural term, HESs, based on the fact that the presentations of all of the cases were heterogeneous [7]. Since then, the terms HES and HESs have increasingly been used interchangeably.

In 1975, Chusid and colleagues [8] reported a case series of 14 patients, and was the first to offer diagnostic criteria for the HES. We now know that HES is indeed described most accurately as a collection of heterogeneous disorders, with many similarities in clinical features, but some differences. Based on recent advances in molecular and genetic diagnostic techniques, and increasing experience with differences in clinical features and prognosis, a number of subtypes have now been identified, including myeloproliferative variants (M-HES) and lymphocytic variants (L-HES) of HES [4]. However, most patients do not fit within these two recently identified subtypes. The 2005 Hypereosinophilic Diseases Working Group (meeting in conjunction with the International Eosinophil Society) [4] designed a classification algorithm intended to capture all the diseases associated with significant and prolonged peripheral blood hypereosinophilia, which is shown in Fig. 1. Most patients who have HES do not adequately meet the features of M-HES or L-HES, and fall under the "undefined" category (authors' clinical experience). Such classification schemes are still a work in progress, and more refining will be needed as more is learned, especially about the additional underlying mechanisms of eosinophilia in all patients who have HES.

The major goal of this article is to give an overview of the clinical features of HES in general and of the various subtypes of HES that have been identified.

Definition of hypereosinophilic syndrome

Chusid and colleagues [8] defined three diagnostic criteria in 1975, which have remained as the basis for the modern definition of HES:

- Peripheral blood eosinophilia with absolute eosinophil count greater than 1500 cells/μL, sustained for more than 6 months
- No other evident cause for eosinophilia, including allergic diseases and parasitic infection
- Signs or symptoms of organ involvement by eosinophilic infiltration

The 6-month time requirement helped exclude short-term episodes of eosinophilia, as exemplified by adverse reactions to medications; however, in the current decade, patients can be considered to have HES without waiting for the 6-month time requirement if the second and third criteria are clearly met and they appear to have a chronic and unremitting clinical course [5]. Also, many investigators now consider that if a patient most closely fits one of the other described eosinophilic diseases (eg, eosinophilic esophagitis, eosinophilic pneumonia, or eosinophilic leukemia) despite the presence of eosinophilia greater than 1500/uL, the patient is not considered to have HES [3]. Patients who have isolated peripheral blood eosinophilia without any organ involvement are not considered to meet the definition of HES as per the third Chusid criteria [3]. Some patients may have long-lasting chronic peripheral blood eosinophilia (in some cases, very high counts) and may never develop any organ involvement or problematic symptoms. However, in some cases, organ involvement may develop later in a patient who initially appeared to have only benign peripheral blood eosinophilia. For this reason, such patients are still included as "undefined benign" in the classification scheme in Fig. 1, despite not meeting Chusid's criteria.

Overview and traditional description of the clinical features of hypereosinophilic syndrome

In general, HES is seen more commonly in men than in women, with a reported male/female ratio of 9:1 [3]. Cases have mostly been described in adults, with the age at diagnosis usually falling between 20 and 50 [3,6,9], but a number of pediatric cases have been reported, encompassing multiple HES subtypes, including M-HES [10,11]. Because we now know that HES is heterogeneous, comprising a number of subtypes, it is not surprising that the clinical features can vary considerably from patient to patient. Affected patients may first present with symptoms related to their particular organ involvement, or the eosinophilia may be detected coincidentally during routine blood testing [9]. Nonspecific constitutional symptoms can be seen as a part of HES; the National Institutes of Health case series reported that fatigue is present in 26% of patients and fever in 12% [9]. Other presenting symptoms included cough (24%), breathlessness (16%), muscle pains (14%), angioedema (14%), rash (12%), and retinal lesions (10%) [9].

Peripheral blood eosinophilia and hematologic manifestations of hypereosinophilic syndrome

As discussed previously, chronic peripheral blood eosinophilia of greater than 1500/uL is present by definition. These peripheral eosinophils are generally mature, but eosinophilic myeloid precursors can occasionally be seen in the peripheral blood [3] (see later discussion that differentiates the M-HES variants from L-HES). Other hematologic laboratory values can also be abnormal, depending on the subtype. In some cases of HES, morphologic abnormalities of the eosinophils can be seen at the gross and ultrastructural levels [12–15]. Any cytogenetic or molecular evidence of eosinophil clonality indicates a diagnosis of chronic eosinophilic leukemia (CEL) [16]. Blasts may or may not be seen on the peripheral smear in CEL. As discussed later, some cases of M-HES (eg, those with the FIP1L1-PDGFRα fusion gene) are really CEL [17]. Splenomegaly can be seen in HES, and hypersplenism may lead to anemia and thrombocytopenia [3]. When the spleen is involved, it can be painful [18]. Pathologic studies have found that eosinophilic accumulation in the spleen does occur [19]. Thrombocytosis and

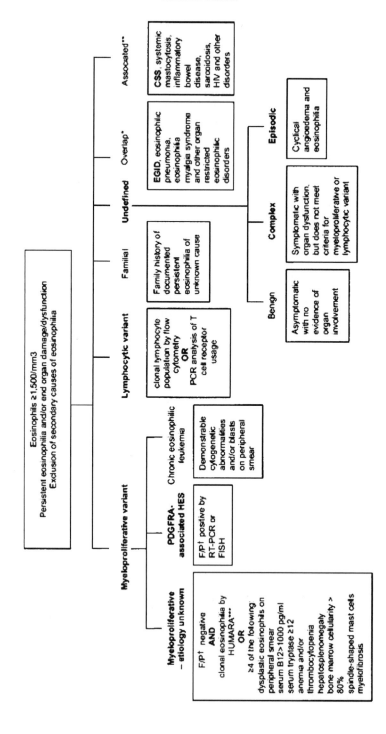

anemia have been reported [20]. Lymphadenopathy is a nonspecific finding that can be seen with HES.

Bone marrow biopsy often shows increased eosinophils and eosinophil precursors. Standard cytogenetic analysis is normal in most patients [9].

Organ system involvement in hypereosinophilic syndrome

A 1994 review of HES [3] reported that 100% of patients have hematologic manifestations (by definition), 58% have cardiovascular manifestations, 56% cutaneous, 54% neurologic, 49% pulmonary, 43% splenic, 30% hepatic, 23% ocular, and 23% gastrointestinal (Table 1). These percentages were determined by combining the data from three patient series [3,9,21,22]. However, recent data suggest that organ involvement may vary considerably, based on the subtype of HES.

Cardiac involvement

The cardiac involvement that can sometimes accompany HES is often the most concerning to both clinicians and patients because it has been, at least in the past, the feature that is associated most often with clinical morbidity and mortality [3,8]. It usually follows three stages:

1. An early acute necrotic stage, with damage occurring to endomyocardial tissue, which is generally asymptomatic clinically and usually escapes diagnosis [2,3,23]
2. The thrombotic stage, during which intramural (or rarely valvular) thrombi develop on the damaged intracardiac tissue [24–27]
3. The fibrotic stage, in which significant intramural fibrosis can lead to impaired cardiac function and output, and significant valvular damage can lead to further problems, such as congestive heart failure [2,23].

This same three-stage pattern of cardiac damage is also seen when cardiac involvement occurs in conjunction with other forms of eosinophilia, including parasitic disease, neoplastic disease, and eosinophilic leukemia [3,23,24,28–32]. Often, however, patients who have HES and other causes of chronic eosinophilia such as parasitic disease can have sustained high

---

Fig. 1. Classification of HES. Specific syndromes discussed at the workshop are indicated in bold. *Incomplete criteria, apparent restriction to specific tissues-organs. **Peripheral eosinophilia 1500/mm³ in association with a defined diagnosis. F/P† Presence of the FIP1L1-PDGFRA mutation. ***Clonality analysis based on the digestion of genomic DNA with methylation-sensitive restriction enzymes followed by PCR amplification of the CAG repeat at the human androgen receptor gene (HUMARA) locus at the X chromosome. CSS, Churg-Strauss syndrome; FISH, fluorescence in situ hybridization; HIV, human immunodeficiency virus; PCR, polymerase chain reaction; RT-PCR, reverse transcriptase polymerase chain reaction. (*From* Klion AD, Bochner BS, Gleich GJ, et al. Approaches to the treatment of HES: a workshop summary report. J Allergy Clin Immunol 2006;117:1292–302; with permission.)

Table 1
General characteristic clinical features of hypereosinophilic syndrome

Organ system (% frequency) [3,9,21,22]	Potential specific findings
Hematologic (100%)	Eosinophilia (100%)
	Anemia
	Thrombocytosis
	Thrombocytopenia
	Lymphadenopathy
Cardiovascular (58%)	Endomyocardial damage/necrosis
	Intramural thrombi
	Endomyocardial fibrosis
	Congestive heart failure
Cutaneous (56%)	Urticaria/angioedema
	Erythematous pruritic papules and nodules
Neurologic (54%)	Primary generalized central nervous system dysfunction
	Peripheral neuropathy
	Thromboembolic neurologic phenomena
Pulmonary (49%)	Nonproductive cough
	Nonspecific infiltrates
	Pulmonary fibrosis
Spleen (43%)	Splenomegaly
	Hypersplenism
Liver (30%)	Chronic active hepatitis
	Hepatic vein obstruction/Budd-Chiari syndrome
Gastrointestinal (23%)	Esophagitis
	Gastroenteritis
	Colitis
Ocular (23%)	Choroidal abnormalities
	Blurry vision

peripheral eosinophil counts but never develop cardiac involvement [3]. The reason that some patients are prone to cardiac damage, but not others, is, so far, unknown. It may well be that chronic eosinophilia-related cardiac damage will only occur if other ill-defined activation and recruitment factors are present [3]. As discussed later, M-HES variants are associated with a higher prevalence of cardiac findings.

Cutaneous involvement

Various patterns of skin involvement can occur with HES. One pattern involves a predominance of urticarial lesions and angioedema, which has traditionally been thought to be associated with a more benign course of HES [9]. If eosinophilia is accompanied by episodic angioedema, the possible diagnosis of episodic angioedema with eosinophilia syndrome, or Gleich's syndrome, should be entertained, which is considered a separate entity. Gleich's syndrome is characterized by recurrent episodes of angioedema, urticaria, pruritus, fever, weight gain, elevated serum IgM, oliguria, and leukocytosis, with peripheral blood eosinophilia and eosinophil degranulation in the dermis [33–36]. Peripheral blood eosinophilia may disappear or drop to a minimal level between attacks. Some patients presenting with Gleich's syndrome, however, may have underlying L-HES [37]. A syndrome similar to Gleich's syndrome is characterized by nonepisodic angioedema with eosinophilia, and is seen predominantly in younger women [36]. This nonepisodic angioedema with eosinophilia syndrome is distinct from HES in that it usually consists of a single, self-limited attack [38–40].

A second pattern of HES cutaneous involvement consists of erythematous pruritic papules and nodules, with a nonvasculitic mixed cellular dermal infiltrate [3,41]. As discussed later, the common patterns of cutaneous involvement are quite prevalent in L-HES variants. A less commonly reported pattern of mucocutaneous involvement is that of debilitating mucosal ulcers that can affect multiple mucosal areas of the body [3,42,43].

Neurologic involvement

Three neurologically related complications can occur in HES: primary generalized central nervous system (CNS) dysfunction, peripheral neuropathies, and thromboembolic phenomena [44]. Primary CNS dysfunction can manifest with encephalopathy and upper motor neuron signs [44]. The mechanism of this dysfunction is unknown and is not well studied. The few autopsies of involved patients that have been done have shown no specific eosinophil-related lesions in the brain [6]. Peripheral neuropathies can include polyneuropathies with sensory or motor components, mononeuritis multiplex, and radiculopathies, with related muscle atrophy [44–52]. The pathology of the affected nerves is usually axonal neuropathy with a few reports of vasculitis, but, as with the primary CNS dysfunction, evidence of direct eosinophilic infiltration usually is not seen and the exact pathophysiology of the neuropathy is unclear [44–49,53,54]. It has been speculated that either specific eosinophil granule proteins, such as eosinophil-derived neurotoxin, may cause direct nerve damage [3,55], or that eosinophil-mediated damage to endothelial cells leads to edema that subsequently causes pressure on nerves and axonal damage [51], although these hypotheses have not been supported or tested adequately [3].

Pulmonary involvement

Lung involvement in HES can be variable. The most common feature is a chronic, nonproductive cough with a normal chest radiograph [3]. Asthma-like wheezing is not common in true HES, and its presence raises the suspicion of Churg-Strauss syndrome as the diagnosis, rather than HES. Of course, pulmonary involvement can also occur secondary to cardiac abnormalities as discussed previously, such as congestive heart failure or pulmonary embolus originating from a right ventricle thrombus. If radiologic findings do occur along with pulmonary involvement, they can consist of various findings, including pleural effusion, diffuse infiltrates, or variably focal infiltrates [8,22,56,57]. If biopsied, infiltrates can be found to contain eosinophilic accumulations [58], and eosinophils may also be seen on bronchoalveolar lavage [59]. Pulmonary infiltrates may or may not improve with corticosteroid therapy [3], and pulmonary fibrosis has been known to develop over time [9]. Overall, pulmonary symptoms can range from mild to severe, and can include development of restrictive or obstructive lung disease and even adult respiratory distress syndrome [60].

Gastrointestinal involvement including hepatic manifestations

Eosinophilic esophagitis, gastritis, enteritis, or colitis can occur in any combination as part of HES, or, as discussed earlier, can be considered separate entities from HES if they occur in isolation without meeting the criteria for HES [61]. Clinical symptoms depend on which part of the gastrointestinal tract is involved, and, in some cases, can be quite similar to inflammatory bowel disease [8,21,62–66]. Specific hepatic involvement can occur, including a chronic, active, hepatitis-like picture [67,68], and hepatic vein obstruction leading to Budd-Chiari syndrome [69,70]. Less common gastrointestinal associations include sclerosing cholangitis and pancreatitis [62,71].

Ocular involvement

Ocular symptoms such as blurry vision can occur in HES, and are thought to be caused by microembolic phenomena or local microthrombosis [9,72,73]. In one study, more than 50% of HES patients were shown to have choroidal abnormalities, such as retinal vessel abnormalities and delayed filling, regardless of whether the patient was symptomatic [72].

Rheumatologic/connective tissue involvement

Although not among the more common HES findings, arthralgias, arthritis, effusions of the large joints, and Raynaud's phenomenon have been reported with HES [3,21,74]. Raynaud's phenomenon can be so severe that digital necrosis can occur [75]. Although myalgias can occur quite commonly in HES along with other constitutional/systemic symptoms [3], focal myositis or diffuse myositis (polymyositis) is rare [74,76,77].

Evolution of the concept of separate myeloproliferative variants of hypereosinophilic syndrome and lymphocytic variants of hypereosinophilic syndrome subtypes

In the 1970s and early 1980s, a number of clinical features were identified that seemed to predict a worse outcome, including very high peripheral blood eosinophil counts of more than 100,000/uL, hepatosplenomegaly, the presence of chromosomal abnormalities or circulating immature precursor cells, increased serum vitamin B12, elevated leukocyte alkaline phosphatase, anemia, or thrombocytopenia [8,18,20]. Because these are clinical features that are seen with myeloproliferative syndromes including chronic myelogenous leukemia, the term "myeloproliferative variant of HES" was created, even though proof of an actual myeloproliferative disease in these HES patients by demonstration of true myeloid clonality was rarely possible with the available technology at that time [5]. Karyotyping of patients was often done, but abnormal karyotypes are rare in HES [5]. No good way existed to detect molecular evidence of a myeloproliferative variant in patients until around 2003, with the discovery of an interstitial deletion on chromosome 4q12 that leads to fusion of the FIP1-like 1 (FIP1L1) and PDGFRα genes, with the fusion product encoding for a protein that has significant constitutive tyrosine kinase activity [78]. The presence of this fusion protein was found to be responsible for pronounced eosinophilia in affected patients. Patients who have this fusion mutation are now known to form most of the so-called M-HES variants [5].

Some early studies of HES patients found that T-cell clones from the patients' peripheral blood displayed eosinophilopoietic activity [5,79,80]. This finding led to the idea that an abnormal T-cell population could be the driving factor in some patients who have HES, with recruitment of eosinophils being a secondary process. The finding of elevated immunoglobulin (Ig)E in some patients who had HES separately suggested that some HES cases may be driven by a Th-2 process [5]. In 1994, a patient who had HES was described who was found to have a clonal T-cell population that secreted elevated IL-5 levels [81]. Since then, about 40 such patients who had identifiable clonal T-cell populations that can secrete IL-5 have been described in the literature [5,82,83]. Such patients, in whom a clonal lymphocyte population can be identified (by flow cytometry or reverse transcriptase polymerase chain reaction [RT-PCR] for T-cell receptor (TCR) usage), are defined as having L-HES subtypes [4].

The question of what proportion of patients falls into M-HES versus L-HES versus other subtypes has been raised. A study of 35 French subjects with HES found 31% with L-HES and 17% with FIPL1-PDGFRα M-HES [37]. A study of 376 patients who had HES in the United Kingdom found 11% with the FIPL1-PDGFRα M-HES variant [84]. Simon and colleagues [83] reported that 27% of 60 HES patients seen principally in dermatology clinics had L-HES; but because skin findings are prevalent in L-HES, this frequency of L-HES might be overrepresented [2]. Affected by differing potential referral biases to medical centers with varying expertise (eg, hematologic, dermatologic, allergic), current information does not provide a definitive measure of the frequencies of L-HES and M-HES, but it does indicate that many with HES remain in the undefined subtype. However, as to male-to-female ratio, the data do indicate that M-HES is, by far, a male-predominant disease, whereas L-HES affects females as often as males [5]. Details of the specific clinical features of M-HES and

L-HES are discussed here, considered in other articles in this issue, and summarized in Boxes 1 and 2.

Specific clinical features of the myeloproliferative variant of hypereosinophilic syndrome

Hematologic involvement

As discussed previously, the ability to differentiate M-HES variants easily was greatly enhanced with the discovery of the FIP1L1-PDGFRα fusion gene mutation, as reported in 2003 [78] and later confirmed by others (see Box 1) [5,85–87]. The gene was found to encode for a protein with strong tyrosine kinase activity that was susceptible to inhibition with imatinib, a tyrosine kinase inhibitor. Consequently, it was found that most patients who had the fusion mutation showed good clinical response when treated with imatinib [85,88]. However, some patients have been identified who show clinical response to imatinib, but do not have a detectable FIP1L1-PDGFRα mutation. It is thought that these patients may have other yet-to-be-defined mutations leading to similar mutant proteins with tyrosine kinase activity. Of patients who respond to imatinib, about two thirds have the FIP1L1-PDGFRα mutation, leaving the other one third who likely have other imatinib-responsive phenotypes [5,78]. Other patients have been described who have features of M-HES but who are imatinib unresponsive. It is unknown whether these patients have either imatinib-resistant mutant proteins with tyrosine kinase activity, or perhaps bone marrow–directed eosinophil expansion involving other molecular mechanisms [5].

Box 1. Characteristic clinical features of the myeloproliferative variant

Affects males predominantly
Often FIP1L1-PDGFRα fusion gene mutation positive
Dysplastic eosinophils on peripheral smear
Elevated serum B12
Elevated serum tryptase
Anemia or thrombocytopenia
Hepatosplenomegaly
Increased bone marrow cellularity
Atypical/spindle-shaped mast cells in bone marrow
Myelofibrosis
Frequently responds to imatinib
Endomyocardial damage/necrosis
Cardiac intramural thrombi
Endomyocardial fibrosis

Box 2. Characteristic clinical features of the lymphocytic variant

Males and females affected equally
FIP1L1-PDGFRα fusion gene mutation negative
Increased serum IgE
May have increased serum IgG, IgM
May have increased serum IL-5
May have increased serum thymus and activation-regulated
  chemokine (TARC)
Abnormal or clonal T-cell populations may be detected
Rarely have cardiac involvement
Frequent cutaneous involvement
Frequent history of atopy
Generally have good response to glucocorticoids

FIP1L1-PDGFRα and related chromosomal mutations associated with HES should be forms of CEL [17]. Because World Health Organization criteria identify eosinophil clonality as the defining feature of CEL, it has been reasoned that any evidence of clonality, including the identification of the FIP1L1-PDGFRα fusion mutation, would classify a patient as having CEL [17]. Future refinements of the classification scheme in Fig. 1 will reflect this new thinking.

As developed by Klion and colleagues [85,88] in 2003, the workshop consensus was that a patient who has HES, in the absence of detectable FIPLI-PDGFRα, related chromosomal mutation, or other evidence of eosinophil clonality, could be considered to fall under M-HES if four or more of the following eight features are present (see Fig. 1) [4]:

Presence of dysplastic eosinophils on peripheral blood smear
Serum B12 level greater than 1000 pg/mL
Serum tryptase greater than or equal to 12 ng/mL
Anemia or thrombocytopenia
Hepatosplenomegaly
Bone marrow biopsy cellularity greater than 80%
Presence of dysplastic mast cells in the bone marrow (defined by Klion
  and colleagues [85] as more than 25% of mast cells being spindle-
  shaped)
Myelofibrosis (presence of antireticulin antibody staining on bone mar-
  row biopsy as per Klion and colleagues [85])

Patients who have elevated serum tryptase are often the ones who have increased and atypical mast cells in the bone marrow. Although HES and mastocytosis can overlap somewhat, HES patients can typically be differentiated from those with mastocytosis by the fact that they do not have the somatic c-kit mutations that can be seen in mastocytosis [85]. (Note that the most common c-kit mutation seen in mastocytosis, the D816V mutation, is characteristically resistant to imatinib) [17,89].

Quite fascinating is the potential reversal of most of the hematologic features of M-HES in patients who are responsive to imatinib, including reduction of serum tryptase, molecular remission of FIP1L1-PDGFRα positivity, disappearance of the bone marrow atypical spindle-shaped mast cells, and improvement of myelofibrosis [88].

Cardiac involvement

In 1983, before the recognition of the M-HES variants of HES, Harley and colleagues [90] reported that the following characteristics were associated with the development of endomyocardial fibrosis:

Male sex
HLA-Bw44 positive
Splenomegaly
Thrombocytopenia
Elevated serum levels of vitamin B12
Presence of dysplastic eosinophils on peripheral blood smear
Presence of abnormal early myeloid precursors on peripheral blood smear
Fibrosis and decreased megakaryocytes in the bone marrow

As we now know, these are, in large part, the clinical features of M-HES, and data have shown an increased frequency of cardiac involvement in FIP1L1-PDGFRα-positive HES patients [4]. The pathophysiologic reason for this increased tendency toward endomyocardial fibrosis in M-HES patients is unknown [85]. Although eosinophilia and other symptoms can often improve in treated M-HES patients (often with imatinib), endomyocardial fibrosis is generally irreversible [86,88], although, rarely, improvement of cardiac findings has been reported with imatinib [91]. This factor makes an argument for early and aggressive treatment of patients thought to have M-HES, to prevent the development of advanced and irreversible cardiac involvement, although it is known that, for unclear reasons, not all patients will develop cardiac involvement.

Cutaneous involvement

Although HES-related cutaneous findings are thought to be more characteristic of L-HES, they can be seen fairly frequently in M-HES [2]. When present, they can rapidly improve in imatinib-responsive patients [5]. One case of lymphomatoid papulosis in a FIP1L1-PDGFRα-positive patient has been described [92].

Pulmonary involvement

Pulmonary involvement can occur in M-HES. Klion and colleagues [85] reported that four out of nine M-HES patients had evidence of restrictive lung disease (in comparison, three patients in this series who had normal tryptase had obstructive disease). Lung involvement in M-HES can rapidly improve in imatinib-responsive patients [5].

Neurologic involvement

Although specific frequency is unknown, neurologic involvement and damage, sometimes severe, can be associated with M-HES.

Specific clinical features of the lymphocytic variant of hypereosinophilic syndrome

L-HES is thought to affect males and females equally. Specific organ system involvement is discussed.

Hematologic involvement

As indicated previously, the identification in 1994 of an IL-5–secreting clonal T-cell population in a patient who had HES led to the subsequent reporting of a number of similar patients who had identifiable IL-5–producing T-cell subpopulations, who make up the L-HES subtype [81]. The abnormal T-cell subpopulations reported tend to have an aberrant surface phenotype. The most common abnormality seen is CD3−CD4+ expression, with rare reports of CD3+CD4−CD8− expression [2]. The abnormal subsets also tend to show an activated (CD25 or HLA−DR+) memory (CD45RO+) pattern [2,5,83,93]. Further investigation of the relatively commonly seen CD3−CD4+ aberrant T-cell subpopulations revealed high expression of CD5 and loss of CD7 or CD27 expression in many cases [93]. These reported associations have been helpful because the reported abnormal marker patterns can be looked for when evaluating a patient who has suspected L-HES, although these specific patterns are not always found. It should be noted that T-cell clonality may not always be detected, because of issues with PCR sensitivity or because of clonal deletion of TCR chain genes [93,94]. The definition of L-HES has been refined to "a primitive lymphoid disorder characterized by nonmalignant expansion of a T-cell population able to produce eosinophilopoietic cytokines (generally IL-5)" [2,5]. The cause of the development of these abnormal T-cell populations in affected patients is unknown.

Other laboratory findings often seen in L-HES include elevated serum IgE, and, occasionally, increased IgM or IgG [82]. However, these are nonspecific for L-HES. Although about 75% of L-HES patients who have clonal CD3−CD4+ cells were found to have high IgE levels [82], increased

IgE has been also seen in FIP1L1-PDGFRα-positive M-HES [87]. Even less specific is serum IL-5, which has often been reported to be elevated in L-HES [2,83], but can also be elevated in M-HES [93].

Although the authors could find no clear data differentiating the frequency of lymphadenopathy in L-HES from that of M-HES, the presence of enlarged lymph nodes has been a common part of the clinical picture of L-HES patients before the development of lymphoma [95–98], and so the presence of enlarging lymph nodes in a patient who has suspected or confirmed L-HES should prompt for evaluation of transformation into lymphoma.

Cardiac involvement

Harley and colleagues [90] reported that the following features predicted patients who remained free of heart disease: female sex, angioedema, hyper-gammaglobulinemia, elevated serum IgE, and circulating immune complexes. This finding suggested that patients who have L-HES are much less likely than those who have M-HES to develop any cardiac involvement, and that has remained true through recent observations.

Cutaneous involvement

In nearly all reported L-HES patients, some sort of cutaneous involvement has been seen, which may include eczematous dermatitis, nonspecific erythroderma, pruritus, urticaria, and angioedema [82,83,93]. This involvement is perhaps not surprising because many patients report a history of atopic disease in the past. Skin biopsies of specific lesions typically show a lymphocytic inflammatory pattern [5]. In the Simon and colleagues cohort, 14 out of 16 patients who had L-HES had cutaneous findings [83].

Some patients who have L-HES have been found to display episodic angioedema in a pattern similar to that seen in Gleich's syndrome [99,100].

Pulmonary involvement

A history of atopic respiratory disease is often seen in L-HES patients [5], so pulmonary findings in such patients may be of typical asthma (and they may also have allergic rhinoconjunctivitis). On the other hand, the typical lung involvement of HES can also be seen in L-HES, although the frequency of this is unclear. Simon and colleagues [83] reported lung disease in 2 out of 16 patients in their L-HES series.

Gastrointestinal involvement

Gastrointestinal tract involvement similar to that seen with the EGIDs often occurs in L-HES.

Rheumatologic/connective tissue involvement

Although generally not one of the more common HES features, arthralgias, arthritis, vasculitis, and tenosynovitis have been reported with L-HES [2,93,101]. However, data are currently inadequate to make detailed prevalence comparisons with M-HES.

Other hypereosinophilic syndrome subtypes

In attempting to design a classification algorithm that captures all of the diseases associated with eosinophilia, the 2005 Hypereosinophilic Diseases Working Group (meeting in conjunction with the International Eosinophil Society) [4] established four separate categories of hypereosinophilic diseases other than M-HES and L-HES: familial eosinophilia, undefined, overlap, and associated (see Fig. 1).

A familial form of HES appears to be a very rare entity. A five-generation kindred with eosinophilia that follows an autosomal dominant pattern has been described [102]. The affected members have chronic high peripheral blood eosinophil counts, yet most remain fairly asymptomatic. It has been suggested that familial eosinophilia can be differentiated from HES by a more benign clinical course that may be related to a relative lack of eosinophil activation [103].

The overlap category is intended to capture cases that do not accurately fit the criteria for HES, but rather, have an apparent restriction of tissue-specific eosinophilia to specific organs. This category includes the EGIDs (including eosinophilic esophagitis and gastroenteritis), eosinophilic pneumonia, and eosinophilia-myalgia syndrome [4].

The associated category is intended to capture cases of peripheral eosinophilia that can occur in association with other defined diagnoses, such as Churg-Strauss syndrome, systemic mastocytosis, inflammatory bowel disease, sarcoidosis, and human immunodeficiency virus (HIV) [4].

The last category is the undefined category [4]. Cases of unexplained eosinophilia that do not meet the three key criteria of HES, but also do not meet the other miscellaneous categories described can be classified under either benign or episodic. Benign cases include patients who have chronic peripheral eosinophilia greater than 1500/uL, but no specific organ involvement. Such patients may have long-lasting chronic peripheral blood eosinophilia (in some cases very high counts) and may never develop any organ involvement or problematic symptom. However, in some cases, organ involvement may develop later in a patient who initially appeared to have only benign peripheral blood eosinophilia. For this reason, such patients are still included as undefined benign in the classification scheme in Fig. 1, despite not meeting Chusid's criteria. Patients who have the episodic angioedema with eosinophilia syndrome (Gleich's syndrome) would fit under the episodic classification. In contrast to most other eosinophilic disorders, Gleich's syndrome is characterized by intermittent episodes of pe-ripheral blood eosinophilia, accompanied by angioedema. In between epi-sodes, the patients are usually asymptomatic, with normal or mildly elevated eosinophil counts.

Cases of HES that do meet the three HES criteria but do not fit into ei-ther the M-HES or L-HES variants can be classified under the complex des-ignation (see Fig. 1) [4]. The clinical features of these with complex HES have not been specifically compiled, but the disease manifestations can be diverse. Also, the frequency of cases that meet the definition of complex HES in comparison to M-HES and L-HES has not been specifically re-ported, but, as noted above, these undefined complex HES patients likely represent most patients who have HES. Because of the previously discussed inadvertent biases in describing the frequency of M-HES and L-HES, the frequency of complex HES may be higher than initially suspected. The au-thors' clinical experience is that most patients who meet Chusid's criteria fall into the complex category, rather than into M-HES or L-HES. Further study of this patient group is clearly needed.

An HES working group will be reconvened in conjunction with the 2007 meeting of the International Eosinophil Society. This working group will re-view the most recent literature and discuss whether any updates are needed to the currently proposed classification scheme (see Fig. 1) [4].

Myeloproliferative variants versus lymphocytic variants: implications for the diagnostic workup and treatment of hypereosinophilic syndrome

Because this issue of *Immunology and Allergy Clinics of North America* contains separate articles covering the evaluation and differential diagnosis of eosinophilia and the management of HES, the authors do not cover these topics in detail here. However, correctly differentiating M-HES, and partic-ularly FIP1L1-PDGFRα M-HES, from the other subtypes is important in determining a patient's prognosis and treatment course, because it is known that FIP1L1-PDGFRα HES patients have good response to imatinib, and even some non-FIP1L1-PDGFRα M-HES patients will respond. In previ-ous decades, the therapeutic regimen focused on using corticosteroids first line, with alternative agents such as hydroxyurea and interferon-alpha (IFN-α) being tried as secondary agents [3], but the selection of therapeutic regimens could not be guided by the nature of particular HES subtypes. All patients who have HES should have an evaluation by RT-PCR or fluores-cence in situ hybridization (FISH) for the presence of the FIP1L1-PDGFRα mutation, to help with classification and guide therapy. The presence of this mutation mandates therapy with imatinib, especially because a number of these M-HES patients may be relatively refractory to corticosteroids [5].

Initially noted clinical features are important because they can help guide the initial and further workup in determining if a patient has M-HES or L-HES. For example, if L-HES is suspected, a thorough examination for the presence of a phenotypically aberrant T-cell subset should be performed [5]. If L-HES is diagnosed, therapy focuses on the use of corticosteroids to reduce eosinophilia but also as an attempt to decrease cytokine production by aberrant T cells [5]. Clinical features that we now know are associated with L-HES have been found to be predictors of a prolonged response to corticosteroid therapy, including the presence of episodic angioedema, a significant and sustained reduction of peripheral eosinophil count 4 to 12 hours after a single dose of prednisone 60 mg or equivalent, an increased serum IgE level, and a lack of hepatosplenomegaly [3,4]. The identification of L-HES might also have implications for the use of IFN-α. Although IFN-α theoretically might help in L-HES by decreasing cytokine production from an abnormal T-cell clone [104], it has also been found to inhibit spontaneous apoptosis of CD3−CD4+ abnormal T cells [105]. Therefore, it has been hypothesized that monotherapy with IFN-α may enhance the potential transformation to lymphoma [2,5], although it has not been observed yet clinically. It is unknown whether such risks would occur if IFN-α were used alongside corticosteroids.

Mepolizumab, an experimental monoclonal antibody to IL-5, is currently under placebo-controlled, multicenter study for the treatment of HES [106]. In theory, this drug is very promising for the treatment of L-HES specifically because L-HES is thought to involve the production of cytokines including IL-5 from abnormal T-cell populations, and early data have supported this theory [107,108]. In contrast, because FIP1L1-PDGFRα HES is a subtype of CEL, mepolizumab will likely not have a significant role in the treatment of FIP1L1-PDGFRα HES patients because these patients will continue to receive first-line treatment with imatinib and, if refractory, will likely be considered for other tyrosine kinase inhibitors. Similarly, other, newer drugs can be considered for study in HES, depending on which subtype they are likely to be helpful for. For example, alemtuzumab (monoclonal antibody to CD52) [109,110], cyclosporine A, and monoclonal antibodies to anti-IL-2R-α might be of benefit theoretically, specifically for L-HES [5], but have not yet undergone formal clinical trials for this purpose.

Long-term prognosis and life expectancy

Previous case series have underscored the fact that with the great variability in underlying pathogenesis and clinical features seen among patients who have HES, the clinical course and long-term prognosis in these patients is also highly variable, ranging from minimal symptoms, requiring little-to-no treatment, to severe disabling disease, leading to either directly related mortality, or, perhaps, transformation to leukemia or lymphoma, with subsequent morbidity or mortality [3,5]. Similarly, the degree of organ involvement and the long-term prognosis of disease do not correlate with the peripheral eosinophil level [5]. Initial studies found that poor prognostic features included very high peripheral blood eosinophil counts of more than 100,000/uL, hepatosplenomegaly, the presence of chromosomal abnormalities or circulating immature precursor cells, increased serum vitamin B12, elevated leukocyte alkaline phosphatase, anemia, or thrombocytopenia [5,18,20]. Of course, it is now known that many of these are features of M-HES. The bad outcomes reported in older case series were often related to issues secondary to severe organ damage (particularly cardiac) or transformation to myelogenous or lymphoid malignancy [5]. M-HES patients can transform to acute myeloid leukemia, including those with the FIP1L1-PDGFRα mutation [1,86,87]. L-HES patients are not necessarily free of worry because these cases may eventually progress to T-cell lymphoma [2,111].

HES mortality and survival rates seem to be improving. Chusid and colleagues [8] originally reported a 12% 3-year survival rate in 1975, whereas Fauci and colleagues [9] reported a 70% 10-year survival rate in 1982, and Lefebvre reported an 80% 5-year survival and 42% 15-year survival in 1989 [22]. More recent survival statistics are not available, but are likely to be better with the new medication options and faster diagnosis of cases. Also, although FIP1L1-PDGFRα-positive M-HES patients appear to have worse overall prognoses because of their risk of cardiac involvement and leukemic transformation [5], clear survival rates for M-HES versus L-HES are not yet available. As the specific cases series are followed over time, this data will soon be clearer.

Summary

HES are disorders characterized by chronic peripheral blood hypereosinophilia with damage to various organs due to eosinophilic infiltration and release of mediators. HES includes various pathophysiologically distinct conditions, with variable clinical features. The diagnosis of HES is made based on meeting three criteria: sustained peripheral hypereosinophilia of more than1500/uL, exclusion of other external causes for hypereosinophilia, and evidence of related organ involvement. Based on recent advances in molecular and genetic diagnostic techniques and increasing experience with differences in clinical features and prognosis, several subtypes have been defined, including M-HES and L-HES. It is to be hoped that other subtypes that likely represent most of the patients who have HES, now lumped together as undefined complex HES, will be further defined in the future, based on new insights into their true causes.

References

[1] Bain BJ. Hypereosinophilia. Curr Opin Hematol 2000;7(1):21–5.
[2] Roufosse F, Cogan E, Goldman M. The hypereosinophilic syndrome revisited. Annu Rev Med 2003;54:169–84.
[3] Weller PF, Bubley GJ. The idiopathic hypereosinophilic syndrome. Blood 1994;83(10): 2759–79.

[4] Klion AD, Bochner BS, Gleich GJ, et al. Approaches to the treatment of hypereosino-philic syndromes: a workshop summary report. J Allergy Clin Immunol 2006;117(6): 1292–302.

[5] Roufosse F, Goldman M, Cogan E. Hypereosinophilic syndrome: lymphoproliferative and myeloproliferative variants. Semin Respir Crit Care Med 2006;27(2):158–70.

[6] Spry C. Eosinophils. A comprehensive review and guide to the scientific and medical liter-ature. Oxford (UK): Oxford Medical Publications; 1988.

[7] Hardy WR, Anderson RE. The hypereosinophilic syndromes. Ann Intern Med 1968;68(6): 1220–9.

[8] Chusid MJ, Dale DC, West BC, et al. The hypereosinophilic syndrome: analysis of fourteen cases with review of the literature. Medicine (Baltimore) 1975;54(1):1–27.

[9] Fauci AS, Harley JB, Roberts WC, et al. NIH conference. The idiopathic hypereosinophilic syndrome. Clinical, pathophysiologic, and therapeutic considerations. Ann Intern Med 1982;97(1):78–92.

[10] Katz HT, Haque SJ, Hsieh FH. Pediatric hypereosinophilic syndrome (HES) differs from adult HES. J Pediatr 2005;146(1):134–6.

[11] Rives S, Alcorta I, Toll T, et al. Idiopathic hypereosinophilic syndrome in children: report of a 7-year-old boy with FIP1L1-PDGFRA rearrangement. J Pediatr Hematol Oncol 2005; 27(12):663–5.

[12] Spry CJ, Tai PC. Studies on blood eosinophils. II. Patients with Loffler's cardiomyopathy. Clin Exp Immunol 1976;24(3):423–34.

[13] Peters MS, Gleich GJ, Dunnette SL, et al. Ultrastructural study of eosinophils from patients with the hypereosinophilic syndrome: a morphological basis of hypodense eosino-phils. Blood 1988;71(3):780–5.

[14] Sokol RJ, Hudson G, Brown MJ, et al. Hypereosinophilic syndrome: case report and mor-phometric study. Acta Haematol 1988;79(2):107–11.

[15] Dvorak A. Subcellular morphology and biochemistry of eosinophils. In: Harris J, editor. Blood cell biochemistry: megakaryocytes, platelets, macrophages and eosinophils. London (UK): Plenum; 1990. p. 237.

[16] Ackerman GA. Eosinophilic leukemia: a morphologic and histochemical study. Blood 1964;24:372–88.

[17] Bain BJ. Relationship between idiopathic hypereosinophilic syndrome, eosinophilic leuke-mia, and systemic mastocytosis. Am J Hematol 2004;77(1):82–5.

[18] Schooley RT, Flaum MA, Gralnick HR, et al. A clinicopathologic correlation of the idio-pathic hypereosinophilic syndrome. II. Clinical manifestations. Blood 1981;58(5):1021–6.

[19] Dale DC, Hubert RT, Fauci A. Eosinophil kinetics in the hypereosinophilic syndrome. J Lab Clin Med 1976;87(3):487–95.

[20] Flaum MA, Schooley RT, Fauci AS, et al. A clinicopathologic correlation of the idio-pathic hypereosinophilic syndrome. I. Hematologic manifestations. Blood 1981;58(5): 1012–20.

[21] Spry CJ, Davies J, Tai PC, et al. Clinical features of fifteen patients with the hypereosino-philic syndrome. Q J Med 1983;52(205):1–22.

[22] Lefebvre C, Bletry O, Degoulet P, et al. [Prognostic factors of hypereosinophilic syndrome. Study of 40 cases]. Ann Med Interne (Paris) 1989;140(4):253–7 [in French].

[23] Brockington IF, Olsen EG. Eosinophilia and endomyocardial fibrosis. Postgrad Med J 1972;48(566):740–1.

[24] Parrillo JE, Borer JS, Henry WL, et al. The cardiovascular manifestations of the hypereo-sinophilic syndrome. Prospective study of 26 patients, with review of the literature. Am J Med 1979;67(4):572–82.

[25] Naito H, Nakatsuka M, Yuki K, et al. [Giant left ventricular thrombi in the hypereosino-philic syndrome: report of two cases]. J Cardiogr 1986;16(2):475–88 [in Japanese].

[26] Hendren WG, Jones EL, Smith MD. Aortic and mitral valve replacement in idiopathic hypereosinophilic syndrome. Ann Thorac Surg 1988;46(5):570–1.

[27] Tanino M, Kitamura K, Ohta G, et al. Hypereosinophilic syndrome with extensive myocardial involvement and mitral valve thrombus instead of mural thrombi. Acta Pathol Jpn 1983;33(6):1233–42.

[28] Davies J, Spry CJ, Sapsford R, et al. Cardiovascular features of 11 patients with eosinophilic endomyocardial disease. Q J Med 1983;52(205):23–39.

[29] Spry CJ, Take M, Tai PC. Eosinophilic disorders affecting the myocardium and endocardium: a review. Heart Vessels Suppl 1985;1:240–2.

[30] Jasim KA, Layzell T, McCulloch AJ. Loffler's eosinophilic endocarditis following carcinoma of the thyroid gland. Br J Clin Pract 1990;44(12):785–6.

[31] Keiser G, Ruttner JR, Wacker H, et al. [Hypereosinophilic syndrome with Loffler's endocarditis in Hodgkin's disease (author's transl)]. Dtsch Med Wochenschr 1974;99(37):1820–2, 1827–29 [in German].

[32] Andy JJ. Helminthiasis, the hypereosinophilic syndrome and endomyocardial fibrosis: some observations and an hypothesis. Afr J Med Med Sci 1983;12(3-4):155–64.

[33] Butterfield JH, Leiferman KM, Abrams J, et al. Elevated serum levels of interleukin-5 in patients with the syndrome of episodic angioedema and eosinophilia. Blood 1992;79(3):688–92.

[34] Ohmoto K, Yamamoto S. Angioedema after interferon therapy for chronic hepatitis C. Am J Gastroenterol 2001;96(4):1311–2.

[35] Gleich GJ, Schroeter AL, Marcoux JP, et al. Episodic angioedema associated with eosinophilia. N Engl J Med 1984;310(25):1621–6.

[36] Banerji A, Weller PF, Sheikh J. Cytokine-associated angioedema syndromes including episodic angioedema with eosinophilia (Gleich's syndrome). Immunol Allergy Clin North Am 2006;26(4):769–81.

[37] Roche-Lestienne C, Lepers S, Soenen-Cornu V, et al. Molecular characterization of the idiopathic hypereosinophilic syndrome (HES) in 35 French patients with normal conventional cytogenetics. Leukemia 2005;19(5):792–8.

[38] Chikama R, Hosokawa M, Miyazawa T, et al. Nonepisodic angioedema associated with eosinophilia: report of 4 cases and review of 33 young female patients reported in Japan. Dermatology 1998;197(4):321–5.

[39] Shimasaki AK. [Five cases of nonepisodic angioedema with eosinophilia]. Rinsho Ketsueki 2001;42(8):639–43 [in Japanese].

[40] Mizukawa Y, Shiohara T. The cytokine profile in a transient variant of angioedema with eosinophilia. Br J Dermatol 2001;144(1):169–74.

[41] Kazmierowski JA, Chusid MJ, Parrillo JE, et al. Dermatologic manifestations of the hypereosinophilic syndrome. Arch Dermatol 1978;114(4):531–5.

[42] Leiferman KM, O'Duffy JD, Perry HO, et al. Recurrent incapacitating mucosal ulcerations. A prodrome of the hypereosinophilic syndrome. JAMA 1982;247(7):1018–20.

[43] Akahoshi M, Hoshino S, Teramura M, et al. [Recurrent oral and genital ulcers as the prodrome of the hypereosinophilic syndrome: report of a probable case]. Nippon Naika Gakkai Zasshi 1987;76(3):421–4 [in Japanese].

[44] Moore PM, Harley JB, Fauci AS. Neurologic dysfunction in the idiopathic hypereosinophilic syndrome. Ann Intern Med 1985;102(1):109–14.

[45] Wichman A, Buchthal F, Pezeshkpour GH, et al. Peripheral neuropathy in hypereosinophilic syndrome. Neurology 1985;35(8):1140–5.

[46] Lupo I, Daniele O, Raimondo D, et al. Peripheral neuropathy in the hypereosinophilic syndrome: a case report. Eur Neurol 1989;29(5):269–72.

[47] Bell D, Mackay IG, Pentland B. Hypereosinophilic syndrome presenting as peripheral neuropathy. Postgrad Med J 1985;61(715):429–32.

[48] Dorfman LJ, Ransom BR, Forno LS, et al. Neuropathy in the hypereosinophilic syndrome. Muscle Nerve 1983;6(4):291–8.

[49] Werner RA, Wolf LL. Peripheral neuropathy associated with the hypereosinophilic syndrome. Arch Phys Med Rehabil 1990;71(6):433–5.

[50] Guidetti D, Gemignani F, Terenziani S, et al. Peripheral neuropathy associated with hyper-eosinophilia. Acta Neurol Belg 1991;91(1):12–9.

[51] Monaco S, Lucci B, Laperchia N, et al. Polyneuropathy in hypereosinophilic syndrome. Neurology 1988;38(3):494–6.

[52] Martin-Gonzalez E, Yebra M, Garcia-Merino A, et al. Neurologic dysfunction in the idiopathic hypereosinophilic syndrome. Ann Intern Med 1986;104(3):448–9.

[53] Grisold W, Jellinger K. Multifocal neuropathy with vasculitis in hypereosinophilic syndrome. An entity or drug-induced effect? J Neurol 1985;231(6):301–6.

[54] Marolda M, Orefice G, Barbieri F, et al. The idiopathic hypereosinophilic syndrome. Clinical, electrophysiological and histological study of a case. Ital J Neurol Sci 1989;10(1):79–84.

[55] Durack DT, Sumi SM, Klebanoff SJ. Neurotoxicity of human eosinophils. Proc Natl Acad Sci U S A 1979;76(3):1443–7.

[56] Epstein DM, Taormina V, Gefter WB, et al. The hypereosinophilic syndrome. Radiology 1981;140(1):59–62.

[57] Cordier JF, Faure M, Hermier C, et al. Pleural effusions in an overlap syndrome of idiopathic hypereosinophilic syndrome and erythema elevatum diutinum. Eur Respir J 1990;3(1):115–8.

[58] Hill R, Wang NS, Berry G. Hypereosinophilic syndrome with pulmonary vascular involvement. Angiology 1984;35(4):238–44.

[59] Slabbynck H, Impens N, Naegels S, et al. Idiopathic hypereosinophilic syndrome-related pulmonary involvement diagnosed by bronchoalveolar lavage. Chest 1992;101(4):1178–80.

[60] Winn RE, Kollef MH, Meyer JI. Pulmonary involvement in the hypereosinophilic syndrome. Chest 1994;105(3):656–60.

[61] Levesque H, Elie-Legrand MC, Thorel JM, et al. [Idiopathic hypereosinophilic syndrome with predominant digestive manifestations or eosinophilic gastroenteritis? Apropos of 2 cases]. Gastroenterol Clin Biol 1990;14(6–7):586–8 [in French].

[62] Scheurlen M, Mork H, Weber P. Hypereosinophilic syndrome resembling chronic inflammatory bowel disease with primary sclerosing cholangitis. J Clin Gastroenterol 1992;14(1):59–63.

[63] Shah AM, Joglekar M. Eosinophilic colitis as a complication of the hypereosinophilic syndrome. Postgrad Med J 1987;63(740):485–7.

[64] Aksnes B, Hammerstrom J, Kleveland PM. [Idiopathic hypereosinophilic syndrome. Enterocolitis–a rare manifestation]. Tidsskr Nor Laegeforen 1989;109(24):2433–5 [in Norwegian].

[65] Vandewiele IA, Maeyaert BM, Van Cutsem EJ, et al. Massive eosinophilic ascites: differential diagnosis between idiopathic hypereosinophilic syndrome and eosinophilic gastroenteritis. Acta Clin Belg 1991;46(1):37–41.

[66] Falade AG, Darbyshire PJ, Raafat F, et al. Hypereosinophilic syndrome in childhood appearing as inflammatory bowel disease. J Pediatr Gastroenterol Nutr 1991;12(2):276–9.

[67] Croffy B, Kopelman R, Kaplan M. Hypereosinophilic syndrome. Association with chronic active hepatitis. Dig Dis Sci 1988;33(2):233–9.

[68] Foong A, Scholes JV, Gleich GJ, et al. Eosinophil-induced chronic active hepatitis in the idiopathic hypereosinophilic syndrome. Hepatology 1991;13(6):1090–4.

[69] Elouaer-Blanc L, Zafrani ES, Farcet JP, et al. Hepatic vein obstruction in idiopathic hypereosinophilic syndrome. Arch Intern Med 1985;145(4):751–3.

[70] Suenaga N, Hayashi F, Miyauhi N, et al. [A case of hypereosinophilic syndrome associated with pulmonary infarction and hepatic vein obstruction (Budd-Chiari syndrome)]. Nihon Kyobu Shikkan Gakkai Zasshi 1991;29(2):239–44 [in Japanese].

[71] Eugene C, Gury B, Bergue A, et al. [Icterus disclosing pancreatic involvement in idiopathic hypereosinophilic syndrome]. Gastroenterol Clin Biol 1984;8(12):966–9 [in French].

[72] Chaine G, Davies J, Kohner EM, et al. Ophthalmologic abnormalities in the hypereosinophilic syndrome. Ophthalmology 1982;89(12):1348–56.

[73] Binaghi M, Perrenoud F, Dhermy P, et al. [Hypereosinophilic syndrome with ocular involvement]. J Fr Ophtalmol 1985;8(4):309–14 [in French].

[74] Layzer RB, Shearn MA, Satya-Murti S. Eosinophilic polymyositis. Ann Neurol 1977;1(1): 65–71.

[75] Takekawa M, Imai K, Adachi M, et al. Hypereosinophilic syndrome accompanied with necrosis of finger tips. Intern Med 1992;31(11):1262–6.

[76] Pye M, Pope R, Jones JH, et al. Eosinophilic polymyositis presenting as a pseudotumour in the hypereosinophilic syndrome. Br J Rheumatol 1987;26(5):384–5.

[77] Peison B, Benisch B, Lim M, et al. Idiopathic hypereosinophilic syndrome with polymyositis. South Med J 1988;81(3):403–6.

[78] Cools J, DeAngelo DJ, Gotlib J, et al. A tyrosine kinase created by fusion of the PDGFRA and FIP1L1 genes as a therapeutic target of imatinib in idiopathic hypereosinophilic syndrome. N Engl J Med 2003;348(13):1201–14.

[79] Raghavachar A, Fleischer S, Frickhofen N, et al. T lymphocyte control of human eosinophilic granulopoiesis. Clonal analysis in an idiopathic hypereosinophilic syndrome. J Immunol 1987;139(11):3753–8.

[80] Schrezenmeier H, Thome SD, Tewald F, et al. Interleukin-5 is the predominant eosinophilopoietin produced by cloned T lymphocytes in hypereosinophilic syndrome. Exp Hematol 1993;21(2):358–65.

[81] Cogan E, Schandene L, Crusiaux A, et al. Brief report: clonal proliferation of type 2 helper T cells in a man with the hypereosinophilic syndrome. N Engl J Med 1994;330(8):535–8.

[82] Roufosse F, Cogan E, Goldman M. Recent advances in pathogenesis and management of hypereosinophilic syndromes. Allergy 2004;59(7):673–89.

[83] Simon HU, Plotz SG, Dummer R, et al. Abnormal clones of T cells producing interleukin-5 in idiopathic eosinophilia. N Engl J Med 1999;341(15):1112–20.

[84] Jovanovic JV, Score J, Waghorn K, et al. Low-dose imatinib mesylate leads to rapid induction of major molecular responses and achievement of complete molecular remission in FIP1L1-PDGFRA-positive chronic eosinophilic leukemia. Blood 2007;109(11):4635–40.

[85] Klion AD, Noel P, Akin C, et al. Elevated serum tryptase levels identify a subset of patients with a myeloproliferative variant of idiopathic hypereosinophilic syndrome associated with tissue fibrosis, poor prognosis, and imatinib responsiveness. Blood 2003;101(12):4660–6.

[86] Vandenberghe P, Wlodarska I, Michaux L, et al. Clinical and molecular features of FIP1L1-PDFGRA (+) chronic eosinophilic leukemias. Leukemia 2004;18(4):734–42.

[87] Griffin JH, Leung J, Bruner RJ, et al. Discovery of a fusion kinase in EOL-1 cells and idiopathic hypereosinophilic syndrome. Proc Natl Acad Sci U S A 2003;100(13):7830–5.

[88] Klion AD, Robyn J, Akin C, et al. Molecular remission and reversal of myelofibrosis in response to imatinib mesylate treatment in patients with the myeloproliferative variant of hypereosinophilic syndrome. Blood 2004;103(2):473–8.

[89] Pardanani A, Brockman SR, Paternoster SF, et al. FIP1L1-PDGFRA fusion: prevalence and clinicopathologic correlates in 89 consecutive patients with moderate to severe eosinophilia. Blood 2004;104(10):3038–45.

[90] Harley JB, Fauci AS, Gralnick HR. Noncardiovascular findings associated with heart disease in the idiopathic hypereosinophilic syndrome. Am J Cardiol 1983;52(3):321–4.

[91] Rotoli B, Catalano L, Galderisi M, et al. Rapid reversion of Loeffler's endocarditis by imatinib in early stage clonal hypereosinophilic syndrome. Leuk Lymphoma 2004;45(12):2503–7.

[92] McPherson T, Cowen EW, McBurney E, et al. Platelet-derived growth factor receptor-alpha-associated hypereosinophilic syndrome and lymphomatoid papulosis. Br J Dermatol 2006;155(4):824–6.

[93] Roufosse F, Schandene L, Sibille C, et al. Clonal Th2 lymphocytes in patients with the idiopathic hypereosinophilic syndrome. Br J Haematol 2000;109(3):540–8.

[94] Brugnoni D, Airo P, Rossi G, et al. A case of hypereosinophilic syndrome is associated with the expansion of a CD3-CD4+ T-cell population able to secrete large amounts of interleukin-5. Blood 1996;87(4):1416–22.

[95] O'Shea JJ, Jaffe ES, Lane HC, et al. Peripheral T cell lymphoma presenting as hypereosinophilia with vasculitis. Clinical, pathologic, and immunologic features. Am J Med 1987; 82(3):539–45.

[96] Moraillon I, Bagot M, Bournerias I, et al. [Hypereosinophilic syndrome with pachyderma preceding lymphoma. Treatment with interferon alpha]. Ann Dermatol Venereol 1991; 118(11):883–5 [in French].

[97] Kim CJ, Park SH, Chi JG. Idiopathic hypereosinophilic syndrome terminating as disseminated T-cell lymphoma. Cancer 1991;67(4):1064–9.

[98] Butterfield JH. Diverse clinical outcomes of eosinophilic patients with T-cell receptor gene rearrangements: the emerging diagnostic importance of molecular genetics testing. Am J Hematol 2001;68(2):81–6.

[99] Zenone T, Felman P, Malcus C, et al. Indolent course of a patient with hypereosinophilic syndrome associated with clonal T-cell proliferation. Am J Med 1999;107(5):509–11.

[100] Morgan SJ, Prince HM, Westerman DA, et al. Clonal T-helper lymphocytes and elevated IL-5 levels in episodic angioedema and eosinophilia (Gleich's syndrome). Leuk Lymphoma 2003;44(9):1623–5.

[101] Bank I, Amariglio N, Reshef A, et al. The hypereosinophilic syndrome associated with CD4+CD3- helper type 2 (Th2) lymphocytes. Leuk Lymphoma 2001;42(1–2):123–33.

[102] Lin AY, Nutman TB, Kaslow D, et al. Familial eosinophilia: clinical and laboratory results on a U.S. kindred. Am J Med Genet 1998;76(3):229–37.

[103] Klion AD, Law MA, Riemenschneider W, et al. Familial eosinophilia: a benign disorder? Blood 2004;103(11):4050–5.

[104] Schandene L, Del Prete GF, Cogan E, et al. Recombinant interferon-alpha selectively inhibits the production of interleukin-5 by human CD4+ T cells. J Clin Invest 1996; 97(2):309–15.

[105] Schandene L, Roufosse F, de Lavareille A, et al. Interferon alpha prevents spontaneous apoptosis of clonal Th2 cells associated with chronic hypereosinophilia. Blood 2000; 96(13):4285–92.

[106] Rosenwasser LJ, Schwartz LB, Sheikh J, et al. Corticosteroid-sparing effects of mepolizumab, an anti-interleukin-5 monoclonal antibody, in patients with hypereosinophilic syndrome. J Allergy Clin Immunol 2007;119:S160.

[107] Plotz SG, Simon HU, Darsow U, et al. Use of an anti-interleukin-5 antibody in the hypereosinophilic syndrome with eosinophilic dermatitis. N Engl J Med 2003;349(24):2334–9.

[108] Garrett JK, Jameson SC, Thomson B, et al. Anti-interleukin-5 (mepolizumab) therapy for hypereosinophilic syndromes. J Allergy Clin Immunol 2004;113(1):115–9.

[109] Pitini V, Teti D, Arrigo C, et al. Alemtuzumab therapy for refractory idiopathic hypereosinophilic syndrome with abnormal T cells: a case report. Br J Haematol 2004;127(5):477.

[110] Sefcick A, Sowter D, DasGupta E, et al. Alemtuzumab therapy for refractory idiopathic hypereosinophilic syndrome. Br J Haematol 2004;124(4):558–9.

[111] Ravoet M, Sibille C, Roufosse F, et al. 6q- is an early and persistent chromosomal aberration in CD3-CD4+ T-cell clones associated with the lymphocytic variant of hypereosinophilic syndrome. Haematologica 2005;90(6):753–65.

ELSEVIER
SAUNDERS

Immunol Allergy Clin N Am
27 (2007) 357–375

IMMUNOLOGY
AND ALLERGY
CLINICS
OF NORTH AMERICA

Mechanisms of Eosinophilia in the Pathogenesis of Hypereosinophilic Disorders

Steven J. Ackerman, PhD[a], Bruce S. Bochner, MD[b],*

[a]*Department of Biochemistry and Molecular Genetics (M/C 669),
Molecular Biology Research Building, Rm. 2074, 900 S. Ashland Avenue,
The University of Illinois at Chicago College of Medicine, Chicago, IL 60607, USA*
[b]*Department of Medicine, Division of Allergy and Clinical Immunology,
Johns Hopkins University School of Medicine, Johns Hopkins Asthma and Allergy Center,
5501 Hopkins Bayview Circle, Room 2B.7a, Baltimore, MD, 21224, USA*

The paradigm that eosinophils play a significant proinflammatory and tissue-damaging role in the pathogenesis of many eosinophil-associated diseases and hypereosinophilic syndromes continues to be supported by an ever-increasing number of definitive animal model and clinical studies. This support includes recent evidence that eosinophils play a pivotal role in the development of tissue remodeling and fibrosis, in part through their potent elaboration of remodeling and fibrogenic growth factors [1–3]. Studies using two different strains of eosinophil-deficient mice strongly support the concept that the eosinophil contributes to the pathophysiology of allergic diseases such as asthma [4,5]. As well, recent clinical trials using a humanized anti-interleukin (IL)-5 antibody (Mepolizumab) to ablate eosinophils in the bone marrow, blood, and tissues of patients show great promise for reversing eosinophilia and aspects of eosinophil-mediated tissue damage, remodeling, and fibrosis in diseases such as asthma [6,7], eosinophilic esophagitis [8], and the hypereosinophilic syndrome (HES) [9]. This article addresses the current understanding of the mechanisms that regulate eosinophil lineage commitment and differentiation in the bone marrow,

This work was supported in part by grants AI033043 (to SJA) and AI041472 (to BSB) from the National Institutes of Health. Dr. Bochner also received support as a Cosner Scholar in Translational Research from Johns Hopkins University.
* Corresponding author.
E-mail address: bbochner@jhmi.edu (B.S. Bochner).

the development of blood and tissue eosinophilia, and their relationships to the pathogenesis and pathophysiology of hypereosinophilic disorders.

Cytokine regulation of eosinophilopoiesis in the bone marrow

Eosinophils differentiate in the bone marrow from stem cell-derived, CD34+, multipotential myeloid progenitors in response to a number of T-cell–derived eosinophilopoietic cytokines and growth factors including IL-3, granulocyte macrophage colony-stimulating factor (GM-CSF), and IL-5. These cytokines affect the eosinophil lineage at three different levels: (1) commitment, proliferation, and differentiation of the hematopoietic progenitors; (2) priming, activation, and survival in the blood and tissues for enhanced functional activities; and (3) recruitment and tissue localization, as discussed later. Activated T cells probably are the primary source for IL-3, IL-5, and GM-CSF pertinent to eosinophil differentiation in the bone marrow and the development of reactive blood and tissue eosinophilia in allergic and parasitic diseases and in some hypereosinophilic syndromes. Other cell types, including mast cells, macrophages, natural killer cells, endothelial cells, epithelial cells, and stromal cells such as fibroblasts, are also producers of these factors (eg, GM-CSF). IL-5, produced primarily by activated T-helper type 2 (Th2) cells [10] and mast cells [11,12], regulates the production of eosinophils both in vitro from purified hematopoietic progenitors and in vivo [13–15]. Both IL-3 and GM-CSF are pluripotent cytokines with activities on other hematopoietic lineages, whereas IL-5 is selective for the eosinophil lineage and plays a crucial role in driving committed eosinophil progenitor-cell proliferation, terminal differentiation, and postmitotic activation [16]. As a late-acting lineage-specific cytokine, IL-5 demonstrates maximum activity on an IL-5-receptor–positive (IL-5R+) eosinophil progenitor pool that first is expanded by earlier-acting multipotential cytokines including IL-3 and GM-CSF [16]. IL-5, however, is both necessary and sufficient for eosinophil development to proceed [16,17]. The expression of the high-affinity IL-5R is a prerequisite and very early lineage-specific event in the hematopoietic program for eosinophil development. Overexpression of IL-5 is observed in many eosinophil-associated diseases [18–20], and IL-5–transgenic mice develop profound eosinophilia [21,22], indicating that IL-5 plays important roles in promoting the production and function of eosinophils in vivo. These early observations have been confirmed and expanded in studies of IL-5–deficient (gene knockout) mice [23,24], which nevertheless produce basal levels of normal eosinophils in the bone marrow but, importantly, fail to develop blood and/or tissue eosinophilia or lung damage, airways hyperreactivity, and airways remodeling in murine allergic asthma models [24,25] and do not develop blood or tissue eosinophilic responses to helminth parasites [23]. The finding that IL-5–deficient (knockout) mice still generate basal levels of eosinophils in the bone marrow is consistent with the current paradigm that basal hematopoiesis occurs independently of the expression of lineage-specific cytokines such as erythropoietin, granulocyte colony-stimulating factor (G-CSF), macrophage colony-stimulating factor (M-CSF), and IL-5 (the "inductive/instructive" model) and instead is regulated at the level of gene transcription through the combinatorial activities of hematopoietic-specific transcription factors that act to resolve lineage-promiscuous gene expression patterns in early uncommitted hematopoietic progenitors [26–28].

Transcriptional regulation of eosinophil lineage commitment and differentiation

During the past 15 years studies of the mechanisms that regulate myeloid gene transcription, hematopoietic lineage specification, and differentiation have provided novel insights into the roles of combinatorial networks of transcription factors in determining progenitor cell fate, including eosinophil lineage commitment and terminal differentiation. Current findings from avian, mouse, and human studies suggest that a handful of transcription factors and their functional interactions are critical in influencing eosinophil lineage specification, development and terminal differentiation [29]. The combinatorial activities of GATA-1, C/EBPα (CCAAT enhancer-binding protein α) and the ets factor PU.1 are required for eosinophil development to proceed, with GATA-1 being the pivotal factor that determines whether granulocyte-macrophage progenitors will differentiate into eosinophils (in the presence of GATA-1) or neutrophils or macrophages (in the absence of GATA-1) (Fig. 1). In contrast, friend of GATA-1 (FOG-1), a coactivator of GATA-1 required for erythroid differentiation, functions as a corepressor that antagonizes GATA-1 activity in eosinophil progenitors [30] and therefore must be down regulated for eosinophil development to proceed in the bone marrow [31]. Convincing data from mouse knockout studies have shown that eosinophils do not develop in GATA-1–null mice [32] and that transgenic deletion of a high-affinity palindromic double-GATA site in the hypersensitivity site 2 (HS2) region of the mouse GATA-1 promoter itself results in a lineage-specific block in eosinophil terminal differentiation [33], suggesting that double-GATA sites may regulate eosinophil lineage-specific expression of GATA-1 itself. Consonant with this finding is the presence of similar high-affinity double-GATA–binding sites in the promoters of a number of hallmark eosinophil genes defining this lineage, including those encoding a number of the secondary granule proteins such as major basic protein-1 (MBP1), the IL-5–binding IL-5Rα subunit [34], and the eotaxin type 3 CC chemokine receptor (CCR3) [35]. The antagonistic activities of GATA-1 and PU.1 have been defined functionally and mechanistically in erythroid versus myeloid differentiation [36], where they may serve to resolve progenitor-cell lineage promiscuity as part of cell fate specification during hematopoietic development [26–28]. In contrast, however, PU.1 and GATA-1 synergize in the eosinophil

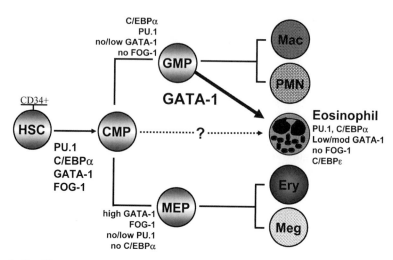

Fig. 1. Combinatorial transcription factor "codes" that specify eosinophil lineage commitment and terminal differentiation. GATA-1 is both necessary and sufficient to drive eosinophil development, and C/EBPε is required for eosinophil terminal differentiation. It remains unclear whether human eosinophils also can develop directly from common myeloid progenitors (CMP). C/EBPα, CCAAT enhancer-binding protein α; Ery, erythrocyte; FOG-1, friend of GATA-1; GMP, granulocyte-macrophage progenitors; HSC, CD34+ hematopoietic stem cells; Mac, macrophage; Meg, megakaryocyte; MEP, megakaryocyte/erythroid progenitors; PMN, polymorphonuclear leukocyte; PU.1, ets factor (identical to Spi-1 oncogene). (*Adapted from* McNagny K, Graf T. Making eosinophils through subtle shifts in transcription factor expression. J Exp Med 2002;195(11):F43–7; with permission.)

lineage for transcription of genes such as *MBP1* [34]. The mechanism for PU.1–GATA-1 synergy may involve PU.1 enhancement rather than antagonism of GATA-1 DNA binding to unique double-GATA sites present in a number of key eosinophil genes [37]. As with GATA-1–null mice, knockout of C/EBPα results in animals that are incapable of producing any granulocytes, including eosinophils [38], and eosinophil terminal differentiation likewise is impaired significantly in PU.1 knockout mice [39,40].

The current consensus regarding the combinatorial transcription factor code that selectively specifies and regulates eosinophilopoiesis as compared with the differentiation of other myeloid lineages is highlighted in Fig. 1. Thus far, the regulation of the relative levels and timing of expression of GATA-1, FOG-1, PU.1, and C/EBPα seems necessary to generate eosinophils, such that the commitment and terminal differentiation of eosinophils from myeloid progenitors requires concomitant expression of C-EBPα, PU.1, a low-to-moderate level of GATA-1, with no expression of FOG-1 [29]. Once myeloid progenitors are committed to the eosinophil lineage, their terminal differentiation and functional maturation in the bone marrow have been shown to require the activity of another member of the C/EBP family of transcription factors, C/EBPε, that is expressed at highest levels during the promyelocyte-to-myelocyte transition. Studies of C/EBPε-null (knockout) mice have shown that eosinophil (and neutrophil) terminal differentiation requires C/EBPε, because these mice lack terminally differentiated, functionally mature granulocytes (both eosinophils and neutrophils) [41,42]. Similarly, patients who have specific granule deficiency have been shown to have a novel mutation in the *C/EBPε* gene that results in loss of function of this transcription factor, the consequence of which is a failure of both neutrophil and eosinophil terminal differentiation and functional maturation, including failed expression of important secondary granule protein genes in both granulocytes [43]. Clearly, greater understanding of the combinatorial and functional interactions of the transcription factors that specify eosinophil lineage commitment and regulate gene transcription and terminal differentiation is needed. Studies in this area ultimately may lead to the identification of novel targets for ablating eosinophil development in general in the bone marrow or selectively knocking down eosinophil expression of key inflammatory mediators, such as the granule cationic proteins, or receptors, such as CCR3, as therapeutic approaches to the treatment of eosinophil-mediated allergic diseases or hypereosinophilic syndromes.

Regulation of eosinophil differentiation by cytokines and exit from the bone marrow

Based on studies with anti-IL-5 antibody, it now is clear that IL-5 is critical for terminal eosinophil differentiation [44,45]. Indeed, one of the key terminal steps in eosinophil hematopoiesis involves surface expression of the IL-5R [46]. Until this point, eosinophils and basophils share maturation pathways. Remnants of these shared differentiation pathways persist even though their divergence is clear when examining their mature circulating counterparts. For example, circulating eosinophils continue to express low levels of the α chain of the high-affinity IgE receptor (FcεRI) [47,48], whereas basophils express low levels of MBP [49], Charcot-Leyden crystal protein (galectin-10) [50], and eosinophil-derived neurotoxin (EDN), eosinophil cationic protein (ECP), and eosinophil peroxidase (EPO) [51]. In the peripheral blood both cell types selectively express the chemokine receptor CCR3 [52], but, at least in mice, its expression on eosinophils in the bone marrow occurs late in differentiation and in conjunction with loss of expression of FIRE (F4/80-related receptor) expressed by mouse eosinophils with an as yet unknown human counterpart [53]. Another terminal differentiation marker is Siglec-8 (and Siglec-F, the latter being its closest functional paralog in the mouse [54,55]), which is expressed more highly on peripheral blood eosinophils than in bone marrow eosinophils and at much higher levels than on basophils [53,56].

IL-5–deficient mice have markedly reduced numbers of bone marrow, tissue, and circulating eosinophils [23]; the opposite is found in IL-5–transgenic mice [21,22]. The exact signals regulating egress from the bone marrow are not entirely understood, however. Studies in mice suggest that, besides IL-5 [57], CCR3 agonists, such as eotaxin-1 (CCL11), are important for eosinophils to leave the bone marrow [58]. Infusion of a β2 integrin–blocking antibody prevented IL-5–mediated marrow release, whereas an antibody to α4 integrin enhanced release. Exactly how this effect occurs is not clear, but it is known that IL-5 and CCR3 agonists alter integrin function in a way that facilitates detachment from various counterligands, as has been observed in vitro in models of endothelial cell adhesion and detachment under flow conditions [59–61]. Separate studies in animals would suggest that eosinophil egress following allergen sensitization and challenge is partially T cell–dependent [62].

Eosinophil trafficking out of the circulation into tissues

Production of IL-5 and/or GM-CSF, as well as administration of these cytokines in humans, results in rapid and sustained peripheral blood eosinophilia [63,64]. Once in the circulation, eosinophils persist there for 18 to 24 hours before migrating to extravascular sites. This circulation time may be even longer in conditions associated with peripheral blood eosinophilia. Diseases associated with eosinophilia, such as hypereosinophilic syndromes, frequently, but not always, are associated with elevations in serum levels of IL-5 or GM-CSF [65–68]. Although the bone marrow is the largest reservoir for eosinophil precursors and their differentiation, their predominant destination beyond the circulation, in normal humans, is the gastrointestinal tract. Based on animal studies, this homing occurs because of constitutive gut epithelial expression of eotaxin-1 (CCL11) [69].

Levels of eosinophils in the circulation undergo diurnal variation, with highest levels in the evening and lowest levels in the early morning, in parallel with diurnal variations of endogenous cortisol levels [70]. Studies with systemically administered adhesion molecule antagonists show that very late antigen-4 (VLA-4, CD49d/CD29), but not leukocyte functional antigen-1 (LFA-1, CD11a/CD18), is involved in constitutive eosinophil trafficking because VLA-4 antibody administration resulted in about a doubling of circulating eosinophil and lymphocyte counts (both express VLA-4), whereas administration of antibodies to LFA-1 had no effect on circulating eosinophil counts [71,72]. The circulating eosinophil half-life under these conditions has not been measured specifically, but the presumption is that VLA-4 blockade interferes with constitutive homing of eosinophils into the gastrointestinal tract and perhaps other sites.

It generally is believed that once eosinophils leave the circulation and migrate into tissue sites, they do not recirculate, although data in animal models suggest that eosinophils exogenously transferred to the lungs may traffic to regional lymph nodes and play a role in antigen presentation [73]. Once in tissues, eosinophil survival depends on local production of cytokines that prevent eosinophil apoptosis. Besides IL-5, other important locally produced survival factors include GM-CSF and, perhaps to a lesser degree, IL-3, tumor necrosis factor-α (TNFα), interferon-γ, leptin [74], CD40 engagement [75], and others (Fig. 2) [76]. Studies show that, in the right local cytokine milieu, eosinophils and their precursors are capable of differentiating and surviving in tissues for several days [77–79]. In addition, eosinophils that are obtained by bronchoalveolar lavage from asthmatics or following segmental lung allergen challenge of allergic subjects display prolonged survival for several days in culture, even in the absence of added cytokines, whereas peripheral blood counterparts do not survive even 24 hours [80,81]. This finding is consistent with the eosinophils having been exposed to survival-promoting cytokines in the inflamed lung or having been induced to generate endogenous survival factors such as GM-CSF [82].

Based primarily on allergic inflammation models [83], selective recruitment of eosinophils to specific tissue sites is regulated effectively by unique patterns of cytokines that activate endothelial cells and induce tissue-resident cells to produce eosinophil-active chemokines and other chemoattractants to facilitate their preferential migration. In the former category, cytokines such as IL-4 and IL-13 selectively induce endothelial expression of vascular cell adhesion molecule 1 (VCAM-1, CD106), therefore providing ligands for α4 integrin–mediated recruitment in a pathway that distinguishes eosinophil responses from neutrophil responses, because neutrophils lack α4 integrins [52,84–86]. Indeed, inhalation of the VLA-4 antagonist IVL745 had modest effects on late-phase sputum eosinophilia in humans but failed to alter the acute or late-phase physiologic response [87]. CCR3-active chemokines, including the eotaxins (CCL11, CCL24, CCL26), RANTES (regulated upon activation, normal T cell expressed and secreted, CCL5), MCP-4 (monocyte chemotactic protein-4, CCL13), and others, derived predominantly from tissue-resident cells such as keratinocytes in the skin and airway epithelium, further facilitate eosinophil adhesion and transendothelial migration [76]. Taking a different approach, it was demonstrated convincingly that lung endothelial Gα_{i2} function, apart from its potential role

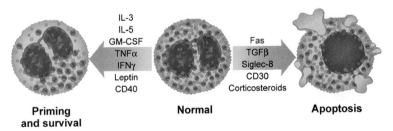

Fig. 2. How eosinophils are influenced to make life-or-death decisions. Stimuli that are known to promote eosinophil priming and survival are displayed and are contrasted with those that facilitate eosinophil apoptosis. Also shown are some of the phenotypic characteristics that accompany the primed state compared with those seen in cells undergoing apoptosis. GM-CSF, granulocyte-macrophage colony-stimulating factor; IL, interleukin; IFNγ, interferon-γ; TGFβ, transforming growth factor-β; TNFα, tumor necrosis factor-α. (Art by Jacqueline Schaffer.)

involving leukocytes, is required for eosinophil recruitment [88]. Given the eosinophil expression of both VLA-4 and VLA-6 (CD49f/CD29), interactions with specific tissue matrix proteins, especially fibronectin and laminin, also may be important, respectively, in localization of these cells and promoting their autocrine GM-CSF–driven prolonged survival within tissues [89,90]. Both TNFα and IL-1 interact synergistically with IL-4 and IL-13 to augment VCAM-1 expression as well as intercellular adhesion molecule-1 (ICAM-1, CD54) expression [91]. This interaction is consistent with the important role of β2 integrins in mediating eosinophil recruitment responses [85,92]. Alpha-4 integrins also can contribute to rolling adhesion, but a more important component of eosinophil rolling adhesion probably is mediated through surface PSGL-1 (P-selectin glycoprotein-1, CD162) on the eosinophil interacting with endothelial P-selectin (CD62P) [93–95]. Unlike their important role in neutrophil recruitment, E-selectin (CD62E) and L-selectin play little or no role in eosinophil recruitment responses [84,96,97]. Nevertheless, a pan-selectin antagonist is in clinical trials and, despite a short half-life, was capable of inhibiting allergen-induced late-phase responses in the airways [98,99]. Whether late-phase lung eosinophilia was affected was not determined. Additional chemoattractants implicated in selective eosinophil migration include complement fragments such as C5a, platelet-activating factor, and sulfidopeptide leukotrienes [100]. Priming, a term used to describe the enhanced responsiveness of a cell to normally active stimuli, occurs in vitro following exposure to cytokines such as GM-CSF and IL-5. In patients who have eosinophilia, eosinophils have a similar functionally primed phenotype, become "hypodense" on density gradients [101,102], and develop a characteristic microscopic appearance with reduced or condensed granules (see Fig. 2) [103], along with enhanced surface expression of activation markers such as CD44 and CD69 [104]. These cells also demonstrate exaggerated adhesion and migration responses to virtually all the stimuli mentioned previously; these exaggerated responses can be a critical aspect of the enhanced eosinophil trafficking seen in hypereosinophilic conditions [105].

For each of these recruitment pathways, there is some degree of tissue specificity regarding homing patterns. For example, constitutive expression of eotaxin as well as β7 integrins seems to be critical, if not absolutely necessary, for gut homing [106], whereas eotaxin-3 is markedly overexpressed in the esophagus in patients who have eosinophilic esophagitis [107]. Based on mouse studies, IL-5, IL-13, CD44 (a receptor for hyaluronic acid), and CCR3-active chemokines are implicated in lung homing of eosinophils [108,109], and the injection of, or the appearance following allergen challenge of, eotaxin-1 (CCL11), eotaxin-2 (CCL24), or RANTES (CCL5) is associated with eosinophil accumulation in the skin [110,111]. Blockade of LFA-1 had only modest effects on eosinophil accumulation in the human lung allergen-challenge model [72], whereas an antibody to eotaxin seems to reduce nasal eosinophilia induced by allergen challenge [112,113]. Also of note is that cysteinyl leukotriene receptor antagonists reduce the number of eosinophils in the airway and blood [114], and mice missing the leukotriene B4 receptor have a profound decrease in lung eosinophils following allergen sensitization and challenge [115]. Finally, eosinophils, along with basophils, mast cells, and Th2 cells, express chemoattractant receptor-homologous molecule expressed on T helper 2 cells (CRTh2), a high-affinity receptor for prostaglandin D2 [116,117], whereas both Th2 cells and eosinophils express the H4 histamine receptor [118]. The relative contribution of these pathways compared with others remains to be delineated when specific antagonists become available.

Activation of eosinophil degranulation and mediator release

For eosinophils to participate in local tissue pathobiology, more must occur than their accumulation; indeed, activation of recruited eosinophils is thought to be a critical aspect of disease pathophysiology. For example, IL-5–transgenic mice have massively increased numbers of eosinophils in the circulation, spleen, and other tissues, but without a second signal these mice are relatively healthy. One of the major pathways by which eosinophils are activated is through cross-linking of surface immunoglobulin receptors, especially those involving IgA and, to a lesser degree, IgG [100]. Although there is general agreement that mouse eosinophils do not express FcεRI, this topic remains controversial for human eosinophils. The preponderance of recent literature suggests that human eosinophils express very low levels, if any, of FcεRI on their surface and that, if present, FcεRI clearly lacks the β chain; therefore, significant, direct activation of eosinophils by means of IgE remains unlikely [119–121]. Stimulation of eosinophils leads to eosinophil granule protein release (eg, ECP, EDN, EPO, MBP), superoxide generation, and synthesis of leukotriene C4 [100,122], although the last is difficult to induce with traditional eosinophil-activating stimuli. Eosinophils also produce platelet-activating factor and a wide range of cytokines and chemokines, not the least of which are IL-1β and transforming growth factor-β (TGF-β), two key players in the eosinophil-mediated tissue remodeling and fibrosis seen in many eosinophil-associated diseases [3,123–125]. Although the quantities of cytokines and chemokines released per eosinophil versus other cells vary widely, GM-CSF is among the cytokines produced in greatest quantities by eosinophils [100]; as noted previously, it functions in part in an autocrine fashion to prolong eosinophil survival once eosinophils are recruited into tissue inflammatory sites. Eosinophil activation in vitro by a number of agonists, including IL-5, interferon-γ, secretory IgA, and others, has been shown to induce secretion of the granule cationic proteins (EPO, MBP1, EDN, ECP) and eosinophil-expressed cytokines (eg, RANTES and IL-4) by a process termed "piecemeal degranulation" [126,127] that involves differential mobilization and vesicular transport of these proteins [114,128,129]. This process is in contrast to secondary granule fusion and classical exocytosis, events rarely observed for eosinophils in inflammatory foci in tissues [130]. Once secreted, the eosinophil granule cationic proteins have multiple potential proinflammatory activities that have been defined in vitro and in vivo, including membrane-, cell-, and tissue-damaging cytotoxicity [131,132], the ability to activate inflammatory cells (eg, mast cells and basophils) selectively, to release inflammatory mediators (eg, histamine) [133], potent blocking activity for inhibitory M2 muscarinic receptors in the airways in asthma models [134], and the ability to augment TGF-β–primed fibroblast elaboration of the inflammatory and profibrotic IL-6 family of cytokines including IL-6 and IL-11 [135], to name just a few. Thus, eosinophils (1) come fully armed with preformed mediators of inflammation, tissue damage, remodeling, and fibrogenesis that are secreted at sites of eosinophilic inflammation in tissues in eosinophil-associated diseases such as the hypereosinophilic syndromes and (2) have the capacity to generate newly formed protein (cytokines, chemokines) and lipid mediators (leukotriene C4, platelet-activating factor) of inflammation when primed and further activated during their recruitment from the bone marrow into the tissue in response to allergic and other stimuli [136].

Regulation of tissue eosinophil survival and activation

Once in tissues, if eosinophils do not encounter the appropriate survival milieu, the lack of exposure to such cytokines normally leads to their prompt apoptosis (see Fig. 2). Separate from this process, however, a number of pathways actively and, to varying degrees, selectively induce eosinophil apoptosis. In humans, corticosteroids markedly and rapidly diminish numbers of circulating and tissue eosinophils. The mechanisms responsible for this action are complex and probably involve a combination of altered release from bone marrow, shortened circulation time, redistribution from the circulation into spleen and other organs, induction of apoptosis, and inhibition of cytokines and chemokines needed for eosinophil survival and recruitment [137–141]. Besides steroids, other proapoptotic molecules for eosinophils include lidocaine [142], TGF-β [143], Siglec-8/Siglec-F [144,145], Fas (CD95) [146], and CD30 [147]. Although prior exposure to survival cytokines or priming conditions tends to improve eosinophil resistance to these death pathways, a unique situation is the Siglec-8 pathway, which actually is augmented by priming cytokines [144,148]. Another drug used to reduce eosinophil numbers is hydroxyurea, although this drug is used to cause a more global inhibitory effect on hematopoiesis. Interferon-α and leukotriene synthesis or receptor blockers also reduce circulating eosinophil numbers [149]. Recently, tyrosine kinase inhibitors such as imatinib mesylate (Gleevec) have been shown to have profound effects on eosinophil numbers because a subset of individuals who have hypereosinophilic syndrome have a deletion mutation on chromosome 4 resulting in the fusion of a gene with unknown function, namely *FIP1L1*, with the *PDGFRα* (platelet-derived growth factor receptor-alpha) gene, resulting in a constitutively active tyrosine kinase [150]. Thus, patients found to be *FIP1L1-PDGFRα* positive, either by fluorescence in situ hybridization or by reverse transcription polymerase chain reaction, now are treated with imatinib mesylate. Other constitutively active tyrosine kinases, including type-2 fibroblast growth factor receptor-1 and PDGFRβ, have been implicated in eosinophilic syndromes [76].

Summary

The heterogeneity of hypereosinophilic syndromes, which ranges from patients who have features of myeloproliferative disorders with cytogenetic abnormalities (eg, *FIP1L1-PDGFRα*–positive chronic eosinophil leukemia, CEL) to patients who have more benign clinical courses (eg, episodic angioedema with eosinophilia), suggests that multiple disease processes are at play that regulate eosinophilopoiesis in the bone marrow, the recruitment of eosinophils to tissues and their survival, the activation and secretion of inflammatory mediators, and pathophysiologic outcomes. Current research aimed at defining the causes of HES and mechanisms that regulate eosinophilia in these diseases and at understanding the development of eosinophil-mediated end-organ damage in eosinophil-associated diseases in general should lead to more selective and improved therapies for hypereosinophilic syndromes. The therapeutic targets for these efforts currently include (1) IL-5 and its high-affinity receptor; (2) underlying T-cell clones (either immunocompetent or occult T-lymphoid malignancies) that elaborate eosinophilopoietins such as IL-5 or GM-CSF [65,68] and tissue- or organ-specific dysfunctional elaboration of eosinophil-active chemoattractant factors such as eosinophil-selective chemokines (eg, eotaxin-3 in the esophagus in eosinophilic esophagitis) [107]; (3) vascular endothelial adhesion molecules (VCAM/VLA-4); and (4) inhibitory receptors such as Siglec-8 [144] and CD300a [151]. The essential absence of end-organ damage in some of the hypereosinophilic syndromes contrasts starkly with the morbidity (and mortality) associated with the development of endomyocardial fibrosis in HES. Because patients who have HES are clearly a heterogeneous group, clinical management based on current knowledge must be tailored specifically to the individual, with the overall goal of controlling the blood and tissue eosinophilia and, in particular, the eosinophil-mediated end-organ damage [152]. Current treatment options permit the control or eradication of eosinophilia and end-organ damage in most patients who have HES [149,152]. The efficacy of imatinib mesylate (Gleevec) in some patients who have HES led to the identification of the *FIP1L1-PDGFRα* gene fusion that encodes a pathogenetically relevant and constitutively active tyrosine kinase [150]. This seminal finding has led to a reclassification of hypereosinophilias into better-defined clinical entities [149,152] and has stimulated new research that ultimately may translate into improved clinical characterization and therapeutic options.

Finally, humanized anti-IL-5 antibody (Mepolizumab) recently has shown clinical efficacy for controlling eosinophilia in HES in clinical trials [9,44,153] and looks highly promising for the treatment of a wide range of patients who have FIP1L1-PDGFRα–negative HES and possibly other eosinophilias [149] (eg, eosinophilic gastrointestinal syndromes such as eosinophilic esophagitis) [8]. Future research on HES and CEL should focus on the molecular basis of imatinib responsiveness in both *FIP1L1-PDGFRα*–positive and –negative patients, addressing how the constitutively activated *FIP1L1-PDGFRα* or other fusion or mutant-activated kinases selectively lead to chronic hypereosinophilia and end-organ damage. Studies of the effects of imatinib on the proliferation and terminal differentiation of bone marrow–derived eosinophil progenitors and the survival and intracellular signaling pathways in eosinophils from imatinib-responsive patients may be particularly revealing in terms of the downstream targets of these novel kinases and the roles of eosinophil-active eosinophilopoietins and survival factors such as IL-5 and GM-CSF [154].

References

[1] Kay AB. The role of eosinophils in the pathogenesis of asthma. Trends Mol Med 2005; 11(4):148–52.

[2] Kay AB, Phipps S, Robinson DS. A role for eosinophils in airway remodelling in asthma. Trends Immunol 2004;25(9):477–82.

[3] Gomes I, Mathur SK, Espenshade BM, et al. Eosinophil-fibroblast interactions induce fibroblast IL-6 secretion and extracellular matrix gene expression: implications in fibrogenesis. J Allergy Clin Immunol 2005;116(4):796–804.

[4] Lee JJ, Dimina D, Macias MP, et al. Defining a link with asthma in mice congenitally deficient in eosinophils. Science 2004;305(5691):1773–6.

[5] Humbles AA, Lloyd CM, McMillan SJ, et al. A critical role for eosinophils in allergic airways remodeling. Science 2004;305(5691):1776–9.

[6] Phipps S, Flood-Page P, Menzies-Gow A, et al. Intravenous anti-IL-5 monoclonal antibody reduces eosinophils and tenascin deposition in allergen-challenged human atopic skin. J Invest Dermatol 2004;122(6):1406–12.

[7] Flood-Page P, Menzies-Gow A, Phipps S, et al. Anti-IL-5 treatment reduces deposition of ECM proteins in the bronchial subepithelial basement membrane of mild atopic asthmatics. J Clin Invest 2003;112(7):1029–36.

[8] Stein ML, Collins MH, Villanueva JM, et al. Anti-IL-5 (Mepolizumab) therapy for eosinophilic esophagitis. J Allergy Clin Immunol 2006;118(6):1312–9.

[9] Rothenberg ME, Gleich GJ, Roufosse FE, et al. Steroid-sparing effects of anti-IL-5 monoclonal antibody (Mepolizumab) therapy in patients with HES: a multicenter, randomized, double-blind, placebo-controlled trial. Blood [ASH Annual Meeting Abstracts] 2006;108: 373.

[10] Takatsu K, Tominaga A, Harada N, et al. T cell-replacing factor (TRF)/interleukin 5 (IL-5): molecular and functional properties. Immunol Rev 1988;102:107–35.

[11] Plaut M, Pierce JH, Watson CJ, et al. Mast cell lines produce lymphokines in response to cross-linkage of Fc epsilon RI or to calcium ionophores. Nature 1989;339(6219):64–7.

[12] Galli SJ, Gordon JR, Wershil BK, et al. Mast cell and eosinophil cytokines in allergy and inflammation. In: Kay AB, Gleich GJ, editors. Eosinophils in allergy and inflammation, vol. 2New York: Marcel Dekker; 1994. p. 255–80.

[13] Palacios R, Karasuyama H, Rolink A. Ly1+ PRO-B lymphocyte clones. Phenotype, growth requirements and differentiation in vitro and in vivo. EMBO J 1987;6(12):3687–93.

[14] Takatsu K, Yamaguchi N, Hitoshi Y, et al. Signal transduction through interleukin-5 receptors. Cold Spring Harb Symp Quant Biol 1989;2:745–51.

[15] Yamaguchi Y, Suda T, Suda J, et al. Purified interleukin 5 supports the terminal differentiation and proliferation of murine eosinophilic precursors. J Exp Med 1988;167(1): 43–56.

[16] Sanderson CJ. Eosinophil differentiation factor (interleukin-5). Immunol Ser 1990;49: 231–56.

[17] Sanderson CJ. Control of eosinophilia. Int Arch Allergy Appl Immunol 1991;94(1–4): 122–6.

[18] Owen WF, Rothenberg ME, Petersen J, et al. Interleukin 5 and phenotypically altered eosinophils in the blood of patients with the idiopathic hypereosinophilic syndrome. J Exp Med 1989;170(1):343–8.

[19] Owen W Jr, Petersen J, Sheff DM, et al. Hypodense eosinophils and interleukin 5 activity in the blood of patients with the eosinophilia-myalgia syndrome. Proc Natl Acad Sci U S A 1990;87(21):8647–51.

[20] Sanderson CJ. Interleukin-5, eosinophils, and disease. Blood 1992;79(12):3101–9.

[21] Dent LA, Strath M, Mellor AL, et al. Eosinophilia in transgenic mice expressing Interleukin-5. J Exp Med 1990;172(5):1425–31.

[22] Tominaga A, Takaki S, Koyama N, et al. Transgenic mice expressing a B-cell growth and differentiation factor gene (interleukin-5) develop eosinophilia and autoantibody production. J Exp Med 1991;173(2):429–37.

[23] Kopf M, Brombacher F, Hodgkin PD, et al. IL-5-deficient mice have a developmental defect in CD5+ B-1 cells and lack eosinophilia but have normal antibody and cytotoxic T cell responses. Immunity 1996;4(1):15–24.

[24] Foster PS, Hogan SP, Ramsay AJ, et al. Interleukin 5 deficiency abolishes airways eosinophilia, airways hyperreactivity, and lung damage in mouse asthma model. J Exp Med 1996; 183:195–201.

[25] Cho JY, Miller M, Baek KJ, et al. Inhibition of airway remodeling in IL-5-deficient mice. J Clin Invest 2004;113(4):551–60.

[26] Cantor AB, Orkin SH. Hematopoietic development: a balancing act. Curr Opin Genet Dev 2001;11(5):513–9.

[27] Miyamoto T, Akashi K. Lineage promiscuous expression of transcription factors in normal hematopoiesis. Int J Hematol 2005;81(5):361–7.

[28] Akashi K. Lineage promiscuity and plasticity in hematopoietic development. Ann N Y Acad Sci 2005;1044:125–31.

[29] McNagny K, Graf T. Making eosinophils through subtle shifts in transcription factor expression. J Exp Med 2002;195(11):F43–7.

[30] Yamaguchi Y, Nishio H, Kishi K, et al. C/EBPbeta and GATA-1 synergistically regulate activity of the eosinophil granule major basic protein promoter: implication for C/EBPbeta activity in eosinophil gene expression. Blood 1999;94(4):1429–39.

[31] Querfurth E, Schuster M, Kulessa H, et al. Antagonism between C/EBPbeta and FOG in eosinophil lineage commitment of multipotent hematopoietic progenitors. Genes Dev 2000;14(19):2515–25.

[32] Hirasawa R, Shimizu R, Takahashi S, et al. Essential and instructive roles of GATA factors in eosinophil development. J Exp Med 2002;195(11):1379–86.

[33] Yu C, Cantor AB, Yang H, et al. Targeted deletion of a high-affinity GATA-binding site in the GATA-1 promoter leads to selective loss of the eosinophil lineage in vivo. J Exp Med 2002;195(11):1387–95.

[34] Du J, Stankiewicz MJ, Liu Y, et al. Novel combinatorial interactions of GATA-1, PU.1, and C/EBPepsilon isoforms regulate transcription of the gene encoding eosinophil granule major basic protein. J Biol Chem 2002;277(45):43481–94.

[35] Zimmermann N, Colyer JL, Koch LE, et al. Analysis of the CCR3 promoter reveals a regulatory region in exon 1 that binds GATA-1. BMC Immunol 2005;6(1):7.

[36] Stopka T, Amanatullah DF, Papetti M, et al. PU.1 inhibits the erythroid program by binding to GATA-1 on DNA and creating a repressive chromatin structure. EMBO J 2005; 24(21):3712–23.

[37] Du J, Vyas D, Xi Q, et al. Double GAT-1 binding sites Specify PU.1 and GATA-1 synergy in transcriptional regulation of myeloid lineage-specific genes. Nucleic Acids Research 2007; submitted for publication.

[38] Zhang DE, Zhang P, Wang ND, et al. Absence of granulocyte colony-stimulating factor signaling and neutrophil development in CCAAT enhancer binding protein alpha- deficient mice. Proc Natl Acad Sci U S A 1997;94(2):569–74.

[39] Ackerman SJ, Du J, Xin F, et al. Eosinophilopoiesis: to be or not to be (an eosinophil)? That is the question: transcriptional themes regulating eosinophil genes and development. Respir Med 2000;94:1135–40.

[40] Du J, Savage MP, Dekoter R, et al. Impaired eosinophilopoiesis and eosinophil gene expression in PU.1 (Spi-1 oncogene) deficient mice. Exp Hematol 2007; in press.

[41] Yamanaka R, Barlow C, Lekstrom-Himes J, et al. Impaired granulopoiesis, myelodysplasia, and early lethality in CCAAT/enhancer binding protein epsilon-deficient mice. Proc Natl Acad Sci U S A 1997;94(24):13187–92.

[42] Yamanaka R, Lekstrom-Himes J, Barlow C, et al. CCAAT/enhancer binding proteins are critical components of the transcriptional regulation of hematopoiesis [review]. Int J Mol Med 1998;1(1):213–21.

[43] Rosenberg HF, Gallin JI. Neutrophil-specific granule deficiency includes eosinophils. Blood 1993;82(1):268–73.

[44] Klion AD, Law MA, Noel P, et al. Safety and efficacy of the monoclonal anti-interleukin-5 antibody SCH55700 in the treatment of patients with hypereosinophilic syndrome. Blood 2004;103(8):2939–41.

[45] Menzies-Gow A, Flood-Page P, Sehmi R, et al. Anti-IL-5 (Mepolizumab) therapy induces bone marrow eosinophil maturational arrest and decreases eosinophil progenitors in the bronchial mucosa of atopic asthmatics. J Allergy Clin Immunol 2003;111(4): 714–9.

[46] Clutterbuck EJ, Hirst EMA, Sanderson CJ. Human interleukin-5 (IL-5) regulates the production of eosinophils in human bone marrow cultures: comparison and interaction with IL-1, IL-3, IL-6, and GMCSF. Blood 1989;73:1504–12.

[47] Seminario M-C, Saini SS, MacGlashan DW Jr, et al. Intracellular expression and release of FceRIa by human eosinophils. J Immunol 1999;162:6893–900.

[48] Smith SJ, Ying S, Meng Q, et al. Blood eosinophils from atopic donors express messenger RNA for the alpha, beta, and gamma subunits of the high-affinity IgE receptor (Fc epsilon RI) and intracellular, but not cell surface, alpha subunit protein. J Allergy Clin Immunol 2000;105(2 Pt 1):309–17.

[49] Ackerman SJ, Kephart GM, Habermann TM, et al. Localization of eosinophil granule major basic protein in human basophils. J Exp Med 1983;158:946–61.

[50] Ackerman SJ, Weil GJ, Gleich GJ. Formation of Charcot-Leyden crystals by human basophils. J Exp Med 1982;155(6):1597–609.

[51] Abu-Ghazaleh RI, Dunnette SL, Loegering DA, et al. Eosinophil granule proteins in peripheral blood granulocytes. J Leukoc Biol 1992;52(6):611–8.

[52] Bochner BS, Schleimer RP. Mast cells, basophils, and eosinophils: distinct but overlapping pathways for recruitment. Immunol Rev 2001;179:5–15.

[53] Voehringer D, van Rooijen N, Locksley RM. Eosinophils develop in distinct stages and are recruited to peripheral sites by alternatively activated macrophages. J Leukoc Biol 2007;81(6):1434–44.

[54] Aizawa H, Zimmermann N, Carrigan PE, et al. Molecular analysis of human Siglec-8 orthologs relevant to mouse eosinophils: identification of mouse orthologs of Siglec-5 (mSiglec-F) and Siglec-10 (mSiglec-G). Genomics 2003;82(5):521–30.

[55] Zhang JQ, Biedermann B, Nitschke L, et al. The murine inhibitory receptor mSiglec-E is expressed broadly on cells of the innate immune system whereas mSiglec-F is restricted to eosinophils. Eur J Immunol 2004;34(4):1175–84.

[56] Kikly KK, Bochner BS, Freeman S, et al. Identification of SAF-2, a novel Siglec expressed on eosinophils, mast cells and basophils. J Allergy Clin Immunol 2000;105:1093–100.

[57] Palframan RT, Collins PD, Severs NJ, et al. Mechanisms of acute eosinophil mobilization from the bone marrow stimulated by interleukin 5: the role of specific adhesion molecules and phosphatidylinositol 3-kinase. J Exp Med 1998;188(9):1621–32.

[58] Palframan RT, Collins PD, Williams TJ, et al. Eotaxin induces a rapid release of eosinophils and their progenitors from the bone marrow. Blood 1998;91(7):2240–8.

[59] Werfel S, Yednock T, Matsumoto K, et al. Functional regulation of b1 integrins and human eosinophils by divalent cations and cytokines. Am J Respir Cell Mol Biol 1996;14:45–52.

[60] Weber C, Kitayama J, Springer TA. Differential regulation of b1 and b2 integrin avidity by chemoattractants in eosinophils. Proc Natl Acad Sci USA 1996;93:10939–44.

[61] Tachimoto H, Burdick M, Hudson SA, et al. CCR3-active chemokines promote rapid detachment of eosinophils from VCAM-1 in vitro. J Immunol 2000;165:2748–54.

[62] Minshall EM, Schleimer R, Cameron L, et al. Interleukin-5 expression in the bone marrow of sensitized Balb/c mice after allergen challenge. Am J Respir Crit Care Med 1998;158(3):951–7.

[63] Groopman JE, Mitsuyasu RT, DeLeo MJ, et al. Effect of recombinant human granulocyte-macrophage colony-stimulating factor on myelopoiesis in the acquired immunodeficiency syndrome. N Engl J Med 1987;317:593–8.

[64] Shi HZ, Xiao CQ, Zhong D, et al. Effect of inhaled interleukin-5 on airway hyperreactivity and eosinophilia in asthmatics. Am J Respir Crit Care Med 1998;157(1):204–9.

[65] Bochner BS, Friedman B, Krishnaswami G, et al. Episodic eosinophilia-myalgia-like syndrome in a patient without L-tryptophan use: association with eosinophil activation and increased serum levels of granulocyte-macrophage colony-stimulating factor. J Allergy Clin Immunol 1991;88(4):629–36.

[66] Butterfield JH, Leiferman KM, Abrams J, et al. Elevated serum levels of interleukin-5 in patients with the syndrome of episodic angioedema and eosinophilia. Blood 1992;79(3): 688–92.

[67] Fang J, Viksman MY, Ebisawa M, et al. Increased circulating levels of interleukin-5 in a case of steroid-resistant hypereosinophilic syndrome with ileal involvement. J Allergy Clin Immunol 1994;94:129–31.

[68] Simon HU, Plotz SG, Dummer R, et al. Abnormal clones of T cells producing interleukin-5 in idiopathic eosinophilia. N Engl J Med 1999;341(15):1112–20.

[69] Mishra A, Hogan SP, Lee JJ, et al. Fundamental signals that regulate eosinophil homing to the gastrointestinal tract. J Clin Invest 1999;103(12):1719–27.

[70] Winkel P, Statland BE, Saunders AM, et al. Within-day physiologic variation of leukocyte types in healthy subjects as assayed by two automated leukocyte differential analyzers. Am J Clin Pathol 1981;75(5):693–700.

[71] Bochner BS. Adhesion molecules as therapeutic targets. Immunol Allergy Clin North Am 2004;24(4):615–30.

[72] Gauvreau GM, Becker AB, Boulet LP, et al. The effects of an anti-CD11a mAb, efalizumab, on allergen-induced airway responses and airway inflammation in subjects with atopic asthma. J Allergy Clin Immunol 2003;112(2):331–8.

[73] Shi HZ, Humbles A, Gerard C, et al. Lymph node trafficking and antigen presentation by endobronchial eosinophils. J Clin Invest 2000;105(7):945–53.

[74] Conus S, Bruno A, Simon HU. Leptin is an eosinophil survival factor. J Allergy Clin Immunol 2005;116(6):1228–34.

[75] Bureau F, Seumois G, Jaspar F, et al. CD40 engagement enhances eosinophil survival through induction of cellular inhibitor of apoptosis protein 2 expression: possible involvement in allergic inflammation. J Allergy Clin Immunol 2002;110:443–9.

[76] Rothenberg ME, Hogan SP. The eosinophil. Annu Rev Immunol 2006;24:147–74.

[77] Simon HU, Yousefi S, Schranz C, et al. Direct demonstration of delayed eosinophil apoptosis as a mechanism causing tissue eosinophilia. J Immunol 1997;158(8):3902–8.

[78] Cameron L, Christodoulopoulos P, Lavigne F, et al. Evidence for local eosinophil differentiation within allergic nasal mucosa: inhibition with soluble IL-5 receptor. J Immunol 2000; 164(3):1538–45.

[79] Denburg JA, Keith PK. Systemic aspects of chronic rhinosinusitis. Immunol Allergy Clin North Am 2004;24(1):87–102.

[80] Broide DH, Lotz M, Cuomo AJ, et al. Cytokines in symptomatic asthma airways. J Allergy Clin Immunol 1992;89(5):958–67.

[81] Kroegel C, Liu MC, Hubbard WM, et al. Blood and bronchoalveolar eosinophils in allergic subjects following segmental antigen challenge: surface phenotype, density heterogeneity, and prostanoid production. J Allergy Clin Immunol 1994;93:725–34.

[82] Esnault S, Malter JS. GM-CSF regulation in eosinophils. Arch Immunol Ther Exp (Warsz) 2002;50(2):121–30.

[83] Rosenberg HF, Phipps S, Foster PS. Eosinophil trafficking in allergy and asthma. J Allergy Clin Immunol 2007;119(6):1303–10.

[84] Fryer AD, Costello RW, Yost BL, et al. Antibody to VLA-4, but not to L-selectin, protects neuronal M2 muscarinic receptors in antigen-challenged guinea pig airways. J Clin Invest 1997;99:2036–44.

[85] Gonzalo JA, Lloyd CM, Kremer L, et al. Eosinophil recruitment to the lung in a murine model of allergic inflammation—the role of T cells, chemokines, and adhesion receptors. J Clin Invest 1996;98(10):2332–45.

[86] Gonzalo JA, Lloyd CM, Wen D, et al. The coordinated action of CC chemokines in the lung orchestrates allergic inflammation and airway hyperresponsiveness. J Exp Med 1998; 188(1):157–67.

[87] Norris V, Choong L, Tran D, et al. Effect of IVL745, a VLA-4 antagonist, on allergen-induced bronchoconstriction in patients with asthma. J Allergy Clin Immunol 2005; 116(4):761–7.

[88] Pero RS, Borchers MT, Spicher K, et al. Galphai2-mediated signaling events in the endothelium are involved in controlling leukocyte extravasation. Proc Natl Acad Sci U S A 2007; 104(11):4371–6.

[89] Anwar ARF, Moqbel R, Walsh GM, et al. Adhesion to fibronectin prolongs eosinophil survival. J Exp Med 1993;177(3):839–43.

[90] Georas SN, McIntyre BW, Ebisawa M, et al. Expression of a functional laminin receptor (a6b1, VLA-6) on human eosinophils. Blood 1993;82:2872–9.

[91] Bochner BS. Cellular adhesion in inflammation. In: Adkinson NF Jr, Yunginger JW, Busse WW, et al, editors. Allergy principles and practice. 6th edition. St. Louis (MO): Mosby; 2003. p. 117–34.

[92] Broide DH, Sullivan S, Gifford T, et al. Inhibition of pulmonary eosinophilia in P-selectin- and ICAM-1-deficient mice. Am J Respir Cell Mol Biol 1998;18(2):218–25.

[93] Bochner BS. Road signs guiding leukocytes along the inflammation superhighway. J Allergy Clin Immunol 2000;106:817–28.

[94] Broide D, Sriramarao P. Eosinophil trafficking to sites of allergic inflammation. Immunol Rev 2001;179:163–72.

[95] Wardlaw AJ. Molecular basis for selective eosinophil trafficking in asthma: a multistep paradigm. J Allergy Clin Immunol 1999;104(5):917–26.

[96] Bochner BS, Sterbinsky SA, Bickel CA, et al. Differences between human eosinophils and neutrophils in the function and expression of sialic acid-containing counterligands for E-selectin. J Immunol 1994;152:774–82.

[97] Broide DH, Miller M, Castaneda D, et al. Core 2 oligosaccharides mediate eosinophil and neutrophil peritoneal but not lung recruitment. Am J Physiol Lung Cell Mol Physiol 2002;282:L259–66.

[98] Beeh KM, Beier J, Meyer M, et al. Bimosiamose, an inhaled small-molecule pan-selectin antagonist, attenuates late asthmatic reactions following allergen challenge in mild asthmatics: a randomized, double-blind, placebo-controlled clinical cross-over-trial. Pulm Pharmacol Ther 2006;19(4):233–41.

[99] Meyer M, Beeh KM, Beier J, et al. Tolerability and pharmacokinetics of inhaled bimosiamose disodium in healthy males. Br J Clin Pharmacol 2007;63(4):451–8.

[100] Kita H, Adolphson CR, Gleich GJ. Biology of eosinophils. In: Adkinson NF Jr, Yunginger JW, Busse WW, et al, editors. Allergy principles and practice. 6th edition. Philadelphia: Mosby; 2003. p. 305–32.

[101] Prin L, Capron M, Tonnel AB, et al. Heterogeneity of human peripheral blood eosinophils: variability in cell density and cytotoxic ability in relation to the level and the origin of hypereosinophilia. Int Arch Allergy Appl Immunol 1983;72(4):336–46.

[102] Fukuda T, Dunnette SL, Reed CE, et al. Increased numbers of hypodense eosinophils in the blood of patients with bronchial asthma. Am Rev Respir Dis 1985;132(5): 981–5.

[103] Caulfield JP, Hein A, Rothenberg ME, et al. A morphometric study of normodense and hypodense human eosinophils that are derived in vivo and in vitro. Am J Pathol 1990;137(1): 27–41.

[104] Matsumoto K, Appiah-Pippim J, Schleimer RP, et al. CD44 and CD69 represent different types of cell surface activation markers for human eosinophils. Am J Respir Cell Mol Biol 1998;18:860–6.

[105] Koenderman L, van der Bruggen T, Schweizer RC, et al. Eosinophil priming by cytokines: from cellular signal to in vivo modulation. Eur Respir J Suppl 1996;22:119s–25s.

[106] Brandt EB, Zimmermann N, Muntel EE, et al. The alpha4bbeta7-integrin is dynamically expressed on murine eosinophils and involved in eosinophil trafficking to the intestine. Clin Exp Allergy 2006;36(4):543–53.

[107] Blanchard C, Wang N, Stringer KF, et al. Eotaxin-3 and a uniquely conserved gene-expression profile in eosinophilic esophagitis. J Clin Invest 2006;116(2):536–47.

[108] Katoh S, Matsumoto N, Kawakita K, et al. A role for CD44 in an antigen-induced murine model of pulmonary eosinophilia. J Clin Invest 2003;111(10):1563–70.

[109] Zimmermann N, Hershey GK, Foster PS, et al. Chemokines in asthma: cooperative interaction between chemokines and IL-13. J Allergy Clin Immunol 2003;111(2): 227–42.

[110] Menzies-Gow A, Ying S, Sabroe I, et al. Eotaxin (CCL11) and eotaxin-2 (CCL24) induce recruitment of eosinophils, basophils, neutrophils, and macrophages as well as features of early- and late-phase allergic reactions following cutaneous injection in human atopic and nonatopic volunteers. J Immunol 2002;169(5):2712–8.

[111] Beck LA, Dalke S, Leiferman KM, et al. Cutaneous injection of RANTES causes eosinophil recruitment: comparison of nonallergic and allergic human subjects. J Immunol 1997; 159(6):2962–72.

[112] Pereira S, Clark T, Darby Y, et al. Effects of anti-eotaxin monoclonal antibody CAT-213 on allergen-induced rhinitis [abstract]. J Allergy Clin Immunol 2003;111:S268.

[113] Main S, Handy R, Wilton J, et al. A potent human anti-eotaxin1 antibody, CAT-213: isolation by phage display and in vitro and in vivo efficacy. J Pharmacol Exp Ther 2006;319(3): 1395–404.

[114] Moqbel R, Lacy P. Exocytotic events in eosinophils and mast cells. Clin Exp Allergy 1999; 29(8):1017–22.

[115] Tager AM, Dufour JH, Goodarzi K, et al. BLTR mediates leukotriene B(4)-induced chemotaxis and adhesion and plays a dominant role in eosinophil accumulation in a murine model of peritonitis. J Exp Med 2000;192(3):439–46.

[116] Nagata K, Hirai H, Tanaka K, et al. CRTH2, an orphan receptor of T-helper-2-cells, is expressed on basophils and eosinophils and responds to mast cell-derived factor(s). FEBS Lett 1999;459(2):195–9.

[117] Hirai H, Tanaka K, Yoshie O, et al. Prostaglandin D2 selectively induces chemotaxis in T helper type 2 cells, eosinophils, and basophils via seven-transmembrane receptor CRTH2. J Exp Med 2001;193(2):255–61.

[118] O'Reilly M, Alpert R, Jenkinson S, et al. Identification of a histamine H4 receptor on human eosinophils–role in eosinophil chemotaxis. J Recept Signal Transduct Res 2002; 22(1–4):431–48.

[119] Sihra BS, Kon OM, Grant JA, et al. Expression of high-affinity IgE receptors (FceRI) on peripheral blood basophils, monocytes, and eosinophils in atopic and nonatopic subjects: relationship to total serum IgE concentrations. J Allergy Clin Immunol 1997;99(5): 699–706.

[120] Kita H, Kaneko M, Bartemes KR, et al. Does IgE bind to and activate eosinophils from patients with allergy? J Immunol 1999;162:6901–11.

[121] Kayaba H, Dombrowicz D, Woerly G, et al. Human eosinophils and human high affinity IgE receptor transgenic mouse eosinophils express low levels of high affinity IgE receptor, but release IL-10 upon receptor activation. J Immunol 2001;167(2):995–1003.

[122] Bandeira-Melo C, Weller PF. Eosinophils and cysteinyl leukotrienes. Prostaglandins Leukot Essent Fatty Acids 2003;69(2–3):135–43.

[123] Gharaee-Kermani M, Phan SH. The role of eosinophils in pulmonary fibrosis [review]. Int J Mol Med 1998;1(1):43–53.

[124] Levi-Schaffer F, Garbuzenko E, Rubin A, et al. Human eosinophils regulate human lung- and skin-derived fibroblast properties in vitro: a role for transforming growth factor beta (TGF-beta). Proc Natl Acad Sci U S A 1999;96(17):9660–5.

[125] Spry CJ. The pathogenesis of endomyocardial fibrosis: the role of the eosinophil. Springer Semin Immunopathol 1989;11(4):471–7.

[126] Dvorak AM, Ackerman SJ, Furitsu T, et al. Mature eosinophils stimulated to develop in human-cord blood mononuclear cell cultures supplemented with recombinant human interleukin-5. II. Vesicular transport of specific granule matrix peroxidase, a mechanism for effecting piecemeal degranulation. Am J Pathol 1992;140(4):795–807.

[127] Melo RC, Perez SA, Spencer LA, et al. Intragranular vesiculotubular compartments are involved in piecemeal degranulation by activated human eosinophils. Traffic 2005;6(10): 866–79.

[128] Logan MR, Odemuyiwa SO, Moqbel R. Understanding exocytosis in immune and inflammatory cells: the molecular basis of mediator secretion. J Allergy Clin Immunol 2003; 111(5):923–32.

[129] Moqbel R, Coughlin JJ. Differential secretion of cytokines. Sci STKE 2006;338:26.

[130] Dvorak AM, Ackerman SJ, Weller PF. Subcellular morphology and biochemistry of eosinophils. In: Harris JR, editor. Blood cell biochemistry: megakaryocytes, platelets, macrophages and eosinophils, vol. 2. London: Plenum Publishing Corporation; 1990. p. 237–344.

[131] Gleich GJ. Mechanisms of eosinophil-associated inflammation. J Allergy Clin Immunol 2000;105(4):651–63.

[132] Martin LB, Kita H, Leiferman KM, et al. Eosinophils in allergy: role in disease, degranulation, and cytokines. Int Arch Allergy Immunol 1996;109(3):207–15.

[133] Thomas LL, Page SM. Inflammatory cell activation by eosinophil granule proteins. Chem Immunol 2000;76:99–117.

[134] Jacoby DB, Costello RM, Fryer AD. Eosinophil recruitment to the airway nerves. J Allergy Clin Immunol 2001;107(2):211–8.

[135] Rochester CL, Ackerman SJ, Zheng T, et al. Eosinophil-fibroblast interactions. Granule major basic protein interacts with IL-1 and transforming growth factor-beta in the stimulation of lung fibroblast IL-6-type cytokine production. J Immunol 1996;156(11):4449–56.

[136] Sedgwick JB, Calhoun WJ, Vrtis RF, et al. Comparison of airway and blood eosinophil function after in vivo antigen challenge. J Immunol 1992;149(11):3710–8.

[137] Gleich GJ, Hunt LW, Bochner BS, et al. Glucocorticoid effects on human eosinophils. In: Schleimer RP, Busse WW, O'Byrne P, editors. Inhaled glucocorticoids in asthma: mechanisms and clinical actions. New York: Marcel Dekker, Inc.; 1996. p. 279–308.

[138] Stellato C, Matsukura S, Fal A, et al. Differential regulation of epithelial-derived C-C chemokine expression by IL-4 and the glucocorticoid budesonide. J Immunol 1999;163(10): 5624–32.

[139] Druilhe A, Letuve S, Pretolani M. Glucocorticoid-induced apoptosis in human eosinophils: mechanisms of action. Apoptosis 2003;8(5):481–95.

[140] Fan J, Heller NM, Gorospe M, et al. The role of post-transcriptional regulation in chemokine gene expression in inflammation and allergy. Eur Respir J 2005;26(5):933–47.

[141] Simon HU. Molecules involved in the regulation of eosinophil apoptosis. Chem Immunol Allergy 2006;91:49–58.

[142] Okada S, Hagan JB, Kato M, et al. Lidocaine and its analogues inhibit IL-5-mediated survival and activation of human eosinophils. J Immunol 1998;160(8):4010–7.

[143] Alam R, Forsythe P, Stafford S, et al. Transforming growth factor beta abrogates the effects of hematopoietins on eosinophils and induces their apoptosis. J Exp Med 1994;179(3): 1041–5.

[144] Nutku E, Aizawa H, Hudson SA, et al. Ligation of Siglec-8: a selective mechanism for induction of human eosinophil apoptosis. Blood 2003;101(12):5014–20.

[145] Zhang M, Angata T, Cho JY, et al. Defining the in vivo function of Siglec-F, a CD33-related Siglec expressed on mouse eosinophils. Blood 2007;109:4280–7.

[146] Matsumoto K, Schleimer RP, Saito H, et al. Induction of apoptosis in human eosinophils by anti-fas antibody treatment in vitro. Blood 1995;86:1437–43.

[147] Matsumoto K, Terakawa M, Miura K, et al. Extremely rapid and intense induction of apoptosis in human eosinophils by anti-CD30 antibody treatment in vitro. J Immunol 2004; 172(4):2186–93.

[148] von Gunten S, Vogel M, Schaub A, et al. Intravenous immunoglobulin preparations contain anti-Siglec-8 autoantibodies. J Allergy Clin Immunol 2007;119(4):1005–11.

[149] Klion AD, Bochner BS, Gleich GJ, et al. Approaches to the treatment of hypereosinophilic syndromes: a workshop summary report. J Allergy Clin Immunol 2006;117(6): 1292–302.

[150] Cools J, DeAngelo DJ, Gotlib J, et al. A tyrosine kinase created by fusion of the PDGFRα and FIP1L1 genes as a therapeutic target of imatinib in idiopathic hypereosinophilic syndrome. N Engl J Med 2003;348(13):1201–14.

[151] Munitz A, Bachelet I, Levi-Schaffer F. Reversal of airway inflammation and remodeling in asthma by a bispecific antibody fragment linking CCR3 to CD300a. J Allergy Clin Immunol 2006;118(5):1082–9.

[152] Ackerman SJ, Butterfield JH. Eosinophilia, eosinophil-associated diseases and the hypereosinophilic syndromes. In: Hoffman RH, Benz EJ, Shattil SJ, et al, editors. Hematology, basic principles and practice. 4th edition. Philadelphia: Churchill Livingstone/W.B. Saunders; 2004. p. 763–86.

[153] Klion AD, Rothenberg ME, Murray JJ, et al. Safety and tolerability of anti-IL-5 monoclonal antibody (Mepolizumab) therapy in patients with HES: a multicenter, randomized, double-blind, placebo-controlled trial. Blood [ASH Annual Meeting Abstracts] 2006;108: 2694.

[154] Yamada Y, Rothenberg ME, Lee AW, et al. The FIP1L1-PDGFRA fusion gene cooperates with IL-5 to induce murine hypereosinophilic syndrome (HES)/chronic eosinophilic leukemia (CEL)-like disease. Blood 2006;107(10):4071–9.

ELSEVIER
SAUNDERS

Immunol Allergy Clin N Am
27 (2007) 377–388

IMMUNOLOGY
AND ALLERGY
CLINICS
OF NORTH AMERICA

Chronic Eosinophilic Leukemias and the Myeloproliferative Variant of the Hypereosinophilic Syndrome

Barbara J. Bain, MBBS, FRACP, FRCPath*,
Sarah H. Fletcher, MBBChir, MRCP

*Department of Haematology, St Mary's Hospital Campus of Imperial College Faculty
of Medicine, St Mary's Hospital, Praed Street, London, W2 1NY, UK*

Eosinophilia can be primary or secondary. Most cases of primary eosinophilia represent a hematological neoplasm; a minority, for example familial eosinophilia, do not. Secondary or reactive eosinophilia can result from a multitude of underlying conditions. In addition to cases of eosinophilia identifiable as primary or secondary, there are patients in whom the cause cannot be discovered and in whom the eosinophilia is therefore referred to as "idiopathic." Among idiopathic cases, a syndrome of persistent unexplained eosinophilia leading to tissue damage has been designated the "idiopathic hypereosinophilic syndrome."

For several decades following Chusid and colleagues' [1] formulation of criteria for the diagnosis of the idiopathic hypereosinophilic syndrome in 1975, the true nature of this condition remained mysterious. Although there were no disease features that identified the condition as "leukemia," there was always a suspicion that in at least some cases the disease represented a hematological neoplasm. A proportion of patients subsequently developed granulocytic sarcoma or acute myeloid leukemia, suggesting that the chronic eosinophilia actually represented a chronic eosinophilic leukemia with the subsequent development of acute myeloid leukemia (AML) representing clonal evolution [2–4], analogous to the acute transformation that can occur in chronic myelogenous leukemia and less often in polycythemia vera and essential thrombocythemia. There have been at least 11 instances of patients with a diagnosis of idiopathic hypereosinophilic syndrome subsequently developing AML, with the time interval being as long as 24 years [4]. There

* Corresponding author.
E-mail address: b.bain@ic.ac.uk (B.J. Bain).

0889-8561/07/$ - see front matter © 2007 Elsevier Inc. All rights reserved.
doi:10.1016/j.iac.2007.06.001 *immunology.theclinics.com*

appear to be some common disease characteristics with 8 of 11 patients having developed a granulocytic sarcoma and 7 of 8 developing central nervous system (CNS) disease. Of four of these patients who were demonstrated to have normal cytogenetic analysis initially, three were restudied at the time of transformation and two of three had become abnormal [3,4].

In the past decade evidence has emerged that suggests that some patients with what would once have been called the idiopathic hypereosinophilic syndrome have a reactive condition and others have a hematological neoplasm.

In some patients with reactive eosinophilia, the cause, eg, parasitic infection, allergic disease, or lymphoma, is readily apparent. In others in whom there is no apparent primary causative condition, subsequent investigation discloses a population of cytokine-secreting T lymphocytes that are driving the eosinophilia [5,6]. The term "lymphocytic variant of hypereosinophilic syndrome" has been used to describe such cases. Sometimes an overt lymphoproliferative disorder subsequently becomes apparent.

FIP1L1-PDGFRA–associated chronic eosinophilic leukemia

An important subset of patients with eosinophilia that would otherwise be unexplained have recently been found to have eosinophilic leukemia, this diagnosis being based on the demonstration of a fusion gene that is a marker of a neoplastic clone of myeloid cells [7]. The term "myeloproliferative variant of hypereosinophilic syndrome" has been used for this condition. The neoplastic nature of the condition in these patients remained undiscovered for a considerable time because most patients had normal chromosomes on conventional cytogenetic analysis. The index patient, who drew attention to the cryptic deletion at 4q12, had t(1;4)(q44;q12) and was found to have an *FIP1L1-PDGFRA* fusion gene. A small number of other patients have had a different translocation with a 4q12 breakpoint, eg, a t(4;10)(q21;p11) in a Japanese man [8] and a few have had an unrelated chromosomal abnormality, such as add(2)(q),del(6)(q),+8,+19 [7] and add(17)(q25) [9]; both of these groups of patients, ie, those with related and those with unrelated clonal chromosomal abnormalities, can be diagnosed as having eosinophilic leukemia using conventional criteria. However, most patients with a normal karyotype could not be recognized as having leukemia before the discovery of the fusion gene and the introduction of tests for its detection.

The *FIP1L1-PDGRA* fusion gene encodes an aberrant, constitutively activated tyrosine kinase that drives the eosinophil proliferation without the need for external growth stimuli. The responsible mutation occurs in a pluripotent lymphoid-myeloid hemopoietic stem cell, able to give rise (at least in some patients) to eosinophils, neutrophils, monocytes, mast cells, B lymphocytes, and T lymphocytes [10]. However, generally abnormal proliferation is confined to eosinophil, mast cell, and, to a lesser extent, neutrophil lineages.

This syndrome has characteristic clinical and pathological features that aid in its recognition. It is predominantly a disease of males with the observed male:female ratio being about 17:1. The age range is wide, from 7 to 77 years, with most patients being between 25 and 55 years [11,12]. Clinical features may be those characteristically associated with leukemia or may be the result of tissue damage attributable to the release of eosinophil granule contents. Leukemia-related disease features include weight loss, fatigue, hepatomegaly, splenomegaly, pruritis, pallor, and bruising. Other patients present with cardiac, respiratory, cutaneous, or gastrointestinal symptoms and signs. The most serious tissue damage is cardiac, with the myocardium, endocardium, and cardiac valves being particularly affected. Other patients suffer from thromboembolic events, both venous and arterial. Respiratory symptoms include dyspnea and cough. Lung disease is usually mainly restrictive but sometimes there is also an obstructive element. Gastrointestinal symptoms often include diarrhea.

The importance of the discovery of the *FIP1L1-PDGFRA* fusion gene is that its aberrant product is a constitutively activated tyrosine kinase, which drives the abnormal proliferation and which can be inhibited by imatinib. Imatinib has already revolutionized the management of chronic myelogenous leukemia. It is now set to revolutionize the management of eosinophilic leukemia resulting from this fusion gene. In fact the FIP1L1-PDGFRA protein is much more readily inhibited than the BCR-ABL1 protein of chronic myelogenous leukemia. Although the same imatinib dose, 400 mg daily, is often used it is also possible to use a dose of 100 mg daily as long as molecular monitoring is possible, thus reducing both the side effects and the cost of treatment.

Timely diagnosis is important because some patients with long-established disease have died from cardiac complications despite effective treatment of the malignancy. Since the fusion gene can be detected in peripheral blood cells, molecular analysis can be performed quite early in the diagnostic process.

FIP1L1-PDGFRA fusion can be identified by the polymerase chain reaction (PCR), the greater sensitivity of nested PCR often being required for detection. It can also be identified by fluorescence in situ hybridization (FISH) analysis, looking for deletion of the *CHIC2* gene (which is located between *FIP1L1* and *PDGFRA* and is lost when this interstitial deletion occurs) or looking for fusion of upstream and downstream signals that are normally separate. The commercial availability of suitable probes means that such analysis is likely to become much more widely available than it has been until now. The detection of a clonal chromosomal abnormality (other than the specific ones described below) is *not* a reason to refrain from *FIP1L1-PDGFRA* analysis; molecular analysis is not needed to establish the diagnosis of chronic eosinophilic leukemia in patients with a clonal karyotypic abnormality but it is still required to identify this particular syndrome and direct therapy.

Patients with *FIP1L1-PDGFRA*–associated chronic eosinophilic leukemia may have cytologically abnormal eosinophils in the blood (eg, hypogranular, hypolobulated, hyperlobulated, or immature with granules having basophilic staining characteristics); however, such abnormalities are neither always present nor specific for the syndrome. The bone marrow aspirate and trephine biopsy may be more helpful. In addition to a marked increase of eosinophils and their precursors, the majority of patients also have an increase of mast cells. These may be scattered and form loose clusters but in some patients there are cohesive clusters of spindle-shaped mast cells, which resemble those of systemic mastocytosis. There is an associated increase in serum mast cell tryptase; this is not usually as high as in systemic mastocytosis but there is some overlap. To avoid misdiagnosis of systemic mastocytosis it is important to look for the fusion gene in such patients. Such misdiagnosis is to be avoided as systemic mastocytosis associated with a *KIT* mutation is rarely responsive to imatinib. Analysis for mutation of the *KIT* gene is best performed on a bone marrow aspirate or needle biopsy specimen since peripheral blood analysis is considerably less sensitive.

The peripheral blood and bone marrow aspirate in *FIP1L1-PDGFRA*–associated chronic eosinophilic leukemia do not usually show any increase of blast cells. If such is found, it is likely to indicate impending transformation. Treatment with imatinib is still appropriate but careful hematological and molecular observation of the response is needed.

Less often *PDGFRA* contributes to other fusion genes. A man with imatinib-responsive chronic eosinophilic leukemia and a complex chromosomal abnormality involving chromosomes 3, 4, and 10 was found to have a *KIF5B-PDGFRA* fusion gene [13] and a woman with ins(9;4)(q33;q12q25) was found to have a *CDK5RAP2-PDGFRA* fusion gene [14].

Two patients (males aged 3 and 37 years) with t(4;22)(q12;q11) and a *BCR-PDGFRA* fusion gene had a myeloproliferative disorder resembling chronic myelogenous leukemia but in both cases eosinophilia was unusually prominent [15]; one of these patients had a T-lymphoblastic transformation and the other developed accelerated phase disease. Imatinib responsiveness, although less than that associated with *FIP1L1-PDGFRA* was subsequently shown in a cell line [16]. Two further patients were subsequently described with t(4;22)(q12;q11), *BCR-PDGFRA* fusion, and chronic myeloid leukemia, one of whom developed B-lymphoblastic transformation; both of these patients were responsive to imatinib [17,18]. One of them did not have peripheral blood eosinophilia but had 13% eosinophils in the bone marrow [18]. This syndrome has disease characteristics intermediate between those of *FIP1L1-PDGFRA*–associated eosinophilic leukemia and those of *BCR-ABL1*-positive chronic myelogenous leukemia; eosinophilia may or may not be prominent.

Other eosinophilic leukemias

There are other forms of eosinophilic leukemia including several specific syndromes that need to be distinguished from other causes of hypereosinophilia. The most important of these is chronic eosinophilic leukemia associated with *ETV6-PDGFRB* or other rearrangements of the *PDGFRB* gene. The importance of this syndrome is that, like *FIP1L1-PDGFRA*–associated chronic eosinophilic leukemia, it is responsive to imatinib.

t(5;12)(q31-33;p12-13) with ETV6-PDGFRB or other PDGFRB rearrangement

This syndrome was first reported by Keene and colleagues [19] in 1987 with Golub and colleagues [20] subsequently demonstrating the presence of an *ETV6-PDGFRB* fusion gene (previously known as *TEL-PDGFRB*). The clinical and hematological features are heterogeneous. The age range is wide but the median age is fairly low and there is a remarkable male predominance. Some patients have splenomegaly, hepatomegaly being less frequent. Cardiac damage leading to cardiac failure can occur [21,22]. Skin infiltration is sometimes seen. The hematological features are quite variable. In the current WHO classification [23], some patients with these rearrangements are classified as having a myeloproliferative disorder (MPD), specifically chronic eosinophilic leukemia. Others are classified as having a myeloproliferative/myelodysplastic syndrome (MPD/MDS), either chronic myelomonocytic leukemia (CMML) or atypical Philadelphia-negative chronic myeloid leukemia (aCML) or even juvenile myelomonocytic leukemia (JMML) [24]. Eosinophilia is usual but not invariable [25]. There may be anemia and thrombocytopenia. In addition to the usual prominent eosinophilia, monocytosis is common and sometimes there is neutrophilia or basophilia. Rarely the hematological features are those of chronic basophilic leukemia [22]. Mast cell infiltration of the bone marrow has been reported and the mast cells can be spindle shaped [22,26] and immunophenotypically abnormal, resembling those of systemic mastocytosis in that they express CD2 and CD25 [22]. Serum tryptase can also be mildly or moderately elevated [22]. As for *FIP1L1-PDGFRA*–associated chronic eosinophilic leukemia, designation as systemic mastocytosis is better avoided despite the probable mast cell involvement, since this condition is quite distinct from systemic mastocytosis with *KIT* mutation. Trephine biopsy may show reticulin fibrosis [22]. Acute transformation can occur after a variable period of time (9 months to 12 years being reported [25]).

Most patients have t(5;12)(q31-33;p12-13) with *ETV6-PDGFRB*. The same fusion gene in one patient resulted from ins(2;12)(p21;q?13q?22) [27]. Other translocations resulting in different fusion genes should be recognized; at least 14 are known (Table 1) [20–22,25–40]. All cases so far described have had a relevant abnormality on standard cytogenetic analysis. The molecular changes can be confirmed by break-apart FISH or, in the case of

Table 1

Cytogenetic abnormalities and fusion genes in chronic myeloproliferative and myeloprolifera-tive/myelodysplastic disorders with t(5;12)(q31-33;p12-13) or related translocations resulting in rearrangement of *PDGFRB* gene

Translocation	Fusion gene	Imatinib response	Reference
Usually t(5;12)(q31~33;p13)	*ETV6-PDGFRB*	Yes	[20,25]
Rarely t(1;3;5)(p36;p21;q33)	*WDR48-PDGFRB*	Yes	[28]
Rarely der(1)t(1;5)(p34;q33), der(5)t(1;5)(p34;q15),der(11) (ins(11;5)(p12;q15q33)	*GP1AP1-PDGRFB*	Yes	[22]
Rarely t(1;5)(q21;q33)	*TPM3-PDGFRB*	Yes	[29]
Rarely t(1;5)(q23;q33)	*PDE4DIP-PDGFRB*	Yes	[30]
Rarely t(3;5)(p21;q31)	*PDGFRB* rearranged	Yes	[27]
Rarely t(4;5)(q21.3;q33)	*PDGFRB* rearranged	Yes	[26]
Rarely t(4;5;5)(q23;q31;q33)	*PRKG2-PDGFRB*	Yes	[22]
Rarely t(3;5)(p21-25;q31-35)	*GOLGA4-PDGFRB*	Yes	[28]
Rarely t(5;7)(q33;q11.2)	*HIP1-PDGFRB*	Likely	[31]
Rarely t(5;10)(q33;q21)	*CCDC6(H4/D10S170)-PDGFRB*	Likely	[32,33]
Rarely t(5;12)(q33;q13)	*PDGFRB* rearranged	Yes	[34]
Rarely t(5;12)(q31-33;q24)	*GIT2-PDGFRB*	Yes	[22]
Rarely t(5;14)(q33;q24)	*NIN-PDGFRB*	Yes	[35]
Rarely t(5;14)(q33;q32)	*KIAA1509-PDGFRB*	Yes	[36]
Rarely t(5;14)(q33;q22)[a]	*TRIP11(CEV14)-PDGFRB*[a]	Not known	[37]
Rarely t(5;15)(q33;q22)	*TP53BP1-PDGFRB*	Yes (transient)	[27,38]
Rarely t(5;16)(q33;p13)	*NDE1-PDGFRB*	Yes	[39]
Rarely t(5;17)(q33;p13)	*RABEP1 (RAB5)-PDGFRB*	Yes	[40]
Rarely t(5;17)(q33;p11.2)	*SPECC1(HCMOGT1)-PDGFRB*	Likely	[24]

[a] New abnormality after relapse of acute myeloid leukemia, associated with appearance of eosinophilia [37].

ETV6-PDGFRB, reverse transcriptase PCR (RT-PCR). Other reported patients have had a translocation with a 5q31 or 5q33 breakpoint and with *PDGFRB* being rearranged but without the fusion partner having been identified (see Table 1).

This diagnosis has major therapeutic relevance because of the imatinib sensitivity and because the median survival was less than 2 years in the pre-imatinib era. Imatinib responsiveness has been demonstrated for the majority of fusion products (see Table 1) and it is predicted that this would also be so for the other variant fusion products. In a series of 12 imatinib-treated patients the median survival was 65 months with 10 of 12 patients being alive at the time of reporting [27].

This syndrome is also responsive to nilotinib [41] and a mouse model has shown sensitivity to the investigational agent, SU11657 [42].

The 8p11 stem cell syndrome

This rare syndrome arises through a mutation in a pluripotent stem cell capable of differentiating into myeloid, T lymphoid, and B lymphoid cells.

Most cases are associated with t(8;13)(p11-12;q12) and a *ZNF198-FGFR1* fusion gene but there are also variant translocations leading to other fusion genes involving *FGFR1* (Table 2) [43–52]. Trisomy 21 is common as a secondary cytogenetic abnormality.

Patients can present in chronic phase with a myeloproliferative disorder with increased neutrophils and neutrophil precursors but usually without any increase in basophils. About 90% of patients have peripheral blood or bone marrow eosinophilia with eosinophil counts up to $40 \times 10^9/L$. Occasional patients have monocytosis. Within a relatively short period of time there is myeloid, T lymphoblastic, or B lymphoblastic transformation. Other patients present with the disease already transformed to acute leukemia or lymphoblastic lymphoma, particularly of T lineage. A single patient may suffer both a lymphoid and a myeloid transformation. Among the patients who present with, or have transformation to, acute myeloid leukemia, granulocytic sarcoma is relatively common.

This condition is resistant to imatinib but other tyrosine kinase inhibitors, eg, PKC412 [53], are under active evaluation and it is likely that a reasonably specific treatment will be developed. Until such time, allogeneic hemopoietic stem cell transplantation is often indicated, as this syndrome otherwise has a very poor prognosis.

Other eosinophilic leukemias

Other patients who present with hypereosinophilia can be recognized as having eosinophilic leukemia on the basis of a clonal molecular or cytogenetic abnormality, more often the latter. Demonstration of clonality by study of X-linked polymorphisms, eg, HUMARA analysis, can indicate that the correct diagnosis is eosinophilic leukemia; however, such analysis is possible only in women. A small number of patients have been found to have the *JAK2* V617F mutation that is more characteristic of polycythemia vera and other classical MPD. A range of cytogenetic abnormalities,

Table 2

Chromosomal rearrangements associated with the 8p11 stem cell syndrome and *FGFR1* rearrangement (previous gene names are in brackets)

Cytogenetics	Molecular genetics
Most often t(8;13)(p11;q12)	*ZNF198-FGFR1* [43,44]
Sometimes t(6;8)(q27;p11-12)	*FGFR1OP1(FOP)-FGFR1* [45]
Sometimes t(7;8)(q34;p11)	*TRIM24(TIF1)-FGFR1* [46]
Sometimes t(8;9)(p11;q33)	*CEP1(CEP110)-FGFR1* [47]
Sometimes t(8;11)(p11;p15)	*FGFR1* rearranged [48]
Sometimes t(8;12)(p11;q15)	*FGFR1* rearranged [48]
Sometimes t(8;17)(p11;q23)	*MYO18A-FGFR1* [49]
Sometimes t(8;17)(p11;q25)	*FGFR1* rearranged [48]
Sometimes t(8;19)(p12;q13.3)	*HERVK-FGFR1* [50]
Sometimes t(8;22)(p11;q11)	*BCR-FGFR1* [51]
Sometimes ins(12;8)(p11p11p22)	*FGFR1OP2-FGFR1* [52]

including some such as trisomy 8 and 20q- that are characteristic of myeloid neoplasms in general, have been recognized in eosinophilic leukemia. Chronic myeloid leukemia associated with *ETV6-ABL1* fusion sometimes has more marked eosinophilic differentiation than is usual in chronic myelogenous leukemia [54,55] and cardiac damage can result from the hypereosinophilia [55].

Investigation of possible eosinophilic leukemia

Any patient with hypereosinophilia and signs of severe tissue damage should be investigated promptly so that specific treatment can be started. In the absence of signs or symptoms of tissue damage, investigation of unexplained hypereosinophilia can proceed in a systematic manner, investigating first the possibilities that appear most probable from the clinical circumstances. If preliminary assessment discloses no reason to suspect allergy or parasitic disease, investigation is needed for an abnormal T-cell population, eosinophilic leukemia, and systemic mastocytosis.

The investigation of hypereosinophilic patients where there is a possibility of eosinophilic leukemia requires a careful history, including a travel history and a drug history; the drug history should elicit any exposure to alternative medications. Symptoms that may be complained of by patients with eosinophilic leukemia include cough, dyspnea, ankle swelling, diarrhea, weight loss, and pruritis. A careful physical examination is equally necessary with lymphadenopathy, hepatomegaly, splenomegaly, rash, or skin infiltration being particularly relevant. When the cause of eosinophilia is not apparent from history, examination, and preliminary investigation, more specific investigations are indicated. These include a CT scan of the chest and abdomen, a bone marrow aspirate and trephine biopsy, cytogenetic analysis on the bone marrow aspirate, peripheral blood analysis for the *FIP1L1-PDGFRA* gene, and peripheral blood immunophenotyping to identify any abnormal T-cell population. Depending on the clinical features, skin biopsy or lymph node biopsy will be indicated in some patients.

The relationship of eosinophilic leukemia to the idiopathic hypereosinophilic syndrome

These diagnoses "eosinophilic leukemia" and "idiopathic hypereosinophilic syndrome" are mutually exclusive [56]. A diagnosis of idiopathic hypereosinophilic syndrome should only be made when a patient has been adequately investigated to exclude not only aberrant T cells but also eosinophilic leukemia. At a minimum, this requires bone marrow aspiration and trephine biopsy, cytogenetic analysis of bone marrow cells, and molecular analysis of peripheral blood cells to demonstrate or exclude *FIP1L1-PDGFRA*–associated chronic eosinophilic leukemia. Use of the term "hypereosinophilic syndrome" should be discouraged since this term reveals nothing of the true nature of the condition. It is more likely to indicate either an imprecise use of language or that the patient has not been adequately investigated. Correct, precise diagnosis and classification are not merely of academic interest but are critical for appropriate management of the patient.

When full investigation reveals no cause for eosinophilia and the patient meets the criteria of Chusid and colleagues [1], a diagnosis of idiopathic hypereosinophilic syndrome remains appropriate. Some patients in whom this diagnosis is legitimately made will have features suggestive, but not diagnostic, of a myeloproliferative/leukemic disorder such as splenomegaly, hypercellularity of the bone marrow, increased serum tryptase, and increased serum B_{12}. When clonality cannot be demonstrated, the true nature of the condition will be revealed only with careful follow-up and perhaps not even then.

The idiopathic hypereosinophilic syndrome has traditionally been managed with corticosteroids, hydroxycarbamide (previously know as hydroxyurea) and interferon. The question now arises as to whether imatinib or other targeted therapy is appropriate in the absence of a demonstrable relevant genetic abnormality. This question is particularly relevant to patients whose clinical and laboratory features suggest a myeloproliferative disorder. In such patients a trial of imatinib is justified if circumstances permit. Data on file by Novartis, the manufacturer of imatinib, based on published and unpublished cases, shows that all of 61 patients with a *FIP1L1-PDGFRA* fusion had a complete hematological response on imatinib [57]. However 12 of 56 patients (21%) with no demonstrable fusion gene also had a complete hematological response and 7 (12%) a partial response. Some responses probably represent patients in whom a fusion gene was present but was not demonstrated because of inadequacy of the techniques applied. Others are likely to represent a response in a patient genuinely lacking the fusion gene. In general, those without *FIP1L1-PDGFRA* fusion are likely to respond less well and need a higher dose of imatinib. If financial constraints limit drug availability, it is desirable to at least give a trial of imatinib in a dose of 100 mg daily for 2 to 4 weeks. This is particularly important if the patient has myeloproliferative features or if there is already cardiac damage. A brief trial of low-dose therapy will serve to identify patients with the fusion gene for whom this therapy is of critical importance.

Other therapeutic measures available or under assessment for the idiopathic hypereosinophilic syndrome include interferon alpha, mepolizumab, and alemtuzumab.

Summary

The precise diagnosis of the myeloproliferative variant of hypereosinophilic syndrome is increasingly important as highly effective targeted therapies become available for a subset of these patients in whom eosinophilic leukemia is the result of a fusion gene encoding an aberrant tyrosine kinase.

References

[1] Chusid ML, Dale DC, West BC, et al. The hypereosinophilic syndrome. Medicine 1975;54: 1–27.

[2] Bain BJ. Eosinophilic leukaemias and the idiopathic hypereosinophilic syndrome. Br J Haematol 1996;95:2–9.

[3] Yoo TJ, Orman SV, Patil SR, et al. Evolution to eosinophilic leukemia with a t(5;11) translocation in a patient with idiopathic hypereosinophilic syndrome. Cancer Genet Cytogenet 1984;11:389–94.

[4] Doorduijn JK, van Lom K, Löwenberg B. Eosinophilia and granulocyte dysplasia terminating in acute myeloid leukaemia after 24 years. Br J Haematol 1996;95:531–4.

[5] Roufosse F, Schandene L, Sibille C, et al. T-cell receptor-independent activation of clonal Th2 cells associated with chronic hypereosinophilia. Blood 1999;94:994–1002.

[6] Simon HU, Plötz SG, Dummer R, et al. Abnormal clones of interleukin-5-producing T cells in idiopathic eosinophilia. N Engl J Med 1999;341:1112–20.

[7] Cools J, DeAngelo DJ, Gotlib J, et al. A tyrosine kinase created by the fusion of the PDGFRA and FIP1L1 genes as a therapeutic target of imatinib in idiopathic hypereosinophilic syndrome. N Engl J Med 2003;348:1201–14.

[8] Tashiro H, Shirasaki R, Noguchi M, et al. Molecular analysis of chronic eosinophilic leukemia with t(4;10) showing good response to imatinib mesylate. Int J Hematol 2006; 83:433–8.

[9] Rotoli B, Catalano L, Galderisi M, et al. Rapid reversion of Loeffler's endocarditis by imatinib in early stage clonal hypereosinophilic syndrome. Leuk Lymphoma 2004;45: 2503–7.

[10] Robyn J, Lemery S, McCoy JP, et al. Multilineage involvement of the fusion gene in patients with FIP1L1/PDGFRA-positive hypereosinophilic syndrome. Br J Haematol 2006;132: 286–92.

[11] Rives S, Alcorta I, Toll T, et al. Idiopathic hypereosinophilic syndrome in children: report of a 7-year-old boy with FIP1L1-PDGFRA rearrangement. J Pediatr Hematol Oncol 2005;27: 663–5.

[12] Klion AD, Noel P, Akin C, et al. Elevated serum tryptase levels identify a subset of patients with a myeloproliferative variant of idiopathic hypereosinophilic syndrome associated with tissue fibrosis, poor prognosis, and imatinib responsiveness. Blood 2003;101:4660–6.

[13] Score J, Curtis C, Waghorn K, et al. Identification of a novel imatinib responsive KIF5B-PDGFRA fusion gene following screening for PDGFRA overexpression in patients with hypereosinophilia. Leukemia 2006;20:827–32.

[14] Walz C, Curtis C, Schnittger S, et al. Transient response to imatinib in a chronic eosinophilic leukemia associated with ins(9;4)(q33;q12q25) and a CDK5RAP2-PDGFRA fusion gene. Genes Chromosomes Cancer 2006;45:950–6.

[15] Baxter EJ, Hochhaus A, Bolufer P, et al. The t(4;22)(q12;q11) in atypical chronic myeloid leukaemia fuses BCR to PDGFRA. Hum Mol Genet 2002;11:1391–7.

[16] Gavrilescu LC, Cross NCP, Van Etten RA. Distinct leukemogenic activity and imatinib responsiveness of a BCR-PDGFRα fusion tyrosine kinase. Blood 2006;108:3634 [abstract].

[17] Trempat P, Villalva C, Laurent G, et al. Chronic myeloproliferative disorders with rearrangement of the platelet-derived growth factor alpha receptor: a new clinical target for STI571/Glivec. Oncogene 2003;22:5702–6.

[18] Safley AM, Sebastian S, Collins TS, et al. Molecular and cytogenetic characterization of a novel translocation t(4;22) involving the breakpoint cluster region and platelet-derived growth factor receptor-alpha genes in a patient with atypical chronic myeloid leukaemia. Genes Chromosomes Cancer 2004;40:44–50.

[19] Keene P, Mendelow B, Pinto MR, et al. Abnormalities of chromosome 12p13 and malignant proliferation of eosinophils: a nonrandom association. Br J Haematol 1987;67:25–31.

[20] Golub TR, Barker GF, Lovett M, et al. Fusion of PDGF receptor beta to a novel ets-like gene, tel, in chronic myelomonocytic leukemia with t(5;12) chromosomal translocation. Cell 1994;77:307–16.

[21] Wittman B, Horan J, Baxter J, et al. A 2-year-old with atypical CML with a t(5;12)(q33;p13) treated successfully with imatinib mesylate. Leuk Res 2004;28(Suppl 1):S65–9.

[22] Walz C, Metzgeroth G, Haferlach C, et al. Characterization of three new imatinib-responsive fusion genes in chronic myeloproliferative disorders generated by disruption of the platelet-derived growth factor receptor beta gene. Haematologica 2007;92:163–9.

[23] Jaffe ES, Harris NL, Stein H, et al, editors. World Health Organization Classification of Tumours: pathology and genetics of tumours of haematopoietic and lymphoid tissues. Lyon: IARC Press; 2001.

[24] Morerio C, Acquila M, Rosanda C, et al. HCMOGT-1 Is a novel fusion partner to PDGFRB in juvenile myelomonocytic leukemia with t(5;17)(q33;p11.2). Cancer Res 2004; 64:2649–51.

[25] Steer EJ, Cross NCP. Myeloproliferative disorders with translocations of chromosome 5q31-35: role of the platelet-derived growth factor receptor beta. Acta Haematol 2002; 107:113–22.

[26] Dalal BI, Horsman DE, Bruyere H, et al. Imatinib mesylate responsiveness in aggressive systemic mastocytosis: novel association with a platelet derived growth factor receptor beta mutation. Am J Hematol 2006;82:77–9.

[27] David M, Cross NC, Burgstaller S, et al. Durable responses to imatinib in patients with PDGFRB fusion gene-positive and BCR-ABL-negative chronic myeloproliferative disorders. Blood 2007;109:61–4.

[28] Curtis C, Apperley JF, Dang R, et al. The platelet derived growth factor receptor beta fuses to two distinct loci at 3p21 in imatinib responsive chronic eosinophilic leukemia. Blood 2005; 106:909a.

[29] Rosati R, La Starza R, Luciano L, et al. TPM3/PDGFRB fusion transcript and its reciprocal in chronic eosinophilic leukemia. Leukemia 2006;20:1623–4.

[30] Wilkinson K, Velloso ERP, Lopes LF, et al. Cloning of the t(1;5)(q23;q33) in a myeloproliferative disorder associated with eosinophilia: involvement of PDGFRB and response to imatinib. Blood 2003;102:4187–90.

[31] Ross TS, Bernard OA, Berger R, et al. Fusion of Huntingtin Interacting Protein 1 to platelet-derived growth factor β receptor (PDGFβR) in chronic myelomonocytic leukemia with t(5;7)(q33;q11.2). Blood 1998;91:4419–26.

[32] Kulkarni S, Heath C, Parker S, et al. Fusion of H4/D10S170 to the platelet-derived growth factor receptor B in BCR-ABL negative myeloproliferative disorders with a t(5;10)(q33;q21). Cancer Res 2000;60:3592–8.

[33] Schwaller J, Anastasiadou E, Cain D, et al. H4(D10S170), a gene frequently rearranged in papillary thyroid carcinoma, is fused to the platelet-derived growth factor receptor β gene in atypical chronic myeloid leukemia with t(5;10)(q33;q22). Blood 2007;97:3910–8.

[34] Apperley JF, Gardenbas M, Melo JV, et al. Chronic myeloproliferative diseases involving rearrangements of the platelet derived growth factor receptor beta (PDGFRB) showing rapid responses to the tyrosine kinase inhibitor STI571 (imatinib mesylate). N Engl J Med 2002;347:481–7.

[35] Vizmanos JL, Novo FJ, Roman JP, et al. NIN, a gene encoding a CEP110-like centrosomal protein, is fused to PDGFRB in a patient with a t(5;14)(q33;q24) and an imatinib-responsive myeloproliferative disorder. Cancer Res 2004;64:2673–6.

[36] Levine RL, Wadleigh M, Sternberg DW, et al. KIAA1509 is a novel PDGFRB fusion partner in imatinib-responsive myeloproliferative disease associated with a t(5;14)(q33;q32). Leukemia 2005;19:27–30.

[37] Abe A, Tanimoto M, Towatari M, et al. Acute myeloblastic leukemia (M2) with translocation followed by marked eosinophilia and additional abnormalities of chromosome 5. Cancer Genet Cytogenet 1995;37:37–41.

[38] Grand FH, Burgstaller S, Kühr T, et al. p53-Binding protein 1 is fused to the platelet-derived growth factor receptor β in a patient with a t(5;15)(q33;q22) and an imatinib-responsive eosinophilic myeloproliferative disorder. Cancer Res 2004;64:7216–9.

[39] Rosati R, La Starza R, Bardi A, et al. PDGFRB fuses to TPM3 in the t(1;5)(q23;q33) of chronic eosinophilic leukemia and to NDE1 in the t(5;16)(q33;p13) of chronic myelomonocytic leukemia. Haematologica 2006;91(Suppl 1):214.

[40] Magnusson MK, Meade KE, Brown KE, et al. Rabaptin-5 is a novel fusion partner to platelet-derived growth factor receptor in chronic myelomonocytic leukemia. Blood 2001;98: 2518–25.

[41] Stover EH, Chen J, Lee BH, et al. The small molecule tyrosine kinase inhibitor AMN107 inhibits TEL-PDGFRβ and FIP1L1-PDGFRα in vitro and in vivo. Blood 2005;106:3206–13.

[42] Cain JA, Grisolano JL, Laird AD, et al. Complete remission of TEL-PDGFRB-induced myeloproliferative disease in mice by receptor tyrosine kinase inhibitor SU11657. Blood 2004;104:561–4.

[43] Xiao S, Nalbolu SR, Aster JC, et al. FGFR1 is fused with a novel zinc-finger gene, ZNF198, in the t(8;13) leukaemia/lymphoma syndrome. Nat Genet 1998;18:84–7.

[44] Macdonald D, Reiter A, Cross NCP. The 8p11 myeloproliferative syndrome: a distinct clinical entity caused by constitutive activation of FGFR1. Acta Haematol 2002;107:101–7.

[45] Popovici C, Zhang B, Grégoire M-J, et al. The t(6;8)(q27;p11) translocation in a stem cell myeloproliferative disorder fuses a novel gene, FOP, to fibroblast growth factor receptor 1. Blood 1999;93:1381–9.

[46] Belloni E, Trubia M, Gasparini P, et al. 8p11 myeloproliferative syndrome with a novel t(7;8) translocation leading to fusion of the FGFR1 and TIF1 genes. Genes Chromosomes Cancer 2005;42:320–5.

[47] Guasch G, Mack GJ, Popovici C, et al. FGFR1 is fused to the centrosome-associated protein CEP110 in the 8p12 stem cell myeloproliferative disorder with t(8;9)(p12;q33). Blood 2000; 95:1788–96.

[48] Sohal J, Chase A, Mould S, et al. Identification of four new translocations involving FGFR1 in myeloid disorders. Genes Chromosomes Cancer 2001;32:155–63.

[49] Walz C, Chase A, Schoch C, et al. The t(8;17)(p11;q23) in the 8p11 myeloproliferative syndrome fuses MYO18A to FGFR1. Leukemia 2005;19:1005–9.

[50] Guasch G, Popovici C, Mugneret F, et al. Endogenous retroviral sequence is fused to FGFR1 kinase in the 8p12 stem-cell myeloproliferative disorder with t(8;19)(p12;q13.3). Blood 2003;101:286–8.

[51] Fioretos T, Panagopoulos J, Larsen C, et al. Fusion of the BCR and the fibroblast growth factor receptor-1 (FGFR1) genes as a result of t(8;22)(p11;q11) in a myeloproliferative disorder: the first fusion gene with BCR but not ABL. Genes Chromosomes Cancer 2001;32: 302–10.

[52] Grand EK, Grand FH, Chase AJ, et al. Identification of a novel gene, FGFR1OP2, fused to FGFR1 in 8p11 myeloproliferative syndrome. Genes Chromosomes Cancer 2004;40:78–83.

[53] Chen J, DeAngelo DJ, Kutok JL, et al. PKC412 inhibits the zinc finger 198-fibroblast growth factor receptor 1 fusion tyrosine kinase and is active in treatment of stem cell myeloproliferative disorder. Proc Natl Acad Sci USA 2004;101:14479–84.

[54] Van Limbergen H, Beverloo HB, van Drunen E, et al. Molecular cytogenetic and clinical findings in ETV6/ABL1-positive leukaemia. Genes Chromosomes Cancer 2001;30:274–82.

[55] Keung YK, Beaty M, Steward W, et al. Chronic myelocytic leukemia with eosinophilia, t(9;12)(q34;p13), and ETV6-ABL gene rearrangement: case report and review of the literature. Cancer Genet Cytogenet 2002;138:139–42.

[56] Bain BJ. Eosinophilic leukemia and idiopathic hypereosinophilic syndrome are mutually exclusive diagnoses. Blood 2004;104:3836–7.

[57] NOVARTIS Pharmaceuticals USA. Available at: http://www.pharma.us.novartis.com/product/pi/pdf/gleevec_tabs.pdf. Accessed April 30, 2007.

IMMUNOLOGY
AND ALLERGY
CLINICS
OF NORTH AMERICA

ELSEVIER
SAUNDERS

Immunol Allergy Clin N Am
27 (2007) 389–413

Lymphocytic Variant Hypereosinophilic Syndromes

Florence Roufosse, MD, PhD[a,b,*],
Elie Cogan, MD, PhD[a],
Michel Goldman, MD, PhD[b]

[a]Department of Internal Medicine, Erasme Hospital, Université Libre de Bruxelles,
808 Route de Lennik, B-1070 Brussels, Belgium
[b]Institute for Medical Immunology, Université Libre de Bruxelles, 8 Rue Adrienne
Bolland, 6040 Gosselies, Belgium

The hypereosinophilic syndrome (HES) is an extremely heterogeneous disorder, in terms of clinical and biologic features, disease course and prognosis, and response to therapy. Recent work dedicated to HES pathogenesis has shown that molecular mechanisms ultimately leading to hypereosinophilia may differ significantly from one patient subgroup to another, providing a basis for clinical heterogeneity. Schematically, two types of pathogenic mechanisms have been described: either eosinophils expand clonally in the setting of a myeloproliferative disorder involving hematopoietic stem cells, with preferential eosinophilic differentiation, or eosinophils proliferate polyclonally in the setting of a cytokine-driven reactive process, with overproduction of eosinophil growth factors by T cells (lymphocytic, or L-HES) [1].

Two major discoveries in the field of fundamental immunology set the stage for suspecting that T cells could play a role in HES pathogenesis: the description of distinct helper (CD4) T cell subsets (ie, Th1 and Th2) according to their cytokine profile [2], and the identification of interleukin (IL)-5 as an essential growth and activation factor for eosinophils [3]. It rapidly emerged that Th2 cells were responsible for hypereosinophilia in allergic and parasitic disorders, through production of IL-5 [4]. Concomitant

This work was supported by grant number 3.4582.05 from the Belgian National Fund for Scientific Research. The Institute for Medical Immunology is supported by the government of the Walloon Region and GSK Biologicals (Rixensart, Belgium).

* Corresponding author. Department of Internal Medicine, Erasme Hospital, Université Libre de Bruxelles, 808 Route de Lennik, B-1070 Brussels, Belgium.

E-mail address: froufoss@ulb.ac.be (F. Roufosse).

production of IL-4 and IL-13 by these cells explained the frequent association of hypereosinophilia with increased serum IgE levels in these disorders.

Pioneers in the field of HES reported increased IgE levels in a significant proportion of patients, and underlined the associated immunoallergic clinical profile observed in most cases [5]. Compared with HES patients with features typically encountered in myeloproliferative disease, those with increased IgE levels were less likely to have life-threatening complications of hypereosinophilia, and were more likely to respond to corticosteroids, explaining that overall disease severity was qualified as benign. Experimental evidence that T cells could be involved in HES pathogenesis was first provided by a study showing that in vitro generated T-cell clones derived from peripheral blood of HES patients were able to stimulate eosinophil colony formation when cultured in presence of bone marrow stem cells [6]. The same group later identified IL-5 as the major eosinophil colony-stimulating factor produced by their T-cell clones [7]. Shortly thereafter, in 1994, a large T-cell population bearing phenotypic abnormalities was identified by flow cytometry, in a routine blood sample from an HES patient with increased serum IgE [8]. This $CD3^-CD4^+$ T-cell subset was shown to be monoclonal, and produced high levels of the Th2 cytokines IL-4 and IL-5 in vitro, suggesting a direct role in disease pathogenesis. This first formal description of a primary T-cell disorder in a patient satisfying Chusid's [9] HES diagnostic criteria was followed by similar observations (Tables 1 and 2), including a large series of 60 patients with persistent unexplained hypereosinophilia, among whom 16 had abnormal T-cell populations [10]. In most reports, T-cell populations associated with HES bear the intriguing $CD3^-CD4^+$ surface phenotype (see Table 1); however, several other phenotypically abnormal T-cell subsets have been observed in small patient subgroups or individual cases (see Table 2). The qualifier "lymphocytic variant" HES (L-HES) was introduced recently to distinguish this proportionally significant pathogenic subgroup from idiopathic HES, and L-HES has been defined as a primitive lymphocytic disorder characterized by nonmalignant expansion of a T-cell population producing IL-5 in patients fulfilling HES diagnostic criteria.

Pathogenic mechanisms of lymphocytic hypereosinophilic syndrome

$CD3^-CD4^+$ T-cell–associated lymphocytic hypereosinophilic syndrome

Phenotypic and functional characterization of $CD3^-CD4^+$ T cells
The T-cell nature of the $CD3^-CD4^+$ subset identified by flow cytometry has been certified by several means, besides morphologic studies. First, monoclonal T-cell receptor (TCR) rearrangement patterns have been observed by Southern blot and polymerase chain reaction analysis for TCRβ and TCRγ chain genes (see Table 1) [8,10–12]. Second, multicolor flow cytometry shows that they stain positively for T-cell surface antigens including CD2, CD5 (generally with a higher fluorescence intensity than normal $CD3^+CD4^+$ cells), and CD28; after permeabilization, they also stain

for intracellular CD3ϵ and the TCRα/β framework [11,12]. Importantly, this phenotype is stable during prolonged in vitro culture, showing that loss of CD3 expression is not a transient response to chronic antigen-dependent stimulation in vivo [13]. Other phenotypic features include CD45RO positivity indicative of memory cells, loss of CD7 or CD27 surface expression, CD95 (Fas-R) positivity, and variable staining intensities for the high affinity IL-2R alpha (CD25) and HLA-DR, reflecting some degree of in vivo activation (see Table 1) [10–12]. In a few reported cases, clonal CD4 T cells have reduced CD3 expression (CD3^{dim}) rather than complete absence of this marker [10]. Decreased or absent CD3 expression on CD4 T cells has been observed in peripheral blood from patients with Sézary syndrome [14], adult T-cell leukemia-lymphoma [15], and angioimmunoblastic T-cell lymphoma [16], all malignant T-cell disorders that must be excluded before considering the diagnosis of HES.

CD3$^-$CD4$^+$ cells are quiescent when cultured in vitro in enriched culture medium; they show no signs of proliferation, and display a high level of spontaneous apoptosis [17]. Although these cells are generally unable to produce measurable amounts of cytokines spontaneously, low levels of IL-5 have been detected in culture supernatants in some cases [10]. Cytokine production is greatly enhanced in presence of classical mitogenic agents, such as phorbol 12-myristate 13-acetate combined with ionophore or with anti-CD28 antibodies [11]. These cells do not respond to stimulation with anti-CD3 + anti-CD28 antibodies [18], and similar observations have been reported with the lectin phytohemagglutinin [19,20], which must bind membrane CD3 to induce T-cell activation. Besides IL-5, which is consistently produced by CD3$^-$CD4$^+$ T cells, reported cytokine profiles show some heterogeneity (see Table 1), but overall they generally also produce the Th2 cytokines IL-4 and IL-13 [8,11,21], favoring polyclonal B-cell activation and IgE synthesis in vivo. Experimental evidence for a direct role of CD3$^-$CD4$^+$ T cells in associated hyper IgE in these patients has been provided in vitro. Indeed, following stimulation with pokeweed mitogen, cultured peripheral blood mononuclear cells from a patient with CD3$^-$CD4$^+$ cells secreted high levels of IgE into supernatants, which decreased if CD4$^+$ T cells (but not if CD3$^+$ T cells) were depleted [22]. Occasionally, patients have normal IgE levels, and this may be caused by the inability of their CD3$^-$CD4$^+$ cells to produce IL-4 and IL-13 [20]. Production of granulocyte-macrophage colony–stimulating factor may synergize with IL-5 for induction of hypereosinophilia [12]. Interestingly, CD3$^-$CD4$^+$ cells may also produce IL-2 and variable amounts of the Th1 cytokine interferon (IFN)-γ [11,21,23]. For investigation of IL-2 production, flow cytometry (combining surface staining for T-cell markers, with intracytoplasmic staining for cytokines) is a more reliable method than measuring concentrations in culture supernatants, caused by possible reuptake by activated CD3$^-$CD4$^+$ cells, which express the CD25 receptor [18].

Table 1
Hypereosinophilic syndrome patients with a CD3⁻CD4⁺ T-cell subset

Ref: Author	Gender	Age[a] (yr)	FU (y)	Skin[b]	Other[c]	Eosino[d] /μL	Lympho[e] /μL	IgE[f] U/mL	Hyperglob[g] (mg/dL)	% gated LC[h]	Surface markers[i]	Clonality[j]	IL-5[k]	Other cytokines[l]	Karyotype
											CD3⁻CD4⁺ subset				
			Clinical features			Biologic features									
O'Shea et al [19]	M	27	7	"Erythem. rash"	Digit necr	5130	7400 (T cells)	518	IgM 3450	~94% (T cells)	25⁻ 7⁻	ND	ND	ND	ND
Bagot et al [41]	M	13	5	PAP, NOD	LN	19,900	5360	12,000	IgG, IgM		2⁺ 5⁺ 7⁻ 25⁻ DR⁻	Y	ND	ND	ND
Cogan et al [8][m]	M	30	6[n]	PAP	Digit necr, LN, pulm infilt, fever	6117	1680	2000	IgM 7200	66% (CD4)	2⁺ TCRα/β⁺	Y	Y	IL4 (no IL-2, IFN-γ)	Chrom 1 breakpoints[n]
Brugnoni et al [20]	M	65	5	PAP	LN	16,600	NL	NL	IgM, IgG	38%	2⁺ 5⁺ RO⁺ TCRα/β⁺	N	Y	No IL-4, IL-2, IFN-γ	NL
Simon et al [10]	F	43	7	URT	—	3195	2656	738	ND	34%	5^hi 25⁺	Y	spon	No spon IL-4, IFN-γ	ND
	M	70	5	PAP	—	3306	2392	56	ND	17.5%	3⁻ 4^lo 5^hi 25⁺	Y	spon	ND	ND
	F	76	7	ERY	—	4532	1854	232	ND	56%	3^lo 4^lo 6^lo 7⁻ 25⁺	Y	no spon	Spon IL-4	ND
	M	55	3	ERY	—	5047	824	1147	ND	33%	3^lo 4⁺ 5^lo 6^lo 7⁻ 25⁺ Vβ6.7⁺	Y	Y	Spon IL-4	ND
Zenone et al [38]	F	32	6	EA	Smeg	2200	4810	NL	—	49%	2⁺ 5⁺ TCRα/β⁺	Y	ND	ND	NL
Roufosse et al [11]	F	16	18[n]	ECZ, sc nod	Synovitis	8920	4630	340	IgM 310	90% (CD4)	7⁻ 27⁻ RO⁺ 95⁺ DR⁺	Y	Y	IL-4, IL-13 IL-2	Partial 6q 10p del

	F	21	12[n]	ECZ, EA	—	9100	3420	15,640	IgM 1250	84% (CD4)	7^- 27^- RO^+ 95^+ DR^+	Y	Y	IL-4, IL-13, IL-2	Partial 6q del
	F	47	19[n]	URT	—	2970	2240	478	IgG 1920	16% (CD4)	7^- 27^- RO^+ 95^+ DR^+	Y	Y	IL-4, IL-13, IL-2, IFN-γ	NL
Bank et al [12]	F	38	6	ECZ, sc nodules	LN	8230	5500	113,000	ND	73%	2^+ 5^+ $TCR\alpha/\beta^-$	N	ND	IL-4, IFN-γ	ND
	M	70	4	NOD, plaques	Pleuritis, DVT, fever	6000	4100	325,000	ND	66%	2^- 5^+ 7^- $TCR\alpha/\beta^-$	Y	Y	IL-4, GM-CSF	ND
	F	46	13	"rash"	Asthma, articul, DVT, fever	6426	8694	NL	ND	95%	2^+ 5^+ 7^- $TCR\alpha/\beta^-$	Y	ND	ND	ND
Sugimoto et al [23]	F	55	10	PAP, ULC	Pulmon infilt	13,700	11,500	11,970	—	98% (CD4)	2^+ 5^+ 7^- RO^+ $TCR\alpha/\beta^-$	Y	ND	IL-4, IFN-γ	t(2;14), t(12;14)
Roumier et al [21]	M	20	—	EA, ECZ	LN	9500	10,900	Incr	+	96%	7^- 27^- $62L^+$ $25RO^+$ DR^+ 95^+	Y (biC)	Y	IL-4, IL-13, IL-2, IFN-γ, TNF	Trisomy 7
Morgan et al [39]	M	44	13	EA, URT	—	27,500	ND	800	IgM 340	ND	2^+ 7^+ 25^+ 95^+	Y	ND	ND	NL
Vaklavas [30]	M	29	20	PAP	Sinus, oronasal, LN	3300	960	10,853	ND	ND	2^+ 5^+ 7^-	Y	ND	ND	NL
Roufosse >2007[n]	M	45	3.5	EA	—	3270	3000	8546	ND	ND	2^+ 7^- RO^+ 95^+ 25^+	Y	ND	ND	ND
	M	36	14	EA	Intestinal, articular	5350	5167	<3.5	IgM 400	31%	5^- 7^- 27^- RO^+ 95^+ 25^+ DR^+	Y	Y	IL-2, IL-4, IL-13	NL
	M	43	2.5	ECZ	—	870	1110	7849	—	9%	5^{hi} 7^- 27^- RO^+ 95^+ 25^+ DR^+	Y	Y	IL-2, IL-4, IL-13, TNF	NL

(continued on next page)

Table 1 (*continued*)

Ref: Author	Clinical features				Biologic features				CD3-CD4+ subset					Karyotype
	Gender	Age[a] FU (yr) (y)	Skin[b]	Other[c]	Eosino[d] /μL	Lympho[e] /μL	IgE[f] U/mL	Hyperglob[g] (mg/dL)	% gated LC[h]	Surface markers[i]	Clonality[j]	IL-5[k]	Other cytokines[l]	
	M	25 9	EA, ECZ URT	LN	9600	1680	22	—	0.6%	5^{hi} 7^{-} 27^{-} RO+ 95^{+} 25^{+}	N	Y	IL-2, IL-4, IL-13	NL

Abbreviations: FU, follow-up; GM-CSF; granulocyte-macrophage colony–stimulating factor IFN, interferon; IL, interleukin; N, no; ND, not done or not available; NL, normal; TNF, tumor necrosis factor; Y, yes.

[a] Age at discovery of eosinophilia or initiation of characteristic symptoms. In a few cases where information on chronology of disease is not available, age at evaluation by authors is given.

[b] Type of cutaneous manifestations is abbreviated as follows: EA, episodic angioedema; ECZ, eczema; ERY, erythroderma; NOD, nodular lesions; sc NOD, subcutaneous nodules; PAP, papular dermatitis; ULC, ulcerative lesions; URT, urticaria.

[c] Involvement of tissues and organs other than the skin are indicated as follows: —, none; DVT, deep vein thrombosis; LN, lymph node.

[d] Highest eosinophil level reported.

[e] Normal values for lymphocytes vary, but are roughly between 1340 and 3950/μL.

[f] Normal serum IgE levels vary among investigators; in general, below 150 U/mL.

[g] Hypergammaglobulinemia is indicated as follows: —, none +, present, but no details available; IgG or IgM indicates the type of immunoglobulin, which is increased in serum, eventually followed by the titre in mg/dL when available.

[h] The proportion of CD3-CD4+ cells is given as the percentage of all lymphocytes in most cases (this includes T cells, B cells, and NK cells); if values are available only as a percentage of a gated lymphocyte subset (eg, on CD4 T cells), this is indicated in the table between parenthesis.

[i] Other phenotypic characteristics of the CD3-CD4+ T cells are indicated when available. The abbreviation for "cluster differentiation" (ie, CD) for the different antigens is not indicated; "CD7" is represented as "7." RO refers to CD45RO, and DR refers to HLA-DR.

[j] T cell clonality is considered present (Y for yes) only when demonstrated using Southern blot or polymerase chain reaction analysis for TCR rearrangement patterns.

[k] Increased IL-5 production in patients with CD3-CD4+ cells is qualified as present (Y for yes) only if this is shown at the single-cell level for the aberrant subset by flow cytometry or immunohistochemistry, or if markedly increased levels are secreted into culture supernatants by stimulated peripheral blood mononuclear cells compared with controls. If low-level IL-5 is detected in culture supernatants of nonstimulated peripheral blood mononuclear cells, this is indicated as "spon."

[l] Production of other cytokines by CD3-CD4+ cells is indicated when assessed.

[m] The long-term follow-up of the patient reported here is found in reference [12] (patient 2).

[n] F. Roufosse, personal unpublished observations, 2007.

Table 2
Lymphocytic-hypereosinophilic syndrome associated with T-cell subsets other than CD3-CD4+

Ref: Author	Gender	Age (y)	FU (y)	Clinical features		Biologic features			Aberrant T-cell subset		Clonality	IL-5	Other cytokines
				Skin	Other	Eosino /μL	Lympho /μL	IgE U/mL	Phenotype	% gated LC			
Simon et al [29]	M	44	20y	—	Liver, intestine, spleen	4420	3888	12	$CD3^+CD4CD8^+CD5^-$ $TCR\alpha/\beta^+$ $CD95^+$	15%	Y	Y	IL-3, IL-2
Kitano et al [28]	M	53	—	—	Cardiac thrombus, liver	6270	1870	ND	$CD3^+CD4CD8^-$	56% (T cells)	Y	Y	No GM-CSF or IL-3
Simon et al [10]	F	47	5	ERY	Lungs	2768	3955	12,050	$CD3^+CD4^+CD2^{lo}$ $CD5^{lo}$	23.3%	Y	Y	No spon IL-4, IFN-γ
	M	71	1	ERY	—	2457	1638	1645	$CD3^+CD4^+V\beta5a^+$	16%	N	Spon	Spon IL-4, IFN-γ
	M	54	0.2	PAP	Spleen	1188	2046	87	$CD3^+CD8^+CD6^{hi}$	6.5%	N	Spon	No spon IL-4, IFN-γ
	M	55	4	—	spleen, lungs	869	2133	<2	$CD2^{lo}CD3^{lo}$ $CD6^{lo}CD7^{lo}$ $CD8^{hi}$	20%	N	—	No spon IL-4
	F	88	13	Poikil.	—	5805	810	5	$CD3^+CD4^+CD7^-$ $V\beta5c^+$	14.5%	N	Y	Spon IL-4
	M	60	2	ERY	—	3180	2438	416	$CD3^+CD4^+CD25^+$	50%	N	Y	Spon IFN-γ, no IL-4
	M	63	8	URT	—	1326	867	36	$CD3^+CD4CD8^-$	25%	N	Spon	Spon IFN-γ, no IL-4
	M	87	1	PAP	—	2323	1314	115	$CD2^{hi}CD3^+CD4^+$ $CD7CD6^{lo}$	18%	N	—	No spon IL-4, IFN-γ
	F	59	5	ERY	—	1332	738	200	$CD3^+CD4^+CD7^-$ and $CD3^+CD4^+CD8^-$ $CD7CD6^{lo}$	20 and 25%	N	Y	ND
Vaklavas 2007	M	5	3	ERY	—	2760	5700	156	$CD3^+CD8^+CD5^{lo}$ $CD7^{lo}$	22%	Y	—	ND
	M	60	10	—	Lungs, LN, kidneys	1150	2640	412	$CD3^+CD8^+CD5^{lo}$	ND	Y	ND	ND
	M	62	5.5	ECZ	—	720	1120	ND	$CD3^+CD4^+CD7^{lo}$	ND	Y	ND	ND
	M	51	4.8	+	—	2500	4100	25,360	$CD3^+CD4^+CD7^-$	ND	Y	ND	ND

See footnotes to Table 1.

Persistent hypereosinophilia in patients with this aberrant T-cell subset indicates sustained IL-5 production in vivo, presumably triggered by T-cell stimuli other than antigen major histocompatibility complex. Interestingly, despite complete absence of membrane TCR/CD3, these cells respond to activating signals provided by antigen-presenting cells in vitro, through engagement of CD2 and CD28 costimulatory receptors [18]. Indeed, CD3⁻CD4⁺ cells cultured in presence of mature dendritic cells proliferate, up-regulate membrane CD25 expression, and secrete Th2 cytokines and IL-2, all of which are inhibited if the cocultures are performed in presence of blocking antibodies interfering with CD2 and CD28 engagement. TCR-independent activation of CD3⁻CD4⁺ cells by antigen-presenting cells in vivo may contribute to IL-5 secretion, and ultimately to hypereosinophilia. In addition, combined IL-2 production and expression of the high-affinity receptor for this cytokine by CD3⁻CD4⁺ cells in these conditions, may be involved in chronic cycling of this T-cell subset and emergence of clonality. In this regard, it is of interest that normal CD4 T cells cultured in the presence of anti-CD2 + anti-CD28 antibodies combinations in vitro were shown to display prolonged IL-2–dependent autocrine proliferation, compared with cells cultured in the presence of the more classical anti-CD3 + anti-CD28 antibodies combination [24]. This finding was associated with increased IL-2Rα (CD25) and IL-2Rβ (CD122) mRNA transcription and stability [25,26].

In vitro findings on CD3⁻CD4⁺ cells have led the authors to hypothesize that acquisition of this unusual phenotype is an early event, which exposes these CD4⁺ T cells to alternative TCR-independent stimuli. The downstream signaling pathways may secondarily be implicated in acquisition of the functional behavior that characterizes this lymphocyte subset, including Th2 cytokine production and prolonged clonal expansion.

Molecular characterization of CD3⁻CD4⁺ T cells

To understand better the pathogenesis of L-HES, mechanisms involved in loss of TCR-CD3 complex expression by CD4 T cells have been explored. A marked decrease of CD3γ chain mRNA was observed in CD3⁻CD4⁺ T cells isolated from HES patients, using Northern blot and microarray analyses [13], contrasting with conserved transcription of the other chains composing the TCR-CD3 complex (TCRα, TCRβ, CD3δ, CD3ε) with the possible exception of CD3ζ. Successful assembly of the TCR-CD3 complex in the endoplasmic reticulum and subsequent membrane translocation depends on the presence of all TCR and CD3 chains; decreased CD3γ chain gene expression has been shown to account for low TCR-CD3 expression on in vitro HIV-infected CD4 T cells [27]. Electromobility shift assays were performed to investigate regulatory mechanisms acting on the CD3γ chain promoter in CD3⁻CD4⁺ cells; nuclear extracts were shown to bind intensely to two NF-AT consensus sequences, NF-ATγ1 and NF-ATγ2 [13]. The latter binds NFATc2 containing complexes and exerts negative regulation on CD3γ gene transcription, whereas the former may exert positive or negative activity, depending on whether NF-ATc1 plus NF-κB p50 or NF-ATc2–containing complexes are bound, respectively. Super-shift assays demonstrated binding of large amounts of NF-ATc2 to the NF-ATγ1 sequence. Inhibitory activity of specific members of the NF-AT family on the CD3γ gene promoter may contribute to acquisition of this unique T-cell phenotype, but upstream primary events remain entirely unknown.

Lymphocytic hypereosinophilic syndrome associated with T-cell abnormalities other than the CD3⁻CD4⁺ phenotype

Besides CD3⁻CD4⁺ T cells, other phenotypically aberrant or clonal T-cell subsets have been described in patients fulfilling HES diagnostic criteria (see Table 2) [10,28–30]. For some, however, formal evidence that they produce IL-5 or other eosinophil growth factors has not been provided. In addition, functional and molecular characteristics of these subsets have not been studied as extensively as for CD3⁻CD4⁺ cells, with the exception of CD3⁺CD4⁻CD8⁻ T cells. Two groups have provided a more detailed analysis of this subset [28,29], showing that the cells express TCRα/β but not TCRγ/δ; are monoclonal; and produce IL-5, IL-3, IL-2 and possibly granulocyte-macrophage colony–stimulating factor. CD3⁺CD4⁻CD8⁻ cells from one patient were shown to display deficient Fas-mediated apoptosis despite normal expression of the Fas-R, CD95 [29]. Reverse transcriptase polymerase chain reaction analysis of Fas-R transcripts demonstrated the existence of two polymerase chain reaction products with different lengths; the shorter splice variant encoded a soluble Fas-R molecule, which interfered with engagement of the membrane-bound receptor, providing a possible explanation for clonal expansion.

Among other T-cell phenotypes associated with HES, CD4 or CD8 subsets with abnormal staining intensities for the lineage-specific T-cell markers CD2, CD5, CD6, and CD7 have been reported [29,30]. In particular, a CD4 T-cell subset with weak or absent membrane CD7 expression seems to be a recurrent abnormality, with five reported cases (see Table 2). Lymphocytes with this phenotype have been observed in affected skin from one HES patient, and stained positively for intracellular IL-5, suggesting a pathogenic role [29]. Clonality was proved by molecular studies in two cases [30], and was highly probable in another given homogenous expression of Vβ5c by the CD4⁺CD7⁻ subset [10]. The relevance of CD4⁺CD7$^{dim/-}$ T cells in HES pathogenesis clearly warrants further investigation.

It is intriguing that the two most frequently encountered aberrant T-cell subsets besides CD3⁻CD4⁺ cells in L-HES patients (ie, CD3⁺TCR$^{α/β+}$CD4⁻CD8⁻ and CD3⁺CD4⁺CD7⁻ cells) are observed in the epidermis of healthy individuals [31,32], and are thought to contribute to the "skin-associated immune system." A modest population of CD4⁺CD7⁻ cells is also found in peripheral blood [33] (representing up to 19% of CD4 T cells) and tends to increase with age. One group has shown that cultured $CD4^+CD7^-$ T cells from healthy subjects produce more IL-4 and less IL-2 than $CD4^+CD7^+$ T cells, after stimulation with anti-CD3 + anti-CD28 antibodies, suggesting that the former are skewed toward a Th2-like profile [34]. Monoclonal $CD3^+TCR^{\alpha/\beta+}CD4^-CD8^-$ and $CD3^+CD4^+CD7^-$ subsets have also been observed in skin from patients with cutaneous T-cell lymphoma [35,36], and high percentages of $CD4^+CD7^-$ cells may be detected in blood of patients with Sézary syndrome [37]. These findings suggest that T cells associated with certain forms of cutaneous T-cell lymphoma may represent the malignant counterpart of T cells that normally contribute to skin defense.

Clinical features and prognosis of lymphocytic hypereosinophilic syndrome

L-HES affects females and males in roughly equivalent proportions, contrasting with the high male/female ratio observed in the overall HES population, which is likely to reflect the overwhelming male predominance of FIP1L1-PDGFRα–associated disease. Age of diagnosis is similar to that of the overall HES population (see Tables 1 and 2).

The clinical profile of patients with $CD3^-CD4^+$ and $CD4^+CD7^-$ T-cell subsets is dominated by cutaneous manifestations, including pruritus, eczema, erythroderma, urticaria, and angioedema. In some cases, the presentation is indistinguishable from that encountered in episodic angioedema with eosinophilia [11,30,38,39], or Gleich's syndrome, a disease characterized by spontaneously remitting episodes of angioedema associated with increased IgM levels. Observed presence of pathogenic $CD3^-CD4^+$ or $CD4^+CD7^-$ T cells together with eosinophils in affected skin from HES patients [10,30] suggests they play a role in cutaneous manifestations. The fact that both populations lack membrane CD7, which is a characteristic of normal epidermal and dermal CD4 T cells [31], may explain preferential homing of pathogenic T cells in the skin, which secondarily attract eosinophils. The respective contributions of these activated T cells versus eosinophils to clinical manifestations remain to be elucidated. Other reported complications associated with $CD3^-CD4^+$ cells include tenosynovitis [11], arthralgia [12], digital arterial occlusion complicated by necrosis [8,19], deep venous thrombosis [12], asthma [12], pulmonary infiltrates [8,23], and eosinophilic pleuritis [12]. Intriguingly, endomyocardial fibrosis or presence of thrombi in cardiac cavities is a rare complication (only one reported case [40]), despite high eosinophil levels.

As for the reported patients with $CD3^+CD4^-CD8^-$ cells (four published cases), skin lesions were the only complication in two [10]: one presented predominant gastrointestinal complications associated with splenic and hepatic eosinophilic infiltrates [29], and one had a thrombus in the left ventricle and hepatomegaly with eosinophilic infiltration of the portal area [28].

Clinical manifestations associated with other less frequent T-cell phenotypes are shown in Table 2.

Biologically, patients with L-HES generally have circulating eosinophil levels well above the defining $1500/\mu L$ cutoff for HES diagnosis, and absolute lymphocyte counts are normal or slightly increased (see Tables 1 and 2). In accordance with the type 2 cytokine profile of the aberrant T cells, serum IgE levels are often increased. Polyclonal hypergammaglobulinemia (increased serum IgM or IgG) may be observed but is less common. This contributes to increased erythrocyte sedimentation rates that are observed in some patients, whereas C-reactive protein levels are generally normal or only slightly increased. Features typically associated with myeloproliferative disease, including anemia or thrombocytopenia, presence of circulating immature myelocytes, and increased vitamin B_{12} levels, are generally absent. Mild lymph node enlargement may be observed, and biopsies show eosinophils and lymphoid hyperplasia [8,20]. Organomegaly is rare, and reflects eosinophilic infiltration. Bone marrow smears contain increased proportions of eosinophil precursors and mature eosinophils.

Short-term prognosis of $CD3^-CD4^+$ T cell–associated HES is clearly better than that of FIP1L1-PDGFRα$^+$ chronic eosinophilic leukemia, given the low incidence of severe or life-threatening end-organ damage and good response to corticosteroid therapy. Long-term prognosis is overshadowed, however, by the possible development of peripheral T-cell lymphoma, many years after HES diagnosis in some cases (Table 3) [10,11,19,30,41]. Malignant progression has been observed in patients with clonal $CD3^-CD4^+$, $CD3^+CD4^-CD8^-$, and $CD4^+CD7^-$ subsets, and in some cases the malignant T cells conserve the initial phenotype, suggesting their premalignant nature. The reported duration of the eosinophilic prodrome is variable, and ranges from 3 to 20 years (mean, 7 years). Few details are available on the histology and grading of lymphomas that develop in this setting. A recent article has described progression toward primary cutaneous peripheral T-cell lymphoma, unspecified, in two HES patients, one with $CD4^+CD7^-$ and the other with $CD3^-CD4^+$ T cells [30]. They both presented with papular dermatitis at HES diagnosis, which progressed to more nodular infiltrative lesions when malignancy was detected. The patient with $CD3^-CD4^+$ cells also developed lymphadenopathy and oronasal involvement.

Diagnosis of lymphocytic hypereosinophilic syndrome

Critical analyses for approaching L-HES diagnosis include both peripheral T-cell phenotyping by flow cytometry, and assessment of T-cell clonality by investigating TCR gene rearrangement patterns. Investigations can be performed on peripheral blood samples, because all abnormal T-cell subsets associated with HES reported have been detected in the circulation. Isolated

Table 3
Malignant T-cell lymphoma in patients with initial diagnosis of lymphocytic-hypereosinophilic syndrome

| Ref | L-HES characteristics | | Duration benign HES (y) | Clinical changes associated with transformation | Characteristics of malignant T-cell lymphoma | | | | |
	T-cell phenotype	Clonality			Diagnostic biopsies	Type of lymphoma	Treatment	Outcome
O'Shea et al [19]	CD3⁻CD4⁺ CD7⁻	ND	7	Modif skin lesions	Skin, lymph node	Diffuse mixed small and large cell	Nitrogen mustard, VCR, PDN, procarbazine	Deceased, *Pneumocystis carinii* infection
Bagot et al [41]	CD3⁻CD4⁺ CD7⁻	Y	5	Extension of skin lesions	Skin, lymph node	Pleiomorphic, large cell	CYP, PDN, Vindesine, total lymphoid irradiation, PUVA	Rapid recurrence; stable under and dependent on IFN-α
Cogan et al [8]ᵃ	CD3⁻CD4⁺ CD7⁻	Y	6	Fever, anorexia, night sweats	Bone marrow, lymph node, liver	Diffuse anaplastic CD30⁺	CYP	Deceased, septicemia
Simon et al [29]	CD3⁺ CD4⁻ CD8⁻	Y	20	Increased lymphocytosis, eosinophils	Not specified	Not specified	Not specified	Deceased, small bowel infarction, peritonitis

Study	Immunophenotype			Clinical features	Site	Diagnosis	Treatment	Response
Simon et al [10]	CD3^{lo}CD4^{lo}CD7$^-$	Y	>7	Increased lymphocytosis, eosinophils	Not specified	Not specified	Not specified	Not specified
	CD3^{lo}CD4$^+$CD7$^-$	Y	>3	Exacerbation skin symptoms	Lymph node	Not specified	Not specified	Not specified
Roufosse et al [11]	CD3$^-$CD4$^+$	Y	6	Subcutaneous nodules, lymphadenopathy, increased lymphocytosis	Lymph node	Diffuse PTCL - pleomorphic, small and medium cell	Fludarabine CHOP-like Allogeneic SCT	Transient partial response No response Complete remission (6 y)
Vaklavas et al [30]	CD3$^+$CD4$^+$CD7^{lo}	Y	3	Infiltrative nodular skin lesions	Skin	Primary cutaneous PTCLu	Multiagent therapy	Partial response
	CD3$^-$CD4$^+$CD7$^-$	Y	>8	Infiltrative nodular skin lesions, lymphadenopathy, oronasal and conjunctival infiltrates	Skin, lymph node	Primary cutaneous PTCLu	Multiagent therapy	Partial response

Abbreviations: CYP, cyclophosphamide; IFN, interferon; PDN, prednisolone; PTCL, peripheral T-cell lymphoma; PUVA, psoralen UVA; VCR, vincristine.
[a] The long-term follow-up of the patient reported here is found in reference [12] (patient 2).

demonstration of clonal TCR rearrangements is by no means sufficient to classify a patient as having L-HES, because this may be observed in healthy subjects or may reflect a reactive condition.

Lymphocyte (T cell) phenotyping may be initiated using markers commonly used in routine practice (ie, CD3, CD4, and CD8), given the large predominance of $CD3^-CD4^+$ and $CD3^+CD4^-CD8^-$ subsets in affected patients. In laboratories unaccustomed to detection of these abnormal populations, quantification of other lymphocytes (staining CD19 for B cells, CD16/CD56 but not CD3 for natural killer cells) may provide indirect evidence for their existence. Indeed, if added percentages of these populations, together with normal $CD3^+$, CD4, and CD8 T cells, amounts to less than 90% of gated lymphocytes, this should raise suspicion of an abnormal T-cell subset in an HES patient. Multicolor flow cytometry, staining CD3, CD4, and CD8 together with other lineage-associated T-cell antigens including CD2, CD5, CD6, CD7, CD27, and CD28, and with CD25 is useful for detecting other less frequent phenotypic abnormalities. Besides the two previously mentioned abnormal T-cell subsets, the only recurrent phenotypic abnormality observed in HES patients is low or absent CD7 on $CD4^+$ T cells, which should be actively searched. This approach is also useful for confirming the diagnosis of $CD3^-CD4^+$ cells when this subset is small or difficult to distinguish from monocytes (ie, if CD4 expression is slightly down-regulated). Indeed, these cells express CD2 and CD28, and membrane expression of several other T-cell markers is almost systematically altered $(CD5^{high}CD7^{neg}CD27^{neg}CD45RO^{pos})$ [11,12,21]. Intracellular staining for $CD3\epsilon$ or the $TCR\alpha/\beta$ framework after permeabilization may further help distinguish this subset from monocytes.

Several pathogenic T-cell subsets have been identified by flow cytometry, by exploring the $TCRV\beta$ repertoire with a panel of antibodies directed against $TCRV\beta$ families [10]. An increased percentage of CD4 T cells that stain for a given $V\beta$ family may arouse suspicion of T-cell clonality. For example, a $CD3^{dim}CD4^+$ T-cell subset was shown to stain positively for the $V\beta6.7$ antigen in one patient [10]. Surface staining for $V\beta$ families is not appropriate for $CD3^-CD4^+$ cells, given the absence of TCR-CD3 on their surface, but intracellular staining after permeabilization is feasible. The authors have attempted to analyze the $TCRV\beta$ repertoire of $CD3^-CD4^+$ cells from HES patients in this fashion, but have not detected specific $V\beta$ subsets using a panel of antibodies that covers roughly 60% of families (F. Roufosse, unpublished data, 2000). It is important to note that identification of a T-cell subset belonging to a given $V\beta$ family does not prove its clonality, which can only be formally demonstrated by molecular analysis of TCR gene rearrangements.

Molecular assessment of T-cell clonality is generally based on Southern blotting for the $TCR\beta$ chain gene, and polymerase chain reaction analysis for the $TCR\gamma$ (and recently, $TCR\beta$) chains. Most reports of $CD3^-CD4^+$ T-cell populations detected in HES patients show clonal TCR rearrangement patterns (see Table 1). In several patients, however, investigators have been unable to demonstrate clonality using these techniques, despite high percentages of abnormal cells in peripheral blood [12,20]. In the same line, molecular analyses confirmed T-cell clonality in only 8 of 16 patients with T-cell subsets bearing various phenotypic abnormalities in one cohort [10]. Several explanations are possible, including lack of sensitivity if the population is small; truly nonclonal nature of the studied population; type of chosen primers relative to the rearrangement, deletion, or translocation of the TCRβ gene; and incomplete rearrangements. The authors have reported one patient with 16% CD3⁻CD4⁺ cells (among gated CD4⁺ lymphocytes) in whom TCR gene rearrangement studies failed to show clonality on whole blood using polymerase chain reaction analysis for the TCRγ chain gene, but a clonal pattern was observed after in vitro purification of the abnormal population [11].

Given the number of observations and reports showing that clonal CD3⁻CD4⁺ cells produce IL-5 (see Table 1), it is reasonable to classify a new patient in whom this particular T-cell subset is detected as L-HES, even if cytokine production has not been investigated. In contrast, other suspected cases of L-HES on the basis of flow cytometry or analysis of TCR gene rearrangement studies should be characterized extensively to assess a causal relationship between presence of aberrant or clonal T cells and hypereosinophilic disease. To this end, T-cell cytokine production should be investigated by culturing peripheral blood mononuclear cells in the absence and presence of T cell–specific stimulating agents for 48 hours, and measuring cytokines in culture supernatants, with a special focus on IL-5. Optimal stimulation is observed using a phorbol ester, such as phorbol 12-myristate 13-acetate, which bypasses proximal signaling events related to cross-linking of membrane receptors, combined with a calcium ionophore or anti-CD28 antibodies. If increased IL-5 concentrations are measured in peripheral blood mononuclear cells supernatants, experiments can be repeated after depletion of specific T-cell subsets (eg, using anti-CD3 or anti-CD4 antibodies) for refining assessment of the type of T cell responsible for IL-5 overproduction [12,20]. If a T-cell subset with a phenotypic abnormality is detected (eg, CD3⁻CD4⁺, CD3⁺CD4⁻CD8⁻, or CD4⁺CD7^{dim/-}), assessment of cytokine production at the single-cell level is possible using flow cytometry, by staining intracellular cytokines together with relevant surface markers, after a short course of in vitro T-cell stimulation with the previously mentioned agents [10,11]. Although these techniques are not standardized (eg, investigators report using different concentrations of cells and reagents, variable culture durations, and so forth), the authors generally run cultures of peripheral blood mononuclear cells from HES patients and from healthy subjects in parallel, and results are generally straightforward, with markedly increased IL-5 levels in supernatants for patients with L-HES.

In routine practice, diagnosis of L-HES is laborious, and may be stalled by the inability to interpret results of flow cytometry or TCR rearrangement patterns, and lack of equipment or expertise to culture T cells and assess cytokine production. Identification of L-HES patients would be facilitated if a straightforward, reproducible, and unique diagnostic test were available. One study has identified increased serum thymus and activation-regulated chemokine (TARC) as a potential biomarker for this variant [42]. Serum TARC levels are indeed over 100-fold higher in patients with L-HES (mean, 56,564 pg/mL; range, 15,459–161,032; N = 10) compared with HES patients with no evidence for an underlying T-cell disorder (mean, 296 pg/mL; range, 91–892; N = 8), whose levels were similar to healthy controls (mean, 265 pg/mL; range, 66–625; N = 38) (F. Roufosse, unpublished data, 2007). In vitro studies have shown that the high-level TARC production observed when $CD3^-CD4^+$ cells are cultured in presence of dendritic cells is inhibited when engagement of the IL-4R is hindered with blocking antibodies [43], indicating that the pathogenic T cells are directly responsible for TARC synthesis by other cell types, through production of IL-4 or IL-13. Similarly, IL-4 has been shown to increase TARC production by human bronchial epithelial cells [44] and murine Langerhans cells [45] in vitro, and serum TARC levels seem to correlate with disease activity in atopic individuals [46], albeit much less dramatically than in L-HES patients. Increased serum TARC may truly be the hallmark of diseases mediated by activated Th2 cells. The fact that this biomarker can be measured in serum (which can easily be stored and shipped) using a commercially available ELISA kit (possibility of standardization, reproducibility) makes it a very appealing diagnostic test. Further studies are required, however, to assess the specificity of this candidate biomarker for L-HES with regard to other patients fulfilling HES diagnostic criteria, and to determine discriminative cutoff values for this variant. To this end, serum TARC should be compared between larger cohorts of L-HES and other HES patients, and healthy subjects and patients with other conditions associated with hypereosinophilia, including atopy, drug allergy, parasitosis, Churg-Strauss syndrome, and organ-specific eosinophil-mediated disorders (eg, eosinophilic gastroenteritis and eosinophilic pneumonia).

Follow-up of patients with lymphocytic hypereosinophilic syndrome

Given the increased risk of developing peripheral T-cell lymphoma, patients with L-HES should be monitored on a regular basis to detect this complication as early as possible. It must be underlined, however, that malignant progression has been observed only in a proportion of patients, whereas most pursue a benign course, with reassuring long-term follow-up in some published cases [11,23,39]. Malignant progression has been observed in association with $CD3^{-/dim}CD4^+$, $CD3^+CD4^-CD8^-$, and $CD4^+CD7^{dim/-}$ subsets several years after detection of monoclonal T cells (see Table 3). This raises the difficult question of when clonal T cells bearing phenotypic abnormalities should be considered malignant. In most reported cases, diagnosis of lymphoma is made when a biopsy (lymph node, skin) reveals the presence of morphologically abnormal lymphocytes. Clinical manifestations associated with malignant transformation include appearance of enlarged lymph nodes [30,47] and progression of skin lesions from papular dermatitis to infiltrative nodules [30]. Hematologically, rapid increases of lymphocytosis (essentially involving the aberrant T cells) and eosinophilia [10], and increased expression of CD25 by CD3$^-$CD4$^+$ cells [47], have been observed.

Another critical question regarding L-HES and malignancy is whether patients who are more likely to develop lymphoma can be singled out on the basis of specific disease characteristics (have any predictive markers been identified). Repeated karyotypes on CD3$^-$CD4$^+$ cells during a period of several years in one patient who eventually developed lymphoma have shown that the nonmalignant CD3$^-$ T cells present at diagnosis contained two distinct partial 6q deletions (6qdel[q13-q22] and 6qdel[q11-q23]), whereas their malignant counterpart 6 years later presented only the short 6qdel(q13-q22) [48]. The fact that this deletion involves chromosomal loci whose absence may be associated with other malignancies (including T-cell and B-cell disorders and solid tumors) strongly suggests that it harbors a tumor suppressor gene, whose nature remains unknown. Parallel investigations in another patient with L-HES have revealed a similar 6q deletion that has remained stable under corticosteroid treatment for 10 years, however, with no evidence of malignancy [48]. Other cytogenetic abnormalities have been reported in L-HES patients, including -16,+der(16)t(16q22;?) in CD3$^+$CD4$^-$CD8$^-$ cells [28] and trisomy 7 in CD3$^-$CD4$^+$ cells [21], but were not associated with malignant progression at time of reporting. Peripheral blood samples from L-HES patients should systematically be subjected to karyotyping, to characterize better the prognostic significance of specific abnormalities, including partial 6q deletions. The fact that CD3$^-$CD4$^+$, CD3$^+$CD4$^-$CD8$^-$, and probably CD4$^+$CD7$^-$ T-cell subsets respond poorly to classical mitogens, such as phytohemagglutinin [19,20,28,34], should be taken into account for interpreting cytogenetic studies performed on cells in metaphase. Indeed, normal T cells proliferate preferentially in these conditions, and the mitoses obtained for karyotyping are not representative of pathogenic T cells. For patients with L-HES, karyotypes should be performed using T-cell growth factors, which induce cell-cycling independently of TCR-CD3–linked signaling, such as IL-2, and eventually IL-7 [49].

Practically, tentative recommendations for follow-up of L-HES patients can be made on the basis of longitudinal observations on a handful of patients, from diagnosis of HES to development of lymphoma. Lymphocytosis should be controlled every 3 to 4 months, and absolute levels and proportions of aberrant T cells should be monitored at least twice a year by flow cytometry. Karyotypes should be performed yearly, with appropriate T-cell mitogens. Appearance of enlarged lymph nodes or modification of skin lesions should prompt biopsies for histologic assessment. Although no data support use of fluorodeoxyglucose positron emission tomography for follow-up of patients with premalignant T cells, the authors perform this yearly in selected patients with CD3⁻CD4⁺ cells.

Therapeutic considerations

The decision to treat a patient with L-HES depends on a critical assessment of clinical disease severity, in light of treatment-related toxicity. Some patients with T-cell clones have very limited cutaneous manifestations, and it may be reasonable to watch and wait despite high eosinophil levels. For instance, one elderly female patient with clonal CD3⁻CD4⁺ T cells, eosinophil levels around 3000/µL, and intermittent episodes of urticaria has not received treatment for 18 years, and has remained stable over time [11]. In others, although clinical manifestations are not life-threatening, they are nonetheless intolerable; typically, extensive pruritic dermatitis requires some form of systemic therapy. In rare instances, preoccupying target-organ involvement represents another indication for treatment. Ideally, therapeutic strategies should target both eosinophils, which are directly involved in end-organ damage and dysfunction, and aberrant T cells, which not only promote hypereosinophilia, but also proliferate clonally and produce mediators other than IL-5, which may contribute partially to disease manifestations. Specific T cell–oriented aims include abrogating production of eosinophilopoietic cytokines or interfering with their effects, and controlling expansion of these cells in hopes of preventing malignant transformation.

Corticosteroids

Corticosteroids (CS) represent first-line therapy for L-HES. Although the response rate in this population remains to be assessed on a well-characterized patient cohort, available data in the literature indicate that satisfactory responses are observed in an important proportion of patients. Apoptosis-inducing effects of CS on eosinophils are well-known, and they also modulate T-cell functions by inhibiting production of type 2 cytokines and IL-2, and by reducing CD25 expression, thereby interfering with clonal IL-2–dependent expansion in vitro [50–52]. In vivo, although CS are very successful in decreasing eosinophil levels in a significant proportion of patients with L-HES, and in controlling clinical manifestations, effects on pathogenic T cells are variable. In most cases, the proportion of CD3⁻CD4⁺ cells is not affected by CS; however, a significant decline of this population has been observed in two patients [11,20].

Practically, it is reasonable to initiate therapy with 20 to 40 mg prednisolone per day, depending on clinical manifestations, followed by progressive tapering so that eosinophil levels and clinical manifestations are controlled using the lowest possible dose. Given the numerous side effects of long-term CS use, therapeutic strategies should aim to minimize overall CS exposure by introducing CS-sparing agents whenever the dose required to control disease is considered unacceptable. Most of the second-line molecules used for treating the overall HES patient population have been administered to patients with L-HES, with variable success. Compounds used for CS-resistant HES patients and for CS-sparing purposes are the same, and include cytotoxic agents (hydroxyurea); immunomodulatory molecules (IFN-α); tyrosine kinase inhibitors (imatinib mesylate); and monoclonal antibodies (alemtuzumb, anti–IL-5). Allogeneic stem cell transplantation is reserved for patients who develop T-cell malignancy.

Cytotoxic agents

There is currently no evidence indicating that hydroxyurea could be useful for treating lymphoproliferative disorders in general, and its effects on pathogenic T cells isolated from L-HES patients (ie, on IL-5-production and clonal expansion) have never been assessed in vitro. Administration of this agent to one patient with CD3⁻CD4⁺ cells was followed by clinical improvement and normalization of eosinophil levels, presumably through a central negative effect on cytokine-driven eosinophil expansion, but the aberrant T-cell clone remained unaffected [23]. Similarly, one group has recently reported use of other cytotoxic compounds (methotrexate and cyclophosphamide) in two patients with clonal T cells, showing successful control of clinical manifestations, but lack of effect on the T-cell clones [30].

Immunomodulatory agents

IFN-α is an interesting alternative for management of patients with L-HES, because it has been shown to antagonize Th2 responses in general, both in vitro and in vivo [53,54], and more specifically to inhibit proliferation of and decrease IL-5 production by CD3⁻CD4⁺ cells isolated from patients with L-HES in a dose-dependent manner in vitro [17,55]. IFN-α also has central inhibitory effects on eosinophil colony formation [56]. Published case reports have shown that treatment with IFN-α was followed by partial regression of pathogenic CD3⁻CD4⁺ T cells in two patients [8,10], and the authors have observed complete disappearance of CD3⁻CD4⁺ cells in one patient treated with combined CS and IFN-α (F. Roufosse, unpublished data, 2004). IFN-α also prolongs survival of clonal CD3⁻CD4⁺ cells in vitro by inhibiting spontaneous apoptosis [17], however, and may provide these cells with a selective advantage. Given the malignant potential of aberrant T cells associated with L-HES, it may be reasonable to avoid IFN-α as monotherapy in this setting, and rather use it in association with a therapeutic agent displaying proapoptotic activity on the clonal T-cell population, such as CS (L. Schaudere, unpublished data).

The dose of IFN-α required to control eosinophilia in the overall HES population is variable, but is generally between 7 and 14 million units per week [57]. There are no published data on efficient doses for patients with L-HES. Therapy should be initiated at low doses, and increased progressively to minimize the debilitating flulike symptoms, which tend to decrease over time. Effects of IFN-α on eosinophil levels and associated symptoms are delayed, meaning that adjustment of optimal dosing may take months.

Tyrosine kinase inhibitors

Imatinib mesylate, the tyrosine kinase inhibitor that targets abl, PDGFRA, PDGFRB, and c-kit, has recently become extremely popular in HES management, given its dramatic effects on cells expressing the F1P1-L1–PDGFRA fusion protein [58]. This agent has been administered briefly to several patients with L-HES, none of which has responded in terms of clinical manifestations or eosinophil levels [30,40,59]. To date, studies on aberrant T cells implicated in L-HES pathogenesis have not revealed abnormal tyrosine kinase activity that justifies a clinical trial with imatinib mesylate or other tyrosine kinase inhibitors in this setting.

Monoclonal antibodies

An interesting therapeutic target in patients with L-HES is the CD52 antigen, which is expressed both on T cells and eosinophils. In a recent report, alemtuzumab, a monoclonal anti-CD52 antibody, was shown to be effective treatment for a patient with a CD3⁻CD4⁺ T-cell subset, inducing rapid normalization of eosinophil levels and clinical remission [40]. Effects on the aberrant T cells were not reported. After an initial treatment period with 30 mg subcutaneous alemtuzumab per week, the interval was increased to every 3 weeks with sustained remission. Some patients with Sézary syndrome have developed cardiac dysfunction during treatment, leading authors to suggest possible treatment-related toxicity [60]. This could be a subject of concern for patients with HES, although the patient reported here actually improved cardiac function with treatment.

Monoclonal anti–IL-5 mAbs target eosinophils by interfering with ligation of IL-5 to the α-chain of the IL-5R on their surface. Several open-label studies evaluating effects of intravenous anti–IL-5 in HES patients showed a rapid decline of blood eosinophil counts shortly after administration, associated with improvement of a range of clinical manifestations, allowing CS tapering in some cases [61–63]. Eosinophil depletion and clinical benefit in response to 750 mg intravenous mepolizumab, the anti–IL-5 mAb produced by GlaxoSmithKline, can be surprisingly long-lasting, and in-between dose intervals may be several months long [62]. Anti–IL-5 treatment is expected to be beneficial for patients with L-HES in terms of eosinophil-mediated clinical manifestations, because eosinophil expansion is clearly driven by exogenous (T cell) production of IL-5, but is unlikely to affect pathogenic T cells. As of yet, patients responding to anti–IL-5 treatment in published reports did not have clear-cut T-cell–mediated HES. Efficacy of mepolizumab as a CS-sparing agent in FIP1L1-PDGFRα⁻ HES patients has very recently been evaluated, however, in the setting of a randomized, double-blind, placebo-controlled clinical trial (manuscript submitted for publication). It is likely that detailed analysis of patient characteristics and study results will disclose whether the L-HES patient subgroup responds to this strategy. Further analyses within the open-label extension of this clinical trial will provide information on long-term safety and tolerance of anti–IL-5 therapy and associated eosinophil depletion.

Strategies warranting future investigation

Future in vitro investigations could explore effects of innovative agents or strategies on pathogenic T cells from patients with L-HES, including cyclosporine A, anti–IL-2R-α mAb, and extracorporeal photochemotherapy. In patients with $CD3^-CD4^+$ cells, cyclosporine A could interfere with nuclear accumulation of NF-ATc2, which is thought to contribute to decreased transcription of CD3γ chain gene and enhanced transcription of Th2 cytokine genes. Furthermore, in vitro studies have shown that IL-2–IL-2R-α interactions are critical for survival and proliferation of $CD3^-CD4^+$ cells, and for production of Th2 cytokines [18], providing rationale for both cyclosporine A and anti–IL-2R-α mAb. As for extracorporeal photochemotherapy, induction of T-cell apoptosis and modulation of cytokine profiles in favor of Th1 responses account for suppressive effects on pathogenic T cells associated with cutaneous T-cell lymphoma, atopic dermatitis, and graft-versus-host disease [64–66]. Because pathogenic T-cell clones in HES are found in peripheral blood, they could represent an ideal target for extracorporeal irradiation. Interestingly, one patient with circulating $CD3^-CD4^+$ T cells and skin lesions harboring T cells with a clonal TCR rearrangement pattern was treated by psoralen plus UVA therapy, and regression of the pathogenic T-cell subset was observed in peripheral blood [12], suggesting that the skin may be an important source of these cells.

Management of T-cell lymphoma in the setting of lymphocytic hypereosinophilic syndrome

Once full-blown peripheral T-cell lymphoma has developed in patients initially diagnosed with L-HES, eradication of malignant T cells is not easily achieved using classical chemotherapeutic regimens [12,30]. The purine nucleoside analogue fludarabine may be effective for controlling indolent lymphoid malignancies [67,68] (eg, Sézary syndrome, peripheral T-cell lymphoma) and potently suppresses $CD4^+$ T cells, making it an interesting candidate for treating malignant $CD3^-CD4^+$ or $CD4^+CD7^-$ T-cell lymphoma. The authors have administered fludarabine to one patient with a $CD3^-CD4^+$ T-cell clone, who experienced temporary benefit in terms of eosinophil levels and cutaneous symptoms (pruritis, eczema). The authors observed very partial regression of the T-cell clone, however, which increased shortly after the sixth cycle of treatment (F. Roufosse, unpublished observation, 1999). She was also resistant to standard CHOP-like chemotherapy. Finally, intensification of chemotherapy followed by transplantation of allogeneic stem cells from an HLA-matched sibling successfully and durably eradicated the malignant CD3$^-$CD4$^+$ T-cell clone, and she is still in complete remission more than 6 years after the procedure.

Summary

The discovery that IL-5–producing T cells are directly involved in hypereosinophilia in a subset of HES patients has been followed by extensive functional characterization of the pathogenic T cells, especially CD3$^-$CD4$^+$ cells, and long-term observation of such patients. These studies have somewhat modified management of this disorder. For example, the former belief that increased serum IgE is associated with a benign disease course has been replaced by concern that patients with phenotypically aberrant T-cell clones may eventually develop peripheral T-cell lymphoma; patient follow-up has been adapted to detect this complication. Although many agree that therapeutic strategies should target T cells and eosinophils, the practical implications remain unclear. The authors are confident that systematic recording of patient responses to currently available therapeutic agents, and identification of novel therapeutic targets through investigation of primary molecular defects underlying L-HES, will result in improved treatment and outcome of this HES variant.

References

[1] Fletcher S, Bain B. Diagnosis and treatment of hypereosinophilic syndromes. Curr Opin Hematol 2007;14(1):37–42.

[2] Mosmann TR, Cherwinski H, Bond MW, et al. Two types of murine helper T cell clone. I. Definition according to profiles of lymphokine activities and secreted proteins. J Immunol 1986;136(7):2348–57.

[3] Campbell HD, Tucker WQ, Hort Y, et al. Molecular cloning, nucleotide sequence, and expression of the gene encoding human eosinophil differentiation factor (interleukin 5). Proc Natl Acad Sci U S A 1987;84(19):6629–33.

[4] Romagnani S. Th1 and Th2 in human diseases. Clin Immunol Immunopathol 1996;80(3 Pt 1): 225–35.

[5] Fauci AS, Harley JB, Roberts WC, et al. NIH conference. The idiopathic hypereosinophilic syndrome: clinical, pathophysiologic, and therapeutic considerations. Ann Intern Med 1982; 97(1):78–92.

[6] Raghavachar A, Fleischer S, Frickhofen N, et al. T lymphocyte control of human eosinophilic granulopoiesis: clonal analysis in an idiopathic hypereosinophilic syndrome. J Immunol 1987;139(11):3753–8.

[7] Schrezenmeier H, Thome SD, Tewald F, et al. Interleukin-5 is the predominant eosinophilopoietin produced by cloned T lymphocytes in hypereosinophilic syndrome. Exp Hematol 1993;21(2):358–65.

[8] Cogan E, Schandene L, Crusiaux A, et al. Brief report: clonal proliferation of type 2 helper T cells in a man with the hypereosinophilic syndrome. N Engl J Med 1994;330(8):535–8.

[9] Chusid MJ, Dale DC, West BC, et al. The hypereosinophilic syndrome: analysis of fourteen cases with review of the literature. Medicine (Baltimore) 1975;54(1):1–27.

[10] Simon HU, Plotz SG, Dummer R, et al. Abnormal clones of T cells producing interleukin-5 in idiopathic eosinophilia. N Engl J Med 1999;341(15):1112–20.

[11] Roufosse F, Schandene L, Sibille C, et al. Clonal Th2 lymphocytes in patients with the idiopathic hypereosinophilic syndrome. Br J Haematol 2000;109(3):540–8.

[12] Bank I, Amariglio N, Reshef A, et al. The hypereosinophilic syndrome associated with CD4+CD3- helper type 2 (Th2) lymphocytes. Leuk Lymphoma 2001;42(1–2):123–33.

[13] Willard-Gallo KE, Badran BM, Ravoet M, et al. Defective CD3gamma gene transcription is associated with NFATc2 overexpression in the lymphocytic variant of hypereosinophilic syndrome. Exp Hematol 2005;33(10):1147–59.

[14] Edelman J, Meyerson HJ. Diminished CD3 expression is useful for detecting and enumerating Sézary cells. Am J Clin Pathol 2000;114(3):467–77.

[15] Yokote T, Akioka T, Oka S, et al. Flow cytometric immunophenotyping of adult T-cell leukemia/lymphoma using CD3 gating. Am J Clin Pathol 2005;124(2):199–204.

[16] Serke S, van Lessen A, Hummel M, et al. Circulating CD4+ T lymphocytes with intracellular but no surface CD3 antigen in five of seven patients consecutively diagnosed with angioimmunoblastic T-cell lymphoma. Cytometry 2000;42(3):180–7.

[17] Schandene L, Roufosse F, de Lavareille A, et al. Interferon alpha prevents spontaneous apoptosis of clonal Th2 cells associated with chronic hypereosinophilia. Blood 2000; 96(13):4285–92.

[18] Roufosse F, Schandene L, Sibille C, et al. T-cell receptor-independent activation of clonal Th2 cells associated with chronic hypereosinophilia. Blood 1999;94(3):994–1002.

[19] O'Shea JJ, Jaffe ES, Lane HC, et al. Peripheral T cell lymphoma presenting as hypereosinophilia with vasculitis: clinical, pathologic, and immunologic features. Am J Med 1987;82(3): 539–45.

[20] Brugnoni D, Airo P, Rossi G, et al. A case of hypereosinophilic syndrome is associated with the expansion of a CD3-CD4+ T-cell population able to secrete large amounts of interleukin-5. Blood 1996;87(4):1416–22.

[21] Roumier AS, Grardel N, Lai JL, et al. Hypereosinophilia with abnormal T cells, trisomy 7 and elevated TARC serum level. Haematologica 2003;88(7):ECR24.

[22] Bank I, Reshef A, Beniaminov M, et al. Role of gamma/delta T cells in a patient with CD4+CD3- lymphocytosis, hypereosinophilia, and high levels of IgE. J Allergy Clin Immunol 1998;102(4 Pt 1):621–30.

[23] Sugimoto K, Tamayose K, Sasaki M, et al. More than 13 years of hypereosinophila associated with clonal CD3-CD4+ lymphocytosis of TH2/TH0 type. Int J Hematol 2002;75(3):281–4.

[24] Costello R, Cerdan C, Pavon C, et al. The CD2 and CD28 adhesion molecules induce long-term autocrine proliferation of CD4+ T cells. Eur J Immunol 1993;23(3):608–13.

[25] Cerdan C, Martin Y, Courcoul M, et al. Prolonged IL-2 receptor alpha/CD25 expression after T cell activation via the adhesion molecules CD2 and CD28. Demonstration of combined transcriptional and post-transcriptional regulation. J Immunol 1992;149(7):2255–61.

[26] Cerdan C, Martin Y, Courcoul M, et al. CD28 costimulation up-regulates long-term IL-2R beta expression in human T cells through combined transcriptional and post-transcriptional regulation. J Immunol 1995;154(3):1007–13.

[27] Willard-Gallo KE, Van de Keere F, Kettmann R. A specific defect in CD3 gamma-chain gene transcription results in loss of T-cell receptor/CD3 expression late after human immunodeficiency virus infection of a CD4+ T-cell line. Proc Natl Acad Sci U S A 1990;87(17):6713–7.

[28] Kitano K, Ichikawa N, Mahbub B, et al. Eosinophilia associated with proliferation of CD(3+)4-(8-) alphabeta(+) T cells with chromosome 16 abnormalities. Br J Haematol 1996;92:315–7.

[29] Simon HU, Yousefi S, Dommann-Scherrer CC, et al. Expansion of cytokine-producing CD4-CD8- T cells associated with abnormal Fas expression and hypereosinophilia. J Exp Med 1996;183(3):1071–82.

[30] Vaklavas C, Tefferi A, Butterfield J, et al. Idiopathic eosinophilia with an occult T-cell clone: prevalence and clinical course. Leuk Res 2007;31:691–4.

[31] Davis AL, McKenzie JL, Hart DN. HLA-DR-positive leucocyte subpopulations in human skin include dendritic cells, macrophages, and CD7-negative T cells. Immunology 1988; 65(4):573–81.

[32] Groh V, Fabbi M, Hochstenbach F, et al. Double-negative (CD4-CD8-) lymphocytes bearing T-cell receptor alpha and beta chains in normal human skin. Proc Natl Acad Sci U S A 1989;86(13):5059–63.

[33] Reinhold U, Abken H, Kukel S, et al. CD7- T cells represent a subset of normal human blood lymphocytes. J Immunol 1993;150(5):2081–9.

[34] Autran B, Legac E, Blanc C, et al. A Th0/Th2-like function of CD4+CD7- T helper cells from normal donors and HIV-infected patients. J Immunol 1995;154(3):1408–17.

[35] Hodak E, David M, Maron L, et al. CD4/CD8 double-negative epidermotropic cutaneous T-cell lymphoma: an immunohistochemical variant of mycosis fungoides. J Am Acad Dermatol 2006;55(2):276–84.

[36] Wood GS, Hong SR, Sasaki DT, et al. Leu-8/CD7 antigen expression by CD3+ T cells: comparative analysis of skin and blood in mycosis fungoides/Sézary syndrome relative to normal blood values. J Am Acad Dermatol 1990;22(4):602–7.

[37] Rappl G, Muche JM, Abken H, et al. CD4(+)CD7(-) T cells compose the dominant T-cell clone in the peripheral blood of patients with Sézary syndrome. J Am Acad Dermatol 2001;44(3):456–61.

[38] Zenone T, Felman P, Malcus C, et al. Indolent course of a patient with hypereosinophilic syndrome associated with clonal T-cell proliferation. Am J Med 1999;107(5):509–11.

[39] Morgan SJ, Prince HM, Westerman DA, et al. Clonal T-helper lymphocytes and elevated IL-5 levels in episodic angioedema and eosinophilia (Gleich's syndrome). Leuk Lymphoma 2003;44(9):1623–5.

[40] Pitini V, Teti D, Arrigo C, et al. Alemtuzumab therapy for refractory idiopathic hypereosinophilic syndrome with abnormal T cells: a case report. Br J Haematol 2004;127(5):477.

[41] Bagot M, Bodemer C, Wechsler J, et al. [Non epidermotropic T lymphoma preceded for several years by hypereosinophilic syndrome]. Ann Dermatol Venereol 1990;117(11):883–5 [in French].

[42] de Lavareille A, Roufosse F, Schmid-Grendelmeier P, et al. High serum thymus and activation-regulated chemokine levels in the lymphocytic variant of the hypereosinophilic syndrome. J Allergy Clin Immunol 2002;110(3):476–9.

[43] de Lavareille A, Roufosse F, Schandene L, et al. Clonal Th2 cells associated with chronic hypereosinophilia: TARC-induced CCR4 down-regulation in vivo. Eur J Immunol 2001; 31(4):1037–46.

[44] Sekiya T, Miyamasu M, Imanishi M, et al. Inducible expression of a Th2-type CC chemokine thymus- and activation-regulated chemokine by human bronchial epithelial cells. J Immunol 2000;165(4):2205–13.

[45] Xiao T, Fujita H, Saeki H, et al. Thymus and activation-regulated chemokine (TARC/CCL17) produced by mouse epidermal Langerhans cells is upregulated by TNF-alpha and IL-4 and downregulated by IFN-gamma. Cytokine 2003;23(4–5):126–32.

[46] Kakinuma T, Nakamura K, Wakugawa M, et al. Thymus and activation-regulated chemokine in atopic dermatitis: serum thymus and activation-regulated chemokine level is closely related with disease activity. J Allergy Clin Immunol 2001;107(3):535–41.

[47] Roufosse F, Cogan E, Goldman M. The hypereosinophilic syndrome revisited. Annu Rev Med 2003;54:169–84.

[48] Ravoet M, Sibille C, Roufosse F, et al. 6q- is an early and persistent chromosomal aberration in CD3-CD4+ T-cell clones associated with the lymphocytic variant of hypereosinophilic syndrome. Haematologica 2005;90(6):753–65.

[49] Thangavelu M, Finn WG, Yelavarthi KK, et al. Recurring structural chromosome abnormalities in peripheral blood lymphocytes of patients with mycosis fungoides/Sézary syndrome. Blood 1997;89(9):3371–7.

[50] Simon HU. Eosinophil apoptosis: pathophysiologic and therapeutic implications. Allergy 2000;55(10):910–5.

[51] Batuman OA, Ferrero AP, Diaz A, et al. Glucocorticoid-mediated inhibition of interleukin-2 receptor alpha and -beta subunit expression by human T cells. Immunopharmacology 1994; 27(1):43–55.

[52] Braun CM, Huang SK, Bashian GG, et al. Corticosteroid modulation of human, antigen-specific Th1 and Th2 responses. J Allergy Clin Immunol 1997;100(3):400–7.

[53] Nakajima H, Nakao A, Watanabe Y, et al. IFN-alpha inhibits antigen-induced eosinophil and CD4+ T cell recruitment into tissue. J Immunol 1994;153(3):1264–70.

[54] Maggi E, Parronchi P, Manetti R, et al. Reciprocal regulatory effects of IFN-gamma and IL-4 on the in vitro development of human Th1 and Th2 clones. J Immunol 1992;148(7):2142–7.

[55] Schandene L, Del Prete GF, Cogan E, et al. Recombinant interferon-alpha selectively inhibits the production of interleukin-5 by human CD4+ T cells. J Clin Invest 1996;97(2): 309–15.

[56] Broxmeyer HE, Lu L, Platzer E, et al. Comparative analysis of the influences of human gamma, alpha and beta interferons on human multipotential (CFU-GEMM), erythroid (BFU-E) and granulocyte-macrophage (CFU-GM) progenitor cells. J Immunol 1983; 131(3):1300–5.

[57] Klion AD, Bochner BS, Gleich GJ, et al. Approaches to the treatment of hypereosinophilic syndromes: a workshop summary report. J Allergy Clin Immunol 2006;117(6):1292–302.

[58] Cools J, DeAngelo DJ, Gotlib J, et al. A tyrosine kinase created by fusion of the PDGFRA and FIP1L1 genes as a therapeutic target of imatinib in idiopathic hypereosinophilic syndrome. N Engl J Med 2003;348(13):1201–14.

[59] Pardanani A, Reeder T, Porrata LF, et al. Imatinib therapy for hypereosinophilic syndrome and other eosinophilic disorders. Blood 2003;101(9):3391–7.

[60] Lenihan DJ, Alencar AJ, Yang D, et al. Cardiac toxicity of alemtuzumab in patients with mycosis fungoides/Sézary syndrome. Blood 2004;104(3):655–8.

[61] Garrett JK, Jameson SC, Thomson B, et al. Anti-interleukin-5 (mepolizumab) therapy for hypereosinophilic syndromes. J Allergy Clin Immunol 2004;113(1):115–9.

[62] Plotz SG, Simon HU, Darsow U, et al. Use of an anti-interleukin-5 antibody in the hypereosinophilic syndrome with eosinophilic dermatitis. N Engl J Med 2003;349(24):2334–9.

[63] Klion AD, Law MA, Noel P, et al. Safety and efficacy of the monoclonal anti-interleukin-5 antibody SCH55700 in the treatment of patients with hypereosinophilic syndrome. Blood 2004;103(8):2939–41.

[64] Prinz B, Michelsen S, Pfeiffer C, et al. Long-term application of extracorporeal photochemotherapy in severe atopic dermatitis. J Am Acad Dermatol 1999;40(4):577–82.

[65] Crovetti G, Carabelli A, Berti E, et al. Photopheresis in cutaneous T-cell lymphoma: five-year experience. Int J Artif Organs 2000;23(1):55–62.

[66] Aubin F, Salard D, Poutier F, et al. La photochimiothérapie extracorporelle. Medicine Science 1999;15:983–9.

[67] Adkins JC, Peters DH, Markham A. Fludarabine: an update of its pharmacology and use in the treatment of haematological malignancies. Drugs 1997;53(6):1005–37.

[68] Quaglino P, Fierro MT, Rossotto GL, et al. Treatment of advanced mycosis fungoides/Sézary syndrome with fludarabine and potential adjunctive benefit to subsequent extracorporeal photochemotherapy. Br J Dermatol 2004;150(2):327–36.

ELSEVIER
SAUNDERS

Immunol Allergy Clin N Am
27 (2007) 415–441

IMMUNOLOGY
AND ALLERGY
CLINICS
OF NORTH AMERICA

Dermatologic Manifestations of the Hypereosinophilic Syndromes

Kristin M. Leiferman, MD[a],*, Gerald J. Gleich, MD[a],
Margot S. Peters, MD[b]

[a]*Department of Dermatology, 4B454 School of Medicine,
University of Utah Health Sciences Center, University of Utah,
30 North 1900 East, Salt Lake City, UT 84132-2409, USA*
[b]*Rochester, Minnesota, USA*

Hypereosinophilic syndromes (HES) may present with cutaneous abnormalities (Box 1). Over 50% of patients have pruritic erythematous macules, papules, plaques, wheals, nodules, or other skin lesions during the course of the disease [1,2], but a diagnosis of HES may be delayed or missed because association between such lesions and HES is not appreciated. Urticaria and angioedema occur in all HES subtypes and are characteristic of certain variant subtypes. Eosinophil granule proteins are deposited diffusely in skin lesions of HES and may mediate increased vasopermeability, resulting in edema and other effects. In addition, there are a variety of cutaneous reaction patterns to consider in evaluating diseases characterized by eosinophilia of peripheral blood and/or tissues (Box 2). The skin diseases discussed in this article are presented based on the classification of HES put forth in the publication resulting from the 2005 workshop summary of the International Eosinophil Society meeting [3].

Sections of this article have been modified from the following documents: Leiferman KM, Peters MS. Eosinophils in cutaneous diseases. In: Wolff K, Goldsmith LA, Katz SI, et al, editors. Fitzpatrick's Dermatology in General Medicine. 7th edition. New York: McGraw-Hill, Inc., in press; and Stetson CL, Leiferman KM. Eosinophilic Dermatoses. In: Bolognia JL, Jorizzo JL, Rapini RP, et al, editors. Dermatology. 2nd edition. St. Louis: Mosby, in press.

Supported in part by Grants AI061097 and AI009728 from the National Institute of Allergy and Infectious Diseases.

* Corresponding author.

E-mail address: kristin.leiferman@hsc.utah.edu (K.M. Leiferman).

Box 1. Hypereosinophilic syndromes: mucocutaneous signs, symptoms, and diagnoses

Angioedema
Eczema
Erosions
Erythema
Erythema annulare centrifugum
Erythroderma
Excoriations
Livedo reticularis
Macules
Mucosal (oral and genital) ulcers
Nail fold infarcts
Necrotizing vasculitis
Nodules
Papules
Patches
Pruritus
Purpuric papules
Splinter hemorrhages
Ulcers
Urticaria
Vasculitis
Wells' syndrome (eosinophilic cellulitis)

Eosinophils and the skin

Normal skin

The presence of eosinophils in normal tissues is surprisingly selective. Eosinophils infiltrate the spleen, lymph node, and thymus, with scant evidence of granule protein deposition. The only organ other than the bone marrow that normally shows both eosinophil infiltration and remarkable degranulation is the gastrointestinal tract [4]. Eosinophil infiltration or degranulation is not seen in skin from normal persons or from normal skin of patients with a variety of disorders [4–6].

Eosinophil infiltration

Mechanisms of eosinophil infiltration in tissues, including skin, have been studied extensively, as reviewed by Bochner and Ackerman elsewhere in this issue. Eosinophils are attracted into tissues and activated by at least three interrelated signals: (1) chemoattractants, (2) adhesion molecules, and (3)

Box 2. Deposition of eosinophil granule proteins in cutaneous diseases

Edema
Chronic urticaria
Solar urticaria
Delayed pressure urticaria
IgE-mediated late phase reaction
Episodic angioedema with eosinophilia (Gleich's syndrome)
Facial edema with eosinophilia
Nodules, eosinophilia, rheumatism, dermatitis,
    swelling syndrome
Granulocyte macrophage colony-stimulating factor reaction
Interleukin-2 capillary leak syndrome

Eczematoid reactions
Atopic dermatitis
Onchocercal dermatitis
Prurigo nodularis
Pachydermatous eosinophilic dermatitis

Vasculitis
Churg-Strauss syndrome
Recurrent cutaneous eosinophilic vasculitis
Eosinophilic vasculitis in connective tissue disease

Blisters
Bullous pemphigoid
Pemphigoid (herpes) gestationis
Bullous morphea
Blisters in Churg-Strauss syndrome
Incontinentia pigmenti

Fibrosis
Eosinophilia myalgia syndrome
Toxic oil syndrome
Eosinophilic fasciitis

Data from Leiferman KM, Peters MS. Eosinophils in cutaneous diseases. In: Wolff K, Goldsmith LA, Katz SI, et al, editors. Fitzpatrick's Dermatology in General Medicine. 7th edition. New York: McGraw-Hill, Inc., in press.

---

activating cytokines [7,8]. Eotaxins 1–3 and "regulated on activation normal T cell–expressed and secreted" (RANTES) are produced by dermal fibroblasts, and RANTES also is produced by keratinocytes. Eosinophil-selective adhesion molecule expression and other eosinophil-activating cytokines also may be induced in skin. Thus, eosinophil signaling is poised for participation in cutaneous inflammation [9,10].

Eosinophil degranulation

As intact cells, eosinophils are readily identified by their tinctorial properties when stained with the acidic dye, eosin. Cytoplasmic granules in eosinophils are distinctive both in composition (namely, cationic proteins that are responsible for their cellular staining properties) and ultrastructural features identified by electron microscopy. Like other granulated cells, eosinophils undergo degranulation. Degranulation refers to the release of eosinophil granule proteins and is defined herein as extracellular deposition of eosinophil granule major basic protein (MBP) or other distinctive granule proteins, which can be detected in tissues by special stains.

Eosinophil degranulation can occur through classical exocytosis or piecemeal degranulation, but, in skin diseases, commonly occurs by cytolysis in skin diseases. A study of lesional skin from patients with atopic dermatitis showed intact eosinophils with abnormal granules and with disrupted cytoplasmic and/or nuclear membranes; membrane-bound granules were present in the dermis near to and in the absence of degenerating eosinophils [11]. There was no evidence of classical granule exocytosis. Disrupted eosinophils have been observed in the dermis of lesional tissue from patients with episodic angioedema associated with eosinophilia [12] and the IgE-mediated late phase reaction [13]. Therefore, deposition of eosinophil granule proteins in skin occurs after eosinophil cytolysis. A similar conclusion was reached through study of involved skin from a patient with HES [14].

Eosinophils and cutaneous edema

Eosinophils may induce cutaneous edema [7] through direct effects on blood vessels or indirectly through mast cells. Topical administration of nanomolar concentrations of eosinophil cationic protein (ECP), eosinophil peroxidase (EPO), and MBP increases vasopermeability in the hamster cheek pouch [15,16]; neither histamine nor nitric oxide appears to participate in this effect [15,17]. Injection of approximately 5 µmol/L of MBP into guinea pig skin increases cutaneous vasopermeability [18]. Intradermal injection of eosinophil granule proteins elicits a wheal-and-flare reaction in human skin [12,19]. In vitro, micromolar concentrations of MBP and ECP inconsistently induce histamine release from mast cells and basophils [20,21]. Stem cell factor is required for MBP to induce histamine release from certain types of human mast cells [22].

The lowest detectable concentrations of eosinophil granule proteins in the skin are 0.05 µmol/L EPO, 0.1 µmol/L MBP, 0.25 µmol/L ECP, and 1 µmol/L eosinophil-derived neurotoxin (EDN) [23]. After injection into guinea pig skin, these proteins persist in vivo for 1 (EPO), 2 (ECP), $2\frac{1}{2}$ (EDN), or

6 (MBP) weeks [23]. Each protein increases cutaneous vasopermeability in a concentration-dependent fashion, with potencies comparable to that of histamine [23]. Pretreatment of guinea pigs with an antihistamine, pyrilamine maleate, does not inhibit the increased vasopermeability induced by ECP and EDN but significantly inhibits that induced by EPO and MBP [23]. Micromolar concentrations of eosinophil granule proteins are commonly deposited in the skin of eosinophil-associated cutaneous disorders (see Box 2), such as atopic dermatitis, and probably increase cutaneous vasopermeability (by histamine-independent and -dependent mechanisms), potentially altering cutaneous function for days to weeks.

Of the skin disorders characterized by swelling [24], eosinophil involvement has been particularly well demonstrated in chronic urticaria [6], pressure urticaria [25], and episodic angioedema (see Box 2) [12]. In addition to intact eosinophils, lesions of urticaria contain prominent extracellular deposition of granule proteins around small blood vessels, dispersed in the dermis, and on connective tissue fibers, in up to 60% of cases [6]. Sequential biopsy specimens from lesions of solar and delayed pressure urticaria, and from lesions elicited by a solar simulator or dermographometer [25,26], demonstrate a pattern of eosinophil and neutrophil degranulation similar to that seen in the IgE-mediated late phase reaction [13], which exhibits erythema, edema, pruritus, warmth, and tenderness. Skin biopsy specimens from patients with episodic angioedema associated with eosinophilia and its localized variant, recurrent facial edema with eosinophilia [12,27], show few eosinophils, but immunofluorescence staining reveals extracellular deposition of eosinophil granule proteins around blood vessels and on collagen bundles [12]. Capillary leak syndromes due to administration of interleukin (IL)-2 and granulocyte macrophage colony-stimulating factor are associated with peripheral blood eosinophilia, increased serum IL-5 levels, and eosinophil degranulation [28,29]. The ability of eosinophils to elaborate vasoactive mediators that elicit cutaneous wheal-and-flare reactions, along with the presence of granule proteins in edematous skin, support a role for eosinophils as key participants in the edema associated with certain cutaneous diseases.

Cutaneous aspects of hypereosinophilic syndrome

Patients who fulfill diagnostic criteria for HES (as reviewed by Sheikh and Weller elsewhere in this issue) develop symptoms related to the organ systems infiltrated by eosinophils. Occurring in over 50% of HES patients, skin lesions, of the trunk and/or extremities, may be the first manifestation of HES [2], and include pruritic erythematous macules, papules, plaques, wheals, and nodules [1]. Urticaria and angioedema occur in all HES subtypes and are characteristic of certain subtypes. HES patients may present with or develop a variety of cutaneous disorders, including erythema annulare centrifugum [30–32], necrotizing vasculitis [33,34], livedo reticularis, purpuric papules [33], and Wells' syndrome (eosinophilic cellulitis) [35,36].

Myeloproliferative hypereosinophilic syndrome variant

The presenting complex of myeloproliferative HES (reviewed by Bain and Fletcher elsewhere in this issue) often includes skin lesions in addition to fever, weight loss, fatigue, malaise, and hepatosplenomegaly [37]. Splinter hemorrhages and/or nail fold infarcts may herald the onset of thromboembolic disease associated with eosinophilic endomyocardial involvement, and this constitutes a medical emergency because of potentially serious sequelae. A distinctive feature of patients with myeloproliferative HES is mucosal ulceration [38,39]. The initial report of this association described two patients who satisfied diagnostic criteria for HES: both had eosinophil counts greater than $1500/mm^3$ for more than 6 months; organ–system involvement, including heart and skin; and no evidence of parasitic, allergic, or other known causes of eosinophilia. In both patients, an initial diagnosis of Behcet's syndrome was based on severe, chronic, and recurrent oral and genital ulcers, but all other major criteria (uveitis, synovitis, cutaneous vasculitis, and meningoencephalitis) for Behcet's syndrome were absent. Furthermore, mucosal ulcers in these patients (Fig. 1) often exceeded the size (1 cm diameter) typically associated with aphthae of Behcet's disease. Both patients died, as did 4 of 7 additional patients. The prognosis of this HES variant remained relatively poor until mucosal ulcers in several patients showed dramatic response to administration of a tyrosine kinase inhibitor, imatinib mesylate (Gleevec) [40]. Furthermore, responsiveness to imatinib is associated with a mutational deletion on chromosome 4, resulting in a fusion gene, Fip1-like-1/platelet-derived growth factor receptor α (FIP1L1-PDGFRα), and generation of an imatinib-sensitive kinase [41,42]. Recently, Klion and colleagues [43] found serum tryptase levels (marking mast cell activity) greater than 12 ng/mL in 9 of 15 patients with HES; 3 of the 9 had mucosal ulcers

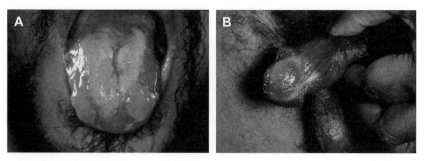

Fig. 1. Mucosal erosions and ulcers of the tongue (A) and glans penis (B) in a patient who has myeloproliferative HES.

and were categorized as having myeloproliferative HES with tissue fibrosis. Overall, these findings suggest that patients with mucosal ulceration and HES are distinctive both in cutaneous manifestations and biologic behavior of their disease. Testing for FIP1L1-PDGFRα should be performed in HES patients because of the striking therapeutic effectiveness of imatinib.

Lymphocytic hypereosinophilic syndrome variant

Lymphocytic HES (reviewed by Roufosse, Cogan, and Goldman elsewhere in this issue) is associated with severe pruritus, eczema, erythroderma, urticaria, and angioedema, as well as lymphadenopathy, and endomyocardial involvement, although cardiac abnormalities occur less commonly than in myeloproliferative HES. Many of these patients have T cell clones that produce IL-5 [44,45]. In contrast to myeloproliferative HES, lymphocytic HES generally follows a benign course, and T cell clones can remain stable for years. Patients should be regarded as having premalignant or malignant T cell proliferation [45], because the disease may evolve into lymphoma. In 3 patients who had lymphocytic HES, repeated infusion of an antibody to IL-5, mepolizumab, effectively controlled their eosinophilic dermatitis [46]; after the first infusion, pruritus decreased and pruritic, eczematous, and urticarial skin lesions regressed; within 24 hours, eosinophil counts dropped to normal, and serum ECP levels became normal during the next 2 days. There was no systemic or local toxicity, including leukopenia or changes in the distribution of lymphocyte subpopulations, indicating that mepolizumab does not cause general immunosuppression. In 2 of 3 patients, mepolizumab was associated with decreased in vitro T helper 2 cytokine production following mitogen stimulation of T cells. These data suggest that eosinophils are able to modulate T cell function, including differentiation and cytokine production, and that treatment of lymphocytic HES with anti–IL-5 should be effective.

Undefined hypereosinophilic syndrome: episodic angioedema associated with eosinophilia

Classified as "undefined" [3], this distinct HES subset is characterized by severe, cyclical attacks of angioedema (Fig. 2) that involve the face, neck, trunk and extremities, urticaria, fever, marked peripheral blood eosinophilia (up to 100,000 cells/μL), and an average increase in body weight of 14% (range, 10%–18%) [12]. Attacks persist for days. Marked leukocytosis and eosinophilia appear to vary in parallel with the clinical severity of the attack. In addition, there is a polyclonal increase in serum IgM levels, and IgE levels may be strikingly high. The disease occurs in children and adults [47,48], and localized variants are described [27].

Serum IL-5 levels are increased in episodic angioedema. During prednisone treatment (administered daily, every other day, or in short [3- to 5-day] courses [7]), IL-5 becomes undetectable as patients improve clinically,

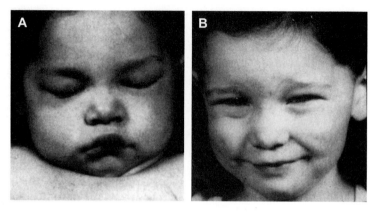

Fig. 2. Episodic angioedema with eosinophilia in a 2-year-old girl with marked edema of the face during an attack (*A*) compared with normal appearance between episodes (*B*). (*From* Katzen DR, Leiferman KM, Weller PF, et al. Hypereosinophilia and recurrent angioneurotic edema in a 2 1/2-year-old girl. Am J Dis Child 1986;140:63; with permission.)

lose weight, and eosinophil counts decrease [49]. In one patient studied over a 3-week period, maximum IL-5 levels and minimum urine output occurred on days 13 and 14; maximum eosinophil counts occurred on days 16 and 17, and peak weight was reached on day 18 [49]. Interestingly, peak eosinophilia lagged behind the peak serum IL-5 level by approximately 3 to 4 days [49]; this may represent the time needed for late stage eosinophil progenitors to fully differentiate into mature eosinophils and gain access to the peripheral blood. IL-5 levels spontaneously decreased during the latter stages of the attacks (Fig. 3). In this patient, intravascular fluid overload developed following prednisone administration, with resultant bradycardia, orthopnea, and bibasilar pulmonary infiltrate, without evidence of cardiac dysfunction. In addition, an increased percentage of activated T helper cells preceded the development of elevated IL-5 levels. A previously reported patient with episodic angioedema and eosinophilia had normal percentages of peripheral blood CD4 helper cells and CD8-positive cells; however, 32% of the CD4 cells expressed the HLA-DR activation antigen (normal value, <2%) [48]. The patient discussed here had a similar percentage (28%) of CD3-positive T cells expressing the HLA-DR activation antigen 10 days before the maximal eosinophil count [49]. Additional markers of T cell activation found in patients with episodic angioedema include IL-1 and soluble IL-2 receptor [50], and patients with this syndrome have developed T cell clones [51,52]. Peripheral blood eosinophils may lack CD69 expression, in contrast to the immunophenotype in other forms of HES [53].

In summary, very high levels of IL-5 are produced in episodic angioedema associated with eosinophilia. IL-5 stimulates bone marrow and activates eosinophils; eosinophils migrate into skin and deposit their granule proteins. These proteins, leukotrienes, and arachidonic acid metabolites contribute to massive increases in vascular permeability. As the stimuli for

IL-5 IN EPISODIC ANGIOEDEMA AND EOSINOPHILIA

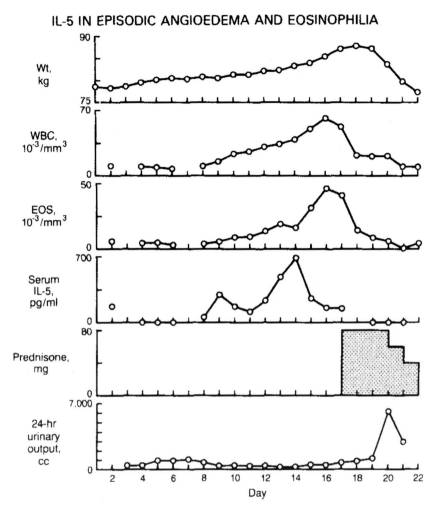

Fig. 3. Episodic angioedema with eosinophilia: clinical and laboratory findings include a biphasic increase in IL-5 levels during an attack, which by day 16 (the day of maximal eosinophilia) was decreasing. Prednisone administration was associated with disappearance of detectable IL-5 in serum. (*From* Butterfield JH, Leiferman KM, Abrams J, et al. Elevated serum levels of interleukin-5 in patients with the syndrome of episodic angioedema and eosinophilia. Blood 1992;79:689; with permission.)

eosinophil production diminish, the clinical abnormalities remit. However, the mechanisms causing the periodic elevations of IL-5 with corresponding eosinophilia are still obscure.

Nodules, eosinophilia, rheumatism, dermatitis, and swelling syndrome

Associated with marked peripheral blood eosinophilia and episodic swelling of the hands and feet, this syndrome was reported initially in 2 patients who also had dermatitis, nontender compressible articular nodules arising from the tenosynovium of extensor tendons, and pain in adjacent muscles and joints [54]. One of the two originally reported patients had dermographism as well as episcleritis. Both patients had increased plasma levels of MBP and EDN and increased serum IgE and IgM levels. Histologic evaluation of nodules revealed tenosynovitis with necrotizing granulomas, nonspecific vasculitis, eosinophil infiltration, and numerous mast cells; immunostaining for MBP provided evidence of degranulation. Lesions responded to low doses of prednisone. One patient had eosinophilia greater than 1500/mL blood for over 15 years without developing cardiovascular disease [54]. Patients with nodules, eosinophilia, rheumatism, dermatitis, and swelling syndrome have activated T cells [55] and also have developed T cell clones [52].

Associated hypereosinophilic syndrome: Churg–Strauss syndrome

Churg-Strauss syndrome (CSS) satisfies the criteria for HES and is classified as "associated HES" [3] because it is a recognized syndrome. Also termed allergic granulomatosis, CSS was described in 1951 as a complex of systemic vasculitis, asthma, and eosinophilia [56]. Cutaneous lesions are characterized by eosinophil infiltration, necrotizing vasculitis, and extravascular granulomas. Eosinophil mediators are prominent in lesions (Fig. 4) [57]. CSS affects respiratory tissues with asthma and sinus disease and is associated with involvement of other organs [58], including the heart and particularly the skin. Patients have cutaneous papules and nodules of the scalp or extremities and hemorrhagic lesions ranging from petechiae to blisters and eschars (Fig. 5). CSS is discussed by Wechsler elsewhere in this issue.

Overlap hypereosinophilic syndrome: eosinophilia myalgia syndrome and the Spanish toxic oil syndrome

Eosinophilia myalgia syndrome (EMS) and toxic oil syndrome (TOS) share many features, particularly cutaneous manifestations. EMS first presented in the fall of 1989 as a novel disease in epidemic form [59]. Although it is not known how long the syndrome had been in existence, a patient with EMS who was first seen in 1986 subsequently confirmed daily use of L-tryptophan for 5 years before onset of symptoms. Essentially all patients had severe myalgias early in the disease [59,60]. In addition to the characteristic features of eosinophilia and disabling myalgias, patients typically suffered multiorgan dysfunction, including fasciitis, pneumonitis, pulmonary hypertension, myocarditis, peripheral neuropathy, encephalopathy, cystitis, and peribiliary inflammatory fibrosis. In some fatal cases, peripheral neuropathy resulted in respiratory paralysis and death. Cutaneous abnormalities consisted of edema, pruritus, faint confluent erythema, hair loss, peau d'orange, and morphea-like skin lesions [61].

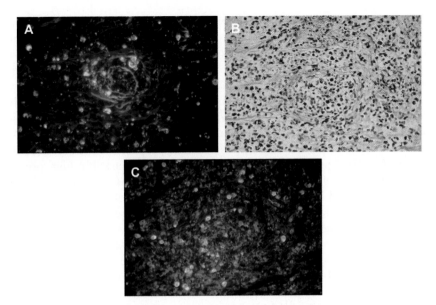

Fig. 4. Cutaneous leukocytoclastic vasculitis in Churg-Strauss syndrome: heavy mixed inflammatory cell infiltrate with numerous eosinophils and eosinophil granule products. MBP in and around a damaged blood vessel (*A*) (original magnification ×400) as demonstrated in the same section counterstained by hematoxylin and eosin (*B*) (original magnification ×400). A serial section (*C*) is stained for EDN and reveals prominent cellular and extracellular EDN in and around the damaged blood vessel (original magnification ×400).

The pathologic hallmarks of EMS are inflammation involving fibrous connective tissue and occlusive microangiopathy. The inflammatory infiltrate consists of mononuclear cells and few to many eosinophils. There is marked deposition of eosinophil granule proteins, often exceeding the degree of infiltration by intact eosinophils [59,62]. The severe myalgias at rest may be related to inflammation of fascial and intramuscular nerves;

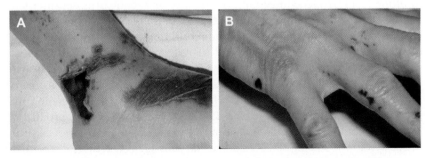

Fig. 5. Skin lesions in Churg-Strauss syndrome. (*A*) Characteristic hemorrhagic bullae and palpable purpura involving the foot. (*B*) Hemorrhagic infarcted lesions of the hand.

irritation or injury of peripheral nerves by EDN, other toxic eosinophil granule proteins and/or eosinophil products such as superoxide ion; or ischemia of nerves caused by occlusive microangiopathy [62]. Ischemia also may be responsible for cramps and increased myalgias on exertion. The denervation atrophy frequently seen in EMS probably is caused by toxic or ischemic peripheral nerve injury. Edema of skin and other soft tissues probably is due to endothelial damage and inflammation of microvessels, resulting in increased vascular permeability.

Association of EMS with ingestion of L-tryptophan was a striking discovery [59,63]. Epidemiologic analyses showed a remarkably high prevalence of L-tryptophan use in 1989 and demonstrated that the EMS outbreak resulted from ingestion of a chemical constituent that, in turn, was associated with specific tryptophan-manufacturing conditions at one company [63]. The L-tryptophan lots ingested by case patients were produced with use of a new strain of *Bacillus amyloliquefaciens* (strain V) for fermentation in a purification process that employed reduced quantities of powdered carbon. High-performance liquid chromatography demonstrated an absorbance peak (peak E) in the implicated lots to a greater degree than in control lots [64,65]. The structure of peak E was subsequently shown to be 1,1'-ethylidenebis[tryptophan] [64,65]. However, it is still not clear whether this contaminant is a marker or the cause of the epidemic.

Resembling EMS, TOS was linked to consumption of adulterated rapeseed oil distributed in the industrial belt around Madrid [66]. Patients had pruritic, erythematous skin lesions, persisting for up to 4 weeks, followed during the next 2 months by subcutaneous edema (mainly of the extremities), myalgias, arthralgias, contractures, and peripheral blood eosinophilia. Over many years, patients developed indurated plaques of the pretibial areas and occasionally the forearms and abdomen, with marked fibrosis extending into subcutaneous fat [66]. Eosinophil infiltration and degranulation were prominent especially in the acute phase of TOS, and serum eosinophil granule protein levels were elevated during all phases [67].

Eosinophils are associated with other fibrotic reactions, including those resulting from parasitic infections, pulmonary or hepatic drug-sensitivity reactions, and in eosinophilic fasciitis [68]. Eosinophilic fasciitis usually presents with pain, erythema, swelling, and induration of the extremities, as well as peripheral blood eosinophilia and hypergammaglobulinemia [69]. Contractures and rippling of the skin may develop. There is infiltration of lymphocytes, plasma cells, mast cells, and eosinophils, as well as increased thickness of the fascia. Eosinophils elaborate mediators that degrade collagen and stimulate dermal fibroblast DNA synthesis and matrix production [70]. MBP and EPO stimulate respiratory epithelial cells to produce profibrotic cytokines, raising the possibility that cells such as keratinocytes might respond similarly [70].

Cutaneous diseases associated with eosinophilia

The distinctive tinctorial properties of eosinophil granules give these cells a prominence in stained tissue sections that contrasts with their lack of diagnostic power and undefined role in pathogenesis. Eosinophils may be seen in skin biopsy specimens from patients with a variety of inflammatory and neoplastic disorders (Box 3), but they are among the diagnostic criteria in a limited number of cutaneous diseases, including Wells' syndrome, Kimura's disease, angiolymphoid hyperplasia with eosinophilia, and eosinophilic pustular folliculitis [71]. Eosinophils also are prominent in immunobullous diseases, particularly pemphigoid.

Wells' syndrome

Wells' syndrome, also termed *eosinophilic cellulitis*, occurs mainly in adults but also may afflict children [72]. Cutaneous edema is characteristic of the disease [71–81] and was the common clinical feature of the first four patients reported by G. C. Wells in 1971 [76]. The four originally

---

Box 3. Eosinophils in cutaneous diseases

Angiolymphoid hyperplasia with eosinophilia
Arthropod bites and sting reactions
Bullous dermatoses
- Pemphigoid
- Pemphigus
- Incontinentia pigmenti
Dermatoses of pregnancy
Drug reactions
Edema
- Angioedema
- Urticaria
Eosinophilic pustular folliculitis
Hypereosinophilic syndromes
Infestations/parasitic diseases
Kimura's disease
Lymphoma
Vasculitis
- Churg-Strauss syndrome
- Eosinophilic vasculitis
Wells' syndrome (eosinophilic cellulitis)

Data from Stetson CL, Leiferman KM. Eosinophilic dermatoses. In: Bolognia JL, Jorizzo JL, Rapini RP, et al, editors. Dermatology. 2nd edition. St. Louis: Mosby, in press.

reported patients had recurrent edematous infiltrative plaques resembling cellulitis at onset and, later, morphea [75]. The disease typically begins with prodromal cutaneous burning or itching, followed by erythema and edema, sometimes in annular or arcuate plaques or nodules. Over several days, lesions evolve into edematous plaques with violaceous borders, sometimes with bullae. The color may gradually change from bright red to brown-red and then to blue-gray or greenish-gray, resembling the fibrotic condition morphea. Uncommon presentations include papules, vesicles, and hemorrhagic bullae. Single or multiple lesions typically involve the extremities and, less often, the trunk. Wells' syndrome usually resolves within weeks to months, without scarring, but recurrences are common. Lesions typically improve after administration of systemic glucocorticoids. For mild disease, topical glucocorticoids may be sufficient.

Skin lesions are characterized by dermal infiltration of eosinophils, histiocytes, and foci of amorphous and/or granular material in association with connective tissue fibers, termed *flame figures* [75]. In early stages, there is dermal edema; later, histiocytes palisade around flame figures. Extracellular deposition of toxic granule proteins in lesions [80] is evidence that eosinophil degranulation contributes to flame figure formation. Approximately 50% of patients have peripheral blood eosinophilia [82]. The severity of skin lesions appears to vary with serum levels of IL-5 and ECP [83], and IL-5 is implicated in hereditary eosinophilic cellulites [82].

Reports of flame figures in lesions from patients with a spectrum of diseases indicate that flame figures are characteristic for, but not diagnostic of, Wells' syndrome [84]. Whether Wells' syndrome is a specific disease triggered by underlying factors such as infection and drugs or a reaction pattern is difficult to ascertain from the literature and clinical experience [84]. Wells' syndrome has been observed in patients with HES [35,36], in addition to a variety of other disorders. Associations with arthropod bites [75,78,85], parasitic infection (onchocerciasis) [86], dental abscess, mastocytoma [87], myeloproliferative disease [87], colon cancer [88], Churg-Strauss syndrome [77], dermographism [89], herpes simplex infection [90], immunobullous disease [75,91], and drug reaction [92,93] suggest that the syndrome is a reactive or hypersensitivity phenomenon [73].

Kimura's disease

In 1948, Kimura and colleagues [94] described "unusual granulation combined with hyperplastic changes in lymphatic tissue" associated with regional lymphadenopathy. Kimura's disease (KD) occurs predominantly in young adult Asian males. Patients have solitary or several asymptomatic, typically chronic and recurrent, nontender, slowly growing subcutaneous nodules that tend to involve the head and neck but may be localized to the extremities, axillae, groin, or trunk. Overlying skin usually appears unaffected. Regional lymphadenopathy is common, and some patients have widespread lymph node enlargement [95,96]. Approximately 16% of KD patients have associated renal disease, including glomerulonephritis and nephrotic syndrome [97].

Peripheral blood eosinophil counts and serum IgE levels are elevated in most patients. Lesions are characterized by lymphoid aggregates, usually lymphoid follicles with germinal centers, numerous eosinophils, and fibrosis; the pattern may include eosinophil abscesses. The combination of peripheral blood eosinophilia, elevated serum IgE level, and histologic findings of lymphoid nodules with numerous eosinophils suggests that KD represents a hypersensitivity reaction.

Angiolymphoid hyperplasia with eosinophilia

Originally described as "subcutaneous angiolymphoid hyperplasia with eosinophilia" [98], angiolymphoid hyperplasia with eosinophilia (ALHE) occurs in both males and females, usually in the third to fifth decade of life. In contrast to KD, which develops mainly in Asians, ALHE has no racial predilection. There may be a history of trauma. Lesions are erythematous, violaceous, or brown papules, plaques or nodules of the dermis and/ or subcutaneous tissues, that typically involve the head and neck region. They may be solitary, few, or multiple; pruritic, painful, or pulsatile; and tend to be chronic, without remission.

The dominant histologic feature is a well-defined area in the dermis and/ or subcutaneous fat of prominent vascular proliferation with large epithelioid or histiocytoid endothelial cells that contain abundant eosinophilic cytoplasm, often with cytoplasmic vacuoles. There are variable numbers of eosinophils and lymphocytes [99], and occasional lymphoid nodules. Approximately 20% of patients have peripheral blood eosinophilia; IgE levels are unremarkable. ALHE may represent a form of arteriovenous shunt [100]. It is considered a reactive phenomenon, possibly developing in response to or in association with an underlying vascular malformation.

Whether ALHE and KD represent separate entities or are part of a single disease spectrum has been debated. The distinction is further blurred by a report of KD and ALHE in the same patient [101]. Both diseases are characterized by persistent lesions that usually involve the head and neck, but each has distinct clinical and histologic features. Although eosinophils may be part of the histologic pattern in both diseases, lymphoid follicles with germinal centers dominate KD, and vascular proliferation with large epithelioid endothelial cells characterizes ALHE. Lesional tissue and peripheral blood eosinophilia are more striking in KD.

Eosinophilic pustular folliculitis

There are three clinical types of eosinophilic pustular folliculitis (EPF) [102]. First reported by Ofuji in 1965, classical EPF is not restricted to

Asians but typically occurs in Japanese individuals during the third to fourth decades of life [103]. Classical EPF is characterized by an annular distribution of recurrent crops or clusters of follicular papules and pustules, which usually resolve in 7 to 10 days. Lesions predominantly involve the face and trunk but may affect the extremities, including palms and soles [103]. In contrast, the second type of EPF, HIV-associated EPF, tends to have an urticarial quality and presents as extremely pruritic discrete follicular papules, typically involving the head, neck, and proximal extremities [104,105]. Described initially in 1986, HIV-associated EPF is now recognized as the most common type. The third type, EPF of infancy, presents during the first year of life; it involves the scalp but also may affect the face and extremities [102,103,105]. EPF of infancy typically resolves completely, while classical and HIV-associated EPF are recurrent. EPF also has been found in association with lymphoma, leukemia, polycythemia vera, and myelodysplastic syndrome, and drug-induced EPF [106] has been reported.

Histologically, the most striking aspect of EPF is infiltration of eosinophils into hair follicles and perifollicular zones, sometimes with follicular damage. Peripheral blood eosinophilia is present in all three types of EPF. Classical EPF patients usually have eosinophilia with leukocytosis, whereas eosinophilia with lymphopenia is a feature of HIV-positive patients. Low CD4 cell counts and high IgE levels are typical of HIV-associated disease [107]. Topical glucocorticoids generally are used first for the treatment of all types of EPF. Nonsteroidal anti-inflammatory drugs, particularly indomethacin, are another first-line therapy; clinical improvement may be observed within 2 weeks and is associated with a decrease in peripheral blood eosinophil counts [108]. Antiretroviral treatment, with resultant increase in CD4 cell counts, often is associated with improvement in HIV-associated EPF, although lesions may develop during antiretroviral therapy.

Autoimmune blistering diseases

Patients with autoimmune blistering diseases often have peripheral blood eosinophilia and prominent infiltration of eosinophils. In 1968, Emmerson and Wilson-Jones [109] introduced the term eosinophilic spongiosis in their report of pemphigus patients who had skin biopsy specimens that showed infiltration of the epidermis with eosinophils and intraepidermal vesicles containing eosinophils. Among the pemphigus subtypes, eosinophilic spongiosis occurs most frequently in pemphigus vulgaris [110]. However, eosinophilic spongiosis is now considered to be a marker more often of bullous pemphigoid (BP) than pemphigus, particularly when patients present with urticarial lesions. Eosinophilic spongiosis also is a feature of other types of pemphigoid, including pemphigoid (herpes) gestationis, and has been noted in lesions of incontinentia pigmenti, acute dermatitis, arthropod bites and incidentally in other disorders. Peripheral blood eosinophilia is variable in these conditions but can be in the HES range.

BP occurs predominantly in older individuals and is characterized clinically by tense cutaneous blisters arising on pruritic, urticarial bases. Blisters also may arise on a background of macular erythema or on normal-appearing skin. Tense blisters or erosions may involve mucosa. In addition to marked peripheral blood eosinophilia, autoantibodies, predominantly IgG class, develop to basement membrane zone (BMZ) antigens. Recently, IgE BMZ antibodies have been implicated in the pathogenesis of BP [111,112].

In addition to eosinophilic spongiosis, lesions of BP show a variable inflammatory cell infiltrate that typically contains eosinophils scattered throughout the upper dermis or clustered at the edge of dermal–epidermal separation. Eosinophils often are present in the blister space, and eosinophil degranulation is massive, with extensive tissue deposition of MBP [113]. Blister fluid contains both MBP and ECP. Deposition of eosinophil granule MBP is associated with blister formation in a related disease, pemphigoid gestationis [114], in the genodermatosis incontinentia pigmenti [115], in blisters of Churg-Strauss syndrome [57] and in bullous morphea [116]. Adhesion molecule expression in lesional tissue, as well as IL-3 and IL-5 in blister fluid, likely contribute to eosinophil activation in pemphigoid [113]. Eosinophils elaborate the 92-kd gelatinase matrix metalloproteinase 9 [117], which probably contributes to dermal–epidermal separation in BP; it is produced by eosinophils at the site of blister formation and has been shown to cleave the extracellular domain of the recombinant 180-kd BP autoantigen, a transmembrane component of the basement membrane zone [117]. There are reports of patients with T cell lymphoma who develop BP, particularly following UV light (UVL) treatments [118]. UVL may induce damage that exposes basement membrane zone antigens and (in conjunction with clonal T cells that generate T helper 2 cytokines IL-4 and IL-5) production of BMZ antibodies ensues. T cell activity in general may be a cofactor with UVL, because pemphigoid has long been associated with psoriasis and UVL treatment [119,120] and also has been reported in UVL-treated morphea [121].

Clinical reaction patterns with eosinophils

There are a variety of cutaneous diseases, with or without associated peripheral blood eosinophilia, in which eosinophil infiltration may be a histologic feature, but either the pattern is unremarkable or eosinophils are not critical for the histologic diagnosis. In many of these dermatoses, eosinophils lose their morphologic integrity after cytolytic disruption and are not identifiable histologically. However, toxic granule proteins and other eosinophil products are deposited in skin and persist for extended periods [23].

Although parasitic infestations typically are associated with eosinophils, the histologic pattern is not diagnostic unless a specific organism is identified in tissue sections [5,122]. Infection with *Onchocerca volvulus* causes pruritic dermatitis with lichenification; there is slight infiltration of eosinophils but extensive extracellular deposition of granule proteins throughout the dermis of lesions [123]; after treatment, extracellular granule proteins are located around degenerating microfilariae [5,124]. Although eosinophils are rarely a prominent histologic feature of atopic dermatitis, extensive extracellular dermal deposition of granule proteins is observed in lesions (Fig. 6); even normal-appearing skin may show scant MBP deposition [123,125–127]. Prurigo nodularis [128,129] and pachydermatous eosinophilic dermatitis [130] exhibit a pattern of dermal extracellular granule protein deposition similar to that seen in atopic dermatitis and onchocercal dermatitis. In both atopic dermatitis and prurigo nodularis, eosinophil granule products are deposited around cutaneous nerves and, although the eosinophil is not recognized as an inducer of itch, there is evidence that eosinophils play a role in itch provocation [131–134].

In addition to pemphigoid gestationis, several other pruritic dermatoses of pregnancy may exhibit tissue eosinophils and peripheral blood eosinophilia [97,135,136]. Polymorphic eruption of pregnancy [137], previously called pruritic urticarial papules and plaques of pregnancy [138], presents in the third trimester with erythematous urticarial lesions involving the abdomen, thighs, buttocks, and upper limbs. Papular dermatitis of pregnancy [139] is an eruption of generalized extremely pruritic wheal-like papules, and autoimmune progesterone dermatitis [140], presents early in pregnancy as follicular and perifollicular papules and pustules predominantly involving the extremities, with the histologic finding of numerous eosinophils (with eosinophil abscesses) in follicles, epidermis, dermis and subcutaneous fat.

Eosinophil granule proteins are toxic to many cell types including endothelial cells, which implicates them in the development of vasculitis, including Churg-Strauss syndrome [57,141,142]. Eosinophils often are

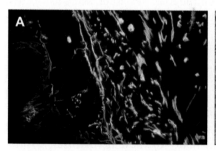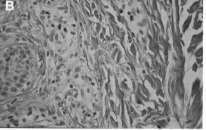

Fig. 6. Atopic dermatitis. (*A*) Skin biopsy section stained for eosinophil granule MBP shows extensive extracellular deposition in the dermis with cellular staining of only three eosinophils (original magnification ×400). (*B*) Hematoxylin-eosin counterstain of the A section shows chronic inflammation (original magnification ×400). (*From* Leiferman KM, Ackerman SJ, Sampson HA, et al. Dermal deposition of eosinophil-granule major basic protein in atopic dermatitis. Comparison with onchocerciasis. N Engl J Med 1985;313:283; with permission. Copyright ©1985 Massachusetts Medical Society. All rights reserved.)

associated with cutaneous allergic drug reactions and urticarial vasculitis. When eosinophils are part of the histologic pattern in leukocytoclastic vasculitis, the eruption is probably drug-induced [143]. Associated with peripheral blood eosinophilia, eosinophilic vasculitis is characterized by widespread chronic, recurrent, pruritic, erythematous, purpuric papules as well as angioedema of the face and hands; the histologic pattern consists of necrotizing small vessel vasculitis with prominent infiltration of eosinophils [141]. Eosinophilic vasculitis may be idiopathic or associated with connective tissue disease [142], Raynaud's phenomenon, or HES [33].

Management

Management is guided by the diagnosis of HES and/or associated diseases. General diagnostic criteria for HES are reviewed by Sheikh and Weller elsewhere in this issue. Obtaining skin biopsies is important, including specimens for histologic evaluation, direct immunofluorescence (DIF) testing, and immunophenotyping. In addition to routine hematoxylin-eosin–stained sections, special stains may be useful. Immunobullous disease, presenting with or without blisters, can be diagnosed by DIF. Immunostains for MBP or other granule proteins can help establish eosinophil involvement when few or no infiltrating eosinophils are present. Giemsa, toluidine blue, and/or tryptase stains will identify mast cells. Immunophenotyping of lymphocytes in cutaneous tissue sections may aid the diagnosis of lymphocytic HES. To detect T cell or B cell clones, skin biopsy tissue also can be subjected to lymphocytoflow and evaluated for T cell receptor and light chain gene rearrangements.

The treatment goal for patients with HES is relief of symptoms and improvement in organ function, while keeping peripheral blood eosinophils at 1000–2000/μL and minimizing side effects [3]. Symptomatic relief is especially important for patients who present with debilitating skin involvement. Moreover, cutaneous lesions and symptoms may reflect underlying disease activity in HES. Therefore, monitoring response of the skin to treatment may be helpful in judging systemic therapeutic efficacy. Myeloproliferative HES is very responsive to imatinib, which usually induces hematologic remission. In the absence of the FIP1L1-PDGFRα genetic mutation, and after *Strongyloides* infection has been excluded [144], first-line therapy is systemic glucocorticoids. Approximately 70% of patients will respond to prednisone, with peripheral eosinophil counts returning to normal. Patients who fail glucocorticoid monotherapy generally have a worse prognosis; in such cases, or when long-term side effects become problematic, other treatments should be used. Patients with features of myeloproliferative HES, but who are FIP1L1-PDGFRα–negative, still may respond to imatinib [41]. Interferon-α has been beneficial in both myeloid and lymphocytic HES types [145]. Other treatment options include: hydroxyurea, dapsone, vincristine sulfate, cyclophosphamide, methotrexate, 6-thioguanine, 2-chlorodeoxyadenosine and cytarabine in combination, pulsed chlorambucil, etoposide, cyclosporine, intravenous immunoglobulin, alemtuzumab, and psoralen ultraviolet A phototherapy [146], extracorporeal photochemotherapy alone or in combination with interferon-α or other therapies, as well as bone marrow and peripheral blood stem cell allogeneic transplantation [147,148]. Two monoclonal antibodies against human IL-5 have been associated with clinical improvement, including decrease in cutaneous symptoms, and reductions in peripheral blood and dermal eosinophils, particularly in patients with lymphocytic HES [46].

Summary

Eosinophils have many biologic effects in skin and other tissues, most of which appear to be deleterious. Eosinophils are not resident cells of the skin and, therefore, when present, are implicated in cutaneous disease. Their involvement may be difficult to recognize because they degranulate and lose morphologic integrity. Cutaneous lesions associated with eosinophil activities particularly include those characterized by edema, eczema, mucosal ulcers, vasculitis, blisters, and fibrosis. All these eosinophil-associated cutaneous lesions are found in HES. Dermatologic disease involving skin and mucous membranes is an important component of all HES variants and may be the presenting signs of HES. Mucosal ulcers and edema are extremely debilitating and may be difficult to treat. Splinter hemorrhages and/or nail fold infarcts may be initial clues to potentially life-threatening thromboembolic disease. In addition to HES, several skin diseases and inflammatory reaction patterns have prominent eosinophil involvement. Many of these are not typically considered in the context of HES, and the diagnosis may be delayed because eosinophil counts are not determined and followed. Recognition of eosinophil participation in cutaneous and extracutaneous diseases is critical, because eosinophilic endomyocardial disease, which can develop in any eosinophil-associated disorder, may have grave consequences.

References

[1] Kazmierowski JA, Chusid MJ, Parrillo JE, et al. Dermatologic manifestations of the hypereosinophilic syndrome. Arch Dermatol 1978;114(4):531–5.
[2] van den Hoogenband HM. Skin lesions as the first manifestation of the hypereosinophilic syndrome. Clin Exp Dermatol 1982;7(3):267–71.
[3] Klion AD, Bochner BS, Gleich GJ, et al. Approaches to the treatment of hypereosinophilic syndromes: a workshop summary report. J Allergy Clin Immunol 2006;117(6):1292–302.
[4] Kato M, Kephart GM, Talley NJ, et al. Eosinophil infiltration and degranulation in normal human tissue. Anat Rec 1998;252(3):418–25.
[5] Ackerman SJ, Kephart GM, Francis H, et al. Eosinophil degranulation. An immunologic determinant in the pathogenesis of the Mazzotti reaction in human onchocerciasis. J Immunol 1990;144(10):3961–9.

[6] Peters MS, Schroeter AL, Kephart GM, et al. Localization of eosinophil granule major basic protein in chronic urticaria. J Invest Dermatol 1983;81(1):39–43.

[7] Kita H, Adolphson CR, Gleich GJ. Biology of eosinophils. In: Adkinson NF, Yunginger JW, Busse WW, editors. Middleton's allergy principles and practice. 6th edition. Philadelphia: Mosby; 2003. p. 305–32.

[8] Rothenberg ME, Hogan SP. The eosinophil. Annu Rev Immunol 2006;24:147–74.

[9] Dulkys Y, Schramm G, Kimmig D, et al. Detection of mRNA for eotaxin-2 and eotaxin-3 in human dermal fibroblasts and their distinct activation profile on human eosinophils. J Invest Dermatol 2001;116(4):498–505.

[10] Petering H, Kluthe C, Dulkys Y, et al. Characterization of the CC chemokine receptor 3 on human keratinocytes. J Invest Dermatol 2001;116(4):549–55.

[11] Cheng JF, Ott NL, Peterson EA, et al. Dermal eosinophils in atopic dermatitis undergo cytolytic degeneration. J Allergy Clin Immunol 1997;99(5):683–92.

[12] Gleich GJ, Schroeter AL, Marcoux JP, et al. Episodic angioedema associated with eosinophilia. N Engl J Med 1984;310(25):1621–6.

[13] Leiferman KM, Fujisawa T, Gray BH, et al. Extracellular deposition of eosinophil and neutrophil granule proteins in the IgE-mediated cutaneous late phase reaction. Lab Invest 1990;62(5):579–89.

[14] Dvorak AM, Weller PF, Monahan-Earley RA, et al. Ultrastructural localization of Charcot-Leyden crystal protein (lysophospholipase) and peroxidase in macrophages, eosinophils, and extracellular matrix of the skin in the hypereosinophilic syndrome. Lab Invest 1990;62(5):590–607.

[15] Minnicozzi M, Duran WN, Gleich GJ, et al. Eosinophil granule proteins increase microvascular macromolecular transport in the hamster cheek pouch. J Immunol 1994;153(6):2664–70.

[16] Minnicozzi M, Gleich GJ, Duran WN, et al. Increased microvascular permeability induced by eosinophil proteins. Int Arch Allergy Immunol 1995;107(1–3):348.

[17] Minnicozzi M, Ramirez MM, Egan RW, et al. Polyarginine and eosinophil-derived major basic protein increase microvascular permeability independently of histamine or nitric oxide release. Microvasc Res 1995;50(1):56–70.

[18] Gleich GJ, Loegering DA, Mann KG, et al. Comparative properties of the Charcot-Leyden crystal protein and the major basic protein from human eosinophils. J Clin Invest 1976;57(3):633–40.

[19] Leiferman KM, Loegering DA, Gleich GJ. Production of wheal-and-flare skin reactions by eosinophil granule proteins. J Invest Dermatol 1984;82:414.

[20] Patella V, de Crescenzo G, Marino I, et al. Eosinophil granule proteins activate human heart mast cells. J Immunol 1996;157(3):1219–25.

[21] Okayama Y, el-Lati SG, Leiferman KM, et al. Eosinophil granule proteins inhibit substance P-induced histamine release from human skin mast cells. J Allergy Clin Immunol 1994;93(5):900–9.

[22] Piliponsky AM, Gleich GJ, Nagler A, et al. Non-IgE-dependent activation of human lung- and cord blood-derived mast cells is induced by eosinophil major basic protein and modulated by the membrane form of stem cell factor. Blood 2003;101(5):1898–904.

[23] Davis MD, Plager DA, George TJ, et al. Interactions of eosinophil granule proteins with skin: limits of detection, persistence, and vasopermeabilization. J Allergy Clin Immunol 2003;112(5):988–94.

[24] Leiferman KM, Peters MS, Gleich GJ. The eosinophil and cutaneous edema. J Am Acad Dermatol 1986;15(3):513–7.

[25] Peters MS, Winkelmann RK, Greaves MW, et al. Extracellular deposition of eosinophil granule major basic protein in pressure urticaria. J Am Acad Dermatol 1987;16(3 Pt 1):513–7.

[26] McEvoy MT, Peterson EA, Kobza-Black A, et al. Immunohistological comparison of granulated cell proteins in induced immediate urticarial dermographism and delayed pressure urticaria lesions. Br J Dermatol 1995;133(6):853–60.

[27] Songsiridej V, Peters MS, Dor PJ, et al. Facial edema and eosinophilia. Evidence for eosinophil degranulation. Ann Intern Med 1985;103(4):503–6.

[28] van Haelst Pisani C, Kovach JS, Kita H, et al. Administration of interleukin-2 (IL-2) results
in increased plasma concentrations of IL-5 and eosinophilia in patients with cancer. Blood
1991;78(6):1538–44.

[29] Mehregan DR, Fransway AF, Edmonson JH, et al. Cutaneous reactions to granulocyte-
monocyte colony-stimulating factor. Arch Dermatol 1992;128(8):1055–9.

[30] Miljkovic J, Bartenjev I. Hypereosinophilic dermatitis-like erythema annulare centrifugum
in a patient with chronic lymphocytic leukaemia. J Eur Acad Dermatol Venereol 2005;
19(2):228–31.

[31] Calux MJ, Valente NY, Pires MC, et al. [Hypereosinophilic syndrome. Cutaneous picture
of "erythema annulare centrifugum"—comparison with ultrastructural study]. Med Cutan
Ibero Lat Am 1988;16(4):299–304.

[32] Shelley WB, Shelley ED. Erythema annulare centrifugum as the presenting sign of the
hypereosinophilic syndrome: observations on therapy. Cutis 1985;35(1):53–5.

[33] Jang KA, Lim YS, Choi JH, et al. Hypereosinophilic syndrome presenting as cutaneous
necrotizing eosinophilic vasculitis and Raynaud's phenomenon complicated by digital
gangrene. Br J Dermatol 2000;143(3):641–4.

[34] Ohtani T, Okamoto K, Kaminaka C, et al. Digital gangrene associated with idiopathic
hypereosinophilia: treatment with allogeneic cultured dermal substitute (CDS). Eur J Dermatol 2004;14(3):168–71.

[35] Tsuji Y, Kawashima T, Yokota K, et al. Wells' syndrome as a manifestation of hypereosinophilic syndrome. Br J Dermatol 2002;147(4):811–2.

[36] Bogenrieder T, Griese DP, Schiffner R, et al. Wells' syndrome associated with idiopathic
hypereosinophilic syndrome. Br J Dermatol 1997;137(6):978–82.

[37] Fauci AS, Harley JB, Roberts WC, et al. NIH conference. The idiopathic hypereosinophilic
syndrome. Clinical, pathophysiologic, and therapeutic considerations. Ann Intern Med
1982;97(1):78–92.

[38] Leiferman KM, Gleich GJ. Hypereosinophilic syndrome: case presentation and update.
J Allergy Clin Immunol 2004;113(1):50–8.

[39] Leiferman KM, O'Duffy JD, Perry HO, et al. Recurrent incapacitating mucosal ulcerations. A prodrome of the hypereosinophilic syndrome. JAMA 1982;247(7):1018–20.

[40] Gleich GJ, Leiferman KM, Pardanani A, et al. Treatment of hypereosinophilic syndrome
with imatinib mesilate. Lancet 2002;359(9317):1577–8.

[41] Cools J, DeAngelo DJ, Gotlib J, et al. A tyrosine kinase created by fusion of the PDGFRA
and FIP1L1 genes as a therapeutic target of imatinib in idiopathic hypereosinophilic syndrome. N Engl J Med 2003;348(13):1201–14.

[42] Griffin JH, Leung J, Bruner RJ, et al. Discovery of a fusion kinase in EOL-1 cells and
idiopathic hypereosinophilic syndrome. Proc Natl Acad Sci U S A 2003;100(13):7830–5.

[43] Klion AD, Noel P, Akin C, et al. Elevated serum tryptase levels identify a subset of patients with a myeloproliferative variant of idiopathic hypereosinophilic syndrome associated with tissue fibrosis, poor prognosis, and imatinib responsiveness. Blood 2003;
101(12):4660–6.

[44] Simon HU, Plotz SG, Dummer R, et al. Abnormal clones of T cells producing interleukin-5
in idiopathic eosinophilia. N Engl J Med 1999;341(15):1112–20.

[45] Roufosse F, Cogan E, Goldman M. Recent advances in pathogenesis and management of
hypereosinophilic syndromes. Allergy 2004;59(7):673–89.

[46] Plotz SG, Simon HU, Darsow U, et al. Use of an anti-interleukin-5 antibody in the
hypereosinophilic syndrome with eosinophilic dermatitis. N Engl J Med 2003;349(24):
2334–9.

[47] Hill DJ, Ekert H, Bryant DH. Episodic angioedema and hypereosinophilia in childhood.
J Allergy Clin Immunol 1986;78(1 Pt 1):122–3.

[48] Katzen DR, Leiferman KM, Weller PF, et al. Hypereosinophilia and recurrent angioneurotic edema in a 2 1/2-year-old girl. Am J Dis Child 1986;140(1):62–4.

[49] Butterfield JH, Leiferman KM, Abrams J, et al. Elevated serum levels of interleukin-5 in patients with the syndrome of episodic angioedema and eosinophilia. Blood 1992;79(3): 688–92.

[50] Putterman C, Barak V, Caraco Y, et al. Episodic angioedema with eosinophilia: a case associated with T cell activation and cytokine production. Ann Allergy 1993;70(3):243–8.

[51] Morgan SJ, Prince HM, Westerman DA, et al. Clonal T-helper lymphocytes and elevated IL-5 levels in episodic angioedema and eosinophilia (Gleich's syndrome). Leuk Lymphoma 2003;44(9):1623–5.

[52] Butterfield JH. Diverse clinical outcomes of eosinophilic patients with T-cell receptor gene rearrangements: the emerging diagnostic importance of molecular genetics testing. Am J Hematol 2001;68(2):81–6.

[53] Kawano M, Muramoto H, Tsunoda S, et al. Absence of CD69 expression on peripheral eosinophils in episodic angioedema and eosinophilia. Am J Hematol 1996;53(1):43–5.

[54] Butterfield JH, Leiferman KM, Gleich GJ. Nodules, eosinophilia, rheumatism, dermatitis and swelling (NERDS): a novel eosinophilic disorder. Clin Exp Allergy 1993; 23(7):571–80.

[55] Zenarola P, Melillo L, Bisceglia M, et al. NERDS syndrome: an additional case report. Dermatology 1995;191(2):133–8.

[56] Churg J, Strauss L. Allergic granulomatosis, allergic angiitis, and periarteritis nodosa. Am J Pathol 1951;27(2):277–301.

[57] Drage LA, Davis MD, De Castro F, et al. Evidence for pathogenic involvementof eosinophils and neutrophilsin Churg-Strauss syndrome. J Am Acad Dermatol 2002;47(2): 209–16.

[58] Keogh KA, Specks U. Churg-Strauss syndrome. Semin Respir Crit Care Med 2006;27(2): 148–57.

[59] Hertzman PA, Blevins WL, Mayer J, et al. Association of the eosinophilia-myalgia syndrome with the ingestion of tryptophan. N Engl J Med 1990;322(13):869–73.

[60] Martin RW, Duffy J, Engel AG, et al. The clinical spectrum of the eosinophilia-myalgia syndrome associated with L-tryptophan ingestion. Clinical features in 20 patients and aspects of pathophysiology. Ann Intern Med 1990;113(2):124–34.

[61] Uitto J, Varga J, Peltonen J, et al. Eosinophilia-myalgia syndrome. Int J Dermatol 1992; 31(4):223–8.

[62] Martin LB, Kita H, Leiferman KM, et al. Eosinophils in allergy: role in disease, degranulation, and cytokines. Int Arch Allergy Immunol 1996;109(3):207–15.

[63] Belongia EA, Hedberg CW, Gleich GJ, et al. An investigation of the cause of the eosinophilia-myalgia syndrome associated with tryptophan use. N Engl J Med 1990;323(6): 357–65.

[64] Mayeno AN, Belongia EA, Lin F, et al. 3-(Phenylamino)alanine, a novel aniline-derived amino acid associated with the eosinophilia-myalgia syndrome: a link to the toxic oil syndrome? Mayo Clin Proc 1992;67(12):1134–9.

[65] Belongia EA, Mayeno AN, Osterholm MT. The eosinophilia-myalgia syndrome and tryptophan. Annu Rev Nutr 1992;12:235–56.

[66] Diggle GE. The toxic oil syndrome: 20 years on. Int J Clin Pract 2001;55(6):371–5.

[67] Ten RM, Kephart GM, Posada M, et al. Participation of eosinophils in the toxic oil syndrome. Clin Exp Immunol 1990;82(2):313–7.

[68] Noguchi H, Kephart GM, Colby TV, et al. Tissue eosinophilia and eosinophil degranulation in syndromes associated with fibrosis. Am J Pathol 1992;140(2):521–8.

[69] Antic M, Lautenschlager S, Itin PH. Eosinophilic fasciitis 30 years after–what do we really know? Report of 11 patients and review of the literature. Dermatology 2006;213(2): 93–101.

[70] Pegorier S, Wagner LA, Gleich GJ, et al. Eosinophil-derived cationic proteins activate the synthesis of remodeling factors by airway epithelial cells. J Immunol 2006;177(7): 4861–9.

[71] Leiferman KM, Peters MS, Gleich GJ. Eosinophils in cutaneous diseases. In: Freedberg IM, Eisen AZ, Wolff K, editors. Fitzpatrick's dermatology in general medicine, vol 1. 6th Edition. New York: McGraw-Hill, Inc.; 2003. p. 959–66.

[72] Gilliam AE, Bruckner AL, Howard RM, et al. Bullous "cellulitis" with eosinophilia: case report and review of Wells' syndrome in childhood. Pediatrics 2005;116(1): e149–55.

[73] Moossavi M, Mehregan DR. Wells' syndrome: a clinical and histopathologic review of seven cases. Int J Dermatol 2003;42(1):62–7.

[74] Spigel GT, Winkelmann RK. Wells' syndrome. Recurrent granulomatous dermatitis with eosinophilia. Arch Dermatol 1979;115(5):611–3.

[75] Wells GC. Recurrent granulomatous dermatitis with eosinophilia. Trans St Johns Hosp Dermatol Soc 1971;57:46–56.

[76] Wells GC, Smith NP. Eosinophilic cellulitis. Br J Dermatol 1979;100(1):101–9.

[77] Schuttelaar ML, Jonkman MF. Bullous eosinophilic cellulitis (Wells' syndrome) associated with Churg-Strauss syndrome. J Eur Acad Dermatol Venereol 2003;17(1):91–3.

[78] Schorr WF, Tauscheck AL, Dickson KB, et al. Eosinophilic cellulitis (Wells' syndrome): histologic and clinical features in arthropod bite reactions. J Am Acad Dermatol 1984; 11(6):1043–9.

[79] Aberer W, Konrad K, Wolff K. Wells' syndrome is a distinctive disease entity and not a histologic diagnosis. J Am Acad Dermatol 1988;18(1 Pt 1):105–14.

[80] Peters MS, Schroeter AL, Gleich GJ. Immunofluorescence identification of eosinophil granule major basic protein in the flame figures of Wells' syndrome. Br J Dermatol 1983; 109(2):141–8.

[81] Brehmer-Andersson E, Kaaman T, Skog E, et al. The histopathogenesis of the flame figure in Wells' syndrome based on five cases. Acta Derm Venereol 1986;66(3):213–9.

[82] Davis MD, Brown AC, Blackston RD, et al. Familial eosinophilic cellulitis, dysmorphic habitus, and mental retardation. J Am Acad Dermatol 1998;38(6 Pt 1):919–28.

[83] Espana A, Sanz ML, Sola J, et al. Wells' syndrome (eosinophilic cellulitis): correlation between clinical activity, eosinophil levels, eosinophil cation protein and interleukin-5. Br J Dermatol 1999;140(1):127–30.

[84] Leiferman KM, Peters MS. Reflections on eosinophils and flame figures: where there's smoke, there's not necessarily Wells' syndrome. Arch Dermatol 2006;142(9):1215–8.

[85] Melski JW. Wells' syndrome, insect bites, and eosinophils. Dermatol Clin 1990;8(2): 287–93.

[86] Van den Hoogenband HM. Eosinophilic cellulitis as a result of onchocerciasis. Clin Exp Dermatol 1983;8:405–8.

[87] Hunt SJ, Santa Cruz DJ. Eosinophilic cellulitis: histologic features in a cutaneous mastocytoma. Dermatologica 1991;182(2):132–4.

[88] Hirsch K, Ludwig RJ, Wolter M, et al. Eosinophilic cellulitis (Wells' syndrome) associated with colon carcinoma. J Dtsch Dermatol Ges 2005;3(7):530–1.

[89] Nguyen NQ, Ma L. Eosinophilic cellulitis and dermographism. Dermatol Online J 2005; 11(4):7.

[90] Ludwig RJ, Grundmann-Kollmann M, Holtmeier W, et al. Herpes simplex virus type 2-associated eosinophilic cellulitis (Wells' syndrome). J Am Acad Dermatol 2003;48 (5 Suppl):S60–1.

[91] Beer TW, Langtry JA, Phillips WG, et al. Flame figures in bullous pemphigoid. Dermatology 1994;188(4):310–2.

[92] Rossini MS, de Souza EM, Cintra ML, et al. Cutaneous adverse reaction to 2-chlorodeoxyadenosine with histological flame figures in patients with chronic lymphocytic leukaemia. J Eur Acad Dermatol Venereol 2004;18(5):538–42.

[93] Winfield H, Lain E, Horn T, et al. Eosinophilic cellulitislike reaction to subcutaneous etanercept injection. Arch Dermatol 2006;142(2):218–20.

[94] Kimura T, Yoshimura S, Ishikawa E. Unusual granulation combined with hyperplastic changes in lymphatic tissue. Transactions of the Japanese Society of Pathology 1948;13: 179–80.

[95] Kung IT, Gibson JB, Bannatyne PM. Kimura's disease: a clinico-pathological study of 21 cases and its distinction from angiolymphoid hyperplasia with eosinophilia. Pathology 1984;16(1):39–44.

[96] Wang TF, Liu SH, Kao CH, et al. Kimura's disease with generalized lymphadenopathy demonstrated by positron emission tomography scan. Intern Med 2006;45(12):775–8.

[97] Connelly A, Powell HR, Chan YF, et al. Vincristine treatment of nephrotic syndrome complicated by Kimura disease. Pediatr Nephrol 2005;20(4):516–8.

[98] Wells GC, Whimster IW. Subcutaneous angiolymphoid hyperplasia with eosinophilia. Br J Dermatol 1969;81(1):1–14.

[99] Helander SD, Peters MS, Kuo TT, et al. Kimura's disease and angiolymphoid hyperplasia with eosinophilia: new observations from immunohistochemical studies of lymphocyte markers, endothelial antigens, and granulocyte proteins. J Cutan Pathol 1995;22(4): 319–26.

[100] Olsen TG, Helwig EB. Angiolymphoid hyperplasia with eosinophilia. A clinicopathologic study of 116 patients. J Am Acad Dermatol 1985;12(5 Pt 1):781–96.

[101] Chong WS, Thomas A, Goh CL. Kimura's disease and angiolymphoid hyperplasia with eosinophilia: two disease entities in the same patient: case report and review of the literature. Int J Dermatol 2006;45(2):139–45.

[102] Nervi SJ, Schwartz RA, Dmochowski M. Eosinophilic pustular folliculitis: a 40 year retrospect. J Am Acad Dermatol 2006;55(2):285–9.

[103] Takematsu H, Nakamura K, Igarashi M, et al. Eosinophilic pustular folliculitis. Report of two cases with a review of the Japanese literature. Arch Dermatol 1985;121(7):917–20.

[104] Soeprono FF, Schinella RA. Eosinophilic pustular folliculitis in patients with acquired immunodeficiency syndrome. Report of three cases. J Am Acad Dermatol 1986;14(6): 1020–2.

[105] Rajendran PM, Dolev JC, Heaphy MR Jr, et al. Eosinophilic folliculitis: before and after the introduction of antiretroviral therapy. Arch Dermatol 2005;141(10):1227–31.

[106] Laing ME, Laing TA, Mulligan NJ, et al. Eosinophilic pustular folliculitis induced by chemotherapy. J Am Acad Dermatol 2006;54(4):729–30.

[107] Rosenthal D, LeBoit PE, Klumpp L, et al. Human immunodeficiency virus-associated eosinophilic folliculitis. A unique dermatosis associated with advanced human immunodeficiency virus infection. Arch Dermatol 1991;127(2):206–9.

[108] Ota T, Hata Y, Tanikawa A, et al. Eosinophilic pustular folliculitis (Ofuji's disease): indomethacin as a first choice of treatment. Clin Exp Dermatol 2001;26(2):179–81.

[109] Emmerson RW, Wilson-Jones E. Eosinophilic spongiosis in pemphigus. A report of an unusual hitological change in pemphigus. Arch Dermatol 1968;97(3):252–7.

[110] Crotty C, Pittelkow M, Muller SA. Eosinophilic spongiosis: a clinicopathologic review of seventy-one cases. J Am Acad Dermatol 1983;8(3):337–43.

[111] Dimson OG, Giudice GJ, Fu CL, et al. Identification of a potential effector function for IgE autoantibodies in the organ-specific autoimmune disease bullous pemphigoid. J Invest Dermatol 2003;120(5):784–8.

[112] Fairley JA, Fu CL, Giudice GJ. Mapping the binding sites of anti-BP180 immunoglobulin E autoantibodies in bullous pemphigoid. J Invest Dermatol 2005;125(3):467–72.

[113] Borrego L, Maynard B, Peterson EA, et al. Deposition of eosinophil granule proteins precedes blister formation in bullous pemphigoid. Comparison with neutrophil and mast cell granule proteins. Am J Pathol 1996;148(3):897–909.

[114] Scheman AJ, Hordinsky MD, Groth DW, et al. Evidence for eosinophil degranulation in the pathogenesis of herpes gestationis. Arch Dermatol 1989;125(8):1079–83.

[115] Thyresson NH, Goldberg NC, Tye MJ, et al. Localization of eosinophil granule major basic protein in incontinentia pigmenti. Pediatr Dermatol 1991;8(2):102–6.

[116] Daoud MS, Su WP, Leiferman KM, et al. Bullous morphea: clinical, pathologic, and immunopathologic evaluation of thirteen cases. J Am Acad Dermatol 1994;30(6):937–43.

[117] Stahle-Backdahl M, Inoue M, Guidice GJ, et al. 92-kD gelatinase is produced by eosinophils at the site of blister formation in bullous pemphigoid and cleaves the extracellular domain of recombinant 180-kD bullous pemphigoid autoantigen. J Clin Invest 1994; 93(5):2022–30.

[118] Patterson JW, Ali M, Murray JC, et al. Bullous pemphigoid. Occurrence in a patient with mycosis fungoides receiving PUVA and topical nitrogen mustard therapy. Int J Dermatol 1985;24(3):173–6.

[119] Koerber WA Jr, Price NM, Watson W. Coexistent psoriasis and bullous pemphigoid: a report of six cases. Arch Dermatol 1978;114(11):1643–6.

[120] Wilczek A, Sticherling M. Concomitant psoriasis and bullous pemphigoid: coincidence or pathogenic relationship? Int J Dermatol 2006;45(11):1353–7.

[121] Sacher C, Konig C, Scharffetter-Kochanek K, et al. Bullous pemphigoid in a patient treated with UVA-1 phototherapy for disseminated morphea. Dermatology 2001;202(1):54–7.

[122] Kephart GM, Andrade ZA, Gleich GJ. Localization of eosinophil major basic protein onto eggs of Schistosoma mansoni in human pathologic tissue. Am J Pathol 1988;133(2): 389–96.

[123] Leiferman KM, Ackerman SJ, Sampson HA, et al. Dermal deposition of eosinophil-granule major basic protein in atopic dermatitis. Comparison with onchocerciasis. N Engl J Med 1985;313(5):282–5.

[124] Kephart GM, Gleich GJ, Connor DH, et al. Deposition of eosinophil granule major basic protein onto microfilariae of Onchocerca volvulus in the skin of patients treated with diethylcarbamazine. Lab Invest 1984;50(1):51–61.

[125] Leiferman KM. Eosinophils in atopic dermatitis. Allergy 1989;44(Suppl 9):20–6.

[126] Leiferman KM. Eosinophils in atopic dermatitis. J Allergy Clin Immunol 1994;94(6 Pt 2): 1310–7.

[127] Leiferman KM. A role for eosinophils in atopic dermatitis. J Am Acad Dermatol 2001;45 (1 Suppl):S21–4.

[128] Perez GL, Peters MS, Reda AM, et al. Mast cells, neutrophils, and eosinophils in prurigo nodularis. Arch Dermatol 1993;129(7):861–5.

[129] Johansson O, Liang Y, Marcusson JA, et al. Eosinophil cationic protein- and eosinophil-derived neurotoxin/eosinophil protein X-immunoreactive eosinophils in prurigo nodularis. Arch Dermatol Res 2000;292(8):371–8.

[130] Jacyk WK, Simson IW, Slater DN, et al. Pachydermatous eosinophilic dermatitis. Br J Dermatol 1996;134(3):469–74.

[131] Chan LS, Robinson N, Xu L. Expression of interleukin-4 in the epidermis of transgenic mice results in a pruritic inflammatory skin disease: an experimental animal model to study atopic dermatitis. J Invest Dermatol 2001;117(4):977–83.

[132] Fang D, Elly C, Gao B, et al. Dysregulation of T lymphocyte function in itchy mice: a role for Itch in TH2 differentiation. Nat Immunol 2002;3(3):281–7.

[133] Tsukuba T, Okamoto K, Okamoto Y, et al. Association of cathepsin E deficiency with development of atopic dermatitis. J Biochem (Tokyo) 2003;134(6):893–902.

[134] Yagi R, Nagai H, Iigo Y, et al. Development of atopic dermatitis-like skin lesions in STAT6-deficient NC/Nga mice. J Immunol 2002;168(4):2020–7.

[135] Sasseville D, Wilkinson RD, Schnader JY. Dermatoses of pregnancy. Int J Dermatol 1981; 20(4):223–41.

[136] Ambros-Rudolph CM, Mullegger RR, Vaughan-Jones SA, et al. The specific dermatoses of pregnancy revisited and reclassified: results of a retrospective two-center study on 505 pregnant patients. J Am Acad Dermatol 2006;54(3):395–404.

[137] Rudolph CM, Al-Fares S, Vaughan-Jones SA, et al. Polymorphic eruption of pregnancy: clinicopathology and potential trigger factors in 181 patients. Br J Dermatol 2006;154(1): 54–60.

[138] Lawley TJ, Hertz KC, Wade TR, et al. Pruritic urticarial papules and plaques of pregnancy. JAMA 1979;241(16):1696–9.

[139] Spangler AS, Reddy W, Bardawil WA, et al. Papular dermatitis of pregnancy. A new clinical entity? JAMA 1962;181:577–81.

[140] Bierman SM. Autoimmune progesterone dermatitis of pregnancy. Arch Dermatol 1973; 107(6):896–901.

[141] Chen KR, Pittelkow MR, Su D, et al. Recurrent cutaneous necrotizing eosinophilic vasculitis. A novel eosinophil-mediated syndrome. Arch Dermatol 1994;130(9):1159–66.

[142] Chen KR, Su WP, Pittelkow MR, et al. Eosinophilic vasculitis in connective tissue disease. J Am Acad Dermatol 1996;35(2 Pt 1):173–82.

[143] Bahrami S, Malone JC, Webb KG, et al. Tissue eosinophilia as an indicator of drug-induced cutaneous small-vessel vasculitis. Arch Dermatol 2006;142(2):155–61.

[144] Scowden EB, Schaffner W, Stone WJ. Overwhelming strongyloidiasis: an unappreciated opportunistic infection. Medicine (Baltimore) 1978;57(6):527–44.

[145] Butterfield JH. Interferon treatment for hypereosinophilic syndromes and systemic mastocytosis. Acta Haematol 2005;114(1):26–40.

[146] Tefferi A. Modern diagnosis and treatment of primary eosinophilia. Acta Haematol 2005; 114(1):52–60.

[147] Halaburda K, Prejzner W, Szatkowski D, et al. Allogeneic bone marrow transplantation for hypereosinophilic syndrome: long-term follow-up with eradication of FIP1L1-PDGFRA fusion transcript. Bone Marrow Transplant 2006;38(4):319–20.

[148] Ueno NT, Anagnostopoulos A, Rondon G, et al. Successful non-myeloablative allogeneic transplantation for treatment of idiopathic hypereosinophilic syndrome. Br J Haematol 2002;119(1):131–4.

ELSEVIER
SAUNDERS

Immunol Allergy Clin N Am
27 (2007) 443–455

IMMUNOLOGY
AND ALLERGY
CLINICS
OF NORTH AMERICA

Gastrointestinal Eosinophilia

Li Zuo, MD, Marc E. Rothenberg, MD, PhD*

*Division of Allergy and Immunology, Department of Pediatrics, Cincinnati Children's Hospital
Medical Center, University of Cincinnati, College of Medicine, 3333 Burnet Avenue,
Cincinnati, OH 45229-3039, USA*

The presence of eosinophils in tissues and blood is a physiological phenomenon. Eosinophils have roles in both host defense and pathological processes, though we are still not certain about their overall function. A unique feature of eosinophils is that they largely reside in the tissues, instead of staying in the blood circulation as neutrophils do. In fact, the gastrointestinal (GI) tract is a primary site for normal eosinophil residence. Significant progress has been made in clarifying that eosinophils are integral members of the GI mucosal immune system. In physiologic states, small numbers of eosinophils are found throughout the GI tract, excepting the esophagus. Gastrointestinal eosinophilia is a broad term for any abnormal eosinophil accumulation in the GI system induced in diverse states.

In this article, the authors group GI eosinophilia into three categories: first is primary GI eosinophilia, also termed eosinophil associated gastrointestinal disorders (EGID). These diseases selectively affect the gastrointestinal tract with eosinophil-rich inflammation in the absence of known causes for eosinophilia. These disorders include eosinophilic esophagitis (EE), eosinophilic gastritis, eosinophilic gastroenteritis, eosinophilic enteritis, and eosinophilic colitis, and are being increasingly recognized. The second is GI eosinophilia resulting from hypereosinophilic syndrome (HES). The third is GI eosinophilia triggered by other known causes of eosinophilia, such as drug reactions, parasitic infections, malignancy, and so on. All three groups of GI eosinophilia are described in this article, although the focus is on primary gastrointestinal eosinophilia, or EGID (Fig. 1).

This work was supported by NIH grants AI 45898-09, NIH AI 070235-02 and T32 DK 07727-12, The Buckeye Foundation, Campaign Urging Research for Eosinophilic Diseases (CURED) Foundation, The Food Allergy Project, and The Food Allergy and Anaphylaxis Network (FAAN).

This article was adapted from: Rothenberg ME. Eosinophilic gastrointestinal disorders (EGID). J Allergy Clin Immunol 2004;113(1):11–28.

* Corresponding author.

E-mail address: rothenberg@cchmc.org (M.E. Rothenberg).

doi:10.1016/j.iac.2007.06.002

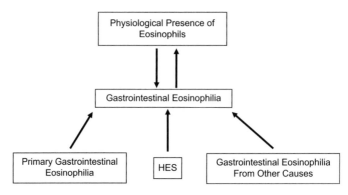

Fig. 1. Gastrointestinal eosinophilia.

Physiological presence of eosinophils in the gastrointestinal tract

Even though eosinophils have been noted to be present at low levels in numerous tissues as well as in the blood circulation, when a large series of biopsy and autopsy specimens were analyzed, the only organs that demonstrated tissue eosinophils (at substantial levels) were the GI tract, spleen, lymph nodes, and thymus [1]. Notably, eosinophil infiltrations were only associated with eosinophil degranulation in the GI tract. Examination of eosinophils throughout the GI tract of conventional healthy mice (untreated mice maintained under pathogen-free conditions) has revealed that eosinophils are normally present in the lamina propria of the stomach, small intestine, cecum, and colon [2]. Unlike intestinal lymphocytes and mast cells, eosinophils are not normally present in Peyer's patches or intraepithelial locations, although they commonly infiltrate these regions in primary GI eosinophilia [3]. Data have suggested that eosinophils respond to distinct stimuli, compared with other intestinal leukocytes [2]; constitutive expression of eotaxin-1 has also been demonstrated to provide the unique signal that promotes localization of eosinophils into the GI tract at baseline. A recent study has shown that tissue-dwelling eosinophils have distinct cytokine expression patterns under inflammatory or noninflammatory conditions, with esophageal eosinophils from eosinophilic esophagitis patients expressing relatively high levels of Th2 cytokines [4].

Function of eosinophilia in the gastrointestinal system

Despite the significant progress in histological studies of GI eosinophilia, the function of eosinophils in the GI tract is still not well understood. In general, eosinophils play both protective and pathologic roles in the GI tract. As part of their protective role, eosinophils are involved in host response against parasitic infections. As part of their involvement in eliciting tissue pathology, allergen-triggered Th2 responses, mediated by IL-5 and

IL-13 (for example) have been shown to elicit esophageal pathology, at least in the setting of experimental models in mice. These pathologic changes can induce fixed structural lesions, such as an esophageal stricture. In vitro studies have shown that eosinophil granule constituents are toxic to a variety of tissues, including intestinal epithelium [5].

Eosinophil granules contain a crystalloid core composed of major basic protein (MBP)-1 (and MBP-2), and a matrix composed of eosinophil cationic protein (ECP), eosinophil-derived neurotoxin (EDN), and eosinophil peroxidase (EPO) [6]. These cationic proteins share certain proinflammatory properties but differ in other ways. For example, MBP, EPO, and ECP have cytotoxic effects on the epithelium, in concentrations similar to those found in biological fluids from patients with eosinophilia. Additionally, ECP and EDN belong to the ribonuclease-A superfamily and possess antiviral and ribonuclease activity [7,8]. Eosinophil cationic protein can insert voltage insensitive, ion-nonselective toxic pores into the membranes of target cells and these pores may facilitate the entry of other toxic molecules [9]. MBP directly increases smooth muscle reactivity by causing dysfunction of vagal muscarinic M2 receptors [10] and also triggers degranulation of mast cells and basophils. Triggering of eosinophils by engagement of receptors for cytokines, immunoglobulins, and complement can lead to the generation of a wide range of inflammatory cytokines, including IL-1, -3, -4, -5, -13, granulocyte macrophage colony stimulating factor, transforming growth factors, tumor necrosis factor-α, regulated on activation normal T-cell expressed and secreted (RANTES), microphage inflammatory protein-1α, vascular endothelial cell growth factor, and eotaxin-1, indicating that they have the potential to modulate multiple aspects of the immune response [11]. In fact, eosinophil-derived transforming growth factor-β is linked with epithelial growth, fibrosis, and tissue remodeling [12,13]. Eosinophils express major histocompatibility complex class-II molecules, relevant costimulatory molecules (CD40, CD28, B7.1, and B7.2) and secrete an array of cytokines capable of promoting lymphocyte proliferation, activation, and Th1 or Th2 polarization (IL-2, IL-4, IL-6, IL-12, IL-10) [11,14–17].

Further eosinophil-mediated damage is caused by toxic hydrogen peroxide and halide acids generated by EPO, and by superoxide generated by the respiratory burst oxidase enzyme pathway in eosinophils. Eosinophils also generate large amounts of the leukotriene (LT) C_4, which is metabolized to LTD_4 and LTE_4. These three lipid mediators increase vascular permeability and mucus secretion, and are potent stimulators of smooth muscle contraction [18]. Clinical investigations have demonstrated extracellular deposition of MBP and ECP in the small bowel of patients with eosinophilic gastroenteritis and have shown a correlation between the level of eosinophils and disease severity. Electron microscopy studies have revealed ultrastructural changes in the secondary granules (indicative of eosinophil degranulation and mediator release) in duodenal samples from patients with eosinophilic gastroenteritis [19]. Furthermore, Charcot-Leyden crystals, remnants of eosinophil degranulation, are commonly found on microscopic examination of stools obtained from patients with eosinophilic gastroenteritis [20,21].

Evidence has also supported the association between eosinophils and the enteric nervous system, contributing to the pathogenesis of disease [22]. A recent human study showed the close association of mucosal eosinophils and their granule proteins with the myenteric ganglia [23]. In vitro study also showed the effect of eosinophils on the activation of nerves as well as on nerve remodeling, including the increase of adhesion molecules, muscarinic M2 receptors, and nerve growth factor production [24,25]. Therefore it is possible that the eosinophil-enteric nerve interaction contribute to the intestinal dysmotility that occurs in EGID.

Primary gastrointestinal eosinophilia

Patients with EGID suffer from a variety of problems, including failure to thrive, abdominal pain, irritability, gastric dysmotility, vomiting, diarrhea, and dysphagia [26]. Even though the term "primary" is used here, evidence is accumulating supporting the concept that EGID arises secondary to the interplay of genetic and environmental factors. A large percentage (approximately 10%) of patients suffering from EGID have an immediate family member with EGID [27]. Several lines of evidence support an allergic etiology, including the finding that approximately 75% of patients with EGID are atopic [21,28–34], that the severity of disease can sometimes be reversed by institution of an allergen-free diet [33–35], and the common finding of mast cell degranulation in tissue specimens [36,37]. Recent models of EGID support a potential allergic etiology for these disorders [38]. Despite the common finding of food-specific immunoglobulin E (IgE) in patients with EGID, food-induced anaphylactic responses occur in only a minority of patients [19,39]. Thus, EGID has properties that fall between pure IgE-mediated food allergy and cellular-mediated hypersensitivity disorders (eg, Celiac disease) [39].

Although the incidence of primary EGID has not been rigorously calculated, a mini-epidemic of these diseases (especially EE) has been noted over the last decade [40,41]. For example, EE is a global health disease now reported in Australia [42], Brazil [43], England [44], Italy [45], Japan [46], Spain [47,48], and Switzerland [49]. Liacouras and colleagues at Children's Hospital of Philadelphia have found that approximately 10% of their pediatric patients with gastroesophageal reflux disease (GERD)-like symptoms, who are unresponsive to acid blockade, have EE [50,51]. Fox and colleagues [40] at Boston Children's Hospital have reported that 6% of their patients with esophagitis have EE. Over a 16-year observation period, Straumann and colleagues [4] have documented a prevalence of approximately one case of EE in every 4000 adults in Switzerland. Croese and colleagues [42] have reported EE to be present in one in 70,000 adults in an Australian provincial city. Finally, the authors have noted that EE occurs in one in 2,000 children in the Cincinnati metropolitan area over a 5-year time period [27]. Collectively, these epidemiological results indicate that EGID is not an uncommon group of diseases, and may have a combined prevalence even higher than pediatric inflammatory bowel disease (IBD).

Evaluation for eosinophil associated gastrointestinal disorders

Patients with EGID present with a variety of clinical problems, most commonly failure to thrive, abdominal pain, irritability, gastric dysmotility, vomiting, diarrhea, dysphagia, microcytic anemia, and hypoproteinemia [27]. A diagnostic evaluation for EGID should be performed on all patients with these refractory problems, especially in individuals with a strong history of allergic diseases, peripheral blood eosinophilia, or a family history of EGID. Depending upon the intestinal segment involved, the frequency of specific symptoms varies (eg, abdominal pain and dysphagia are most common in eosinophilic gastroenteritis and EE, respectively), but there are no pathognomonic symptoms or blood tests for diagnosing EGID. Notably, blood eosinophil counts are normal in the majority of patients. If EGID is suspected (based on clinical presentation or evaluation of endoscopic biopsies), then additional testing should be considered to rule out the possibility that there may be another primary disease process, such as drug hypersensitivity, collagen-vascular disease, malignancy, or infection.

The evaluation for EGID starts with a comprehensive history and physical examination. Evaluation for intestinal parasites by examination of stool samples, intestinal aspirates obtained during colonoscopy, or specific blood antibody titres should be performed, especially when patients have high-risk exposure (eg, living on farms or drinking well water). For example, in one series of patients with eosinophilic enteritis, the common dog hookworm *Ancylostoma caninum* (identified by endoscopic detection) has been shown to be the cause of eosinophilic enteritis in 15% of patients [52], raising the possibility that other occult infections may be involved in the pathogenesis of other apparent cases of EGID. As a precaution, before using systemic immunosuppression for EGID, infection with *Strongyloides stercoralis* should be ruled out, because this infection can become life threatening in the setting of systemic immunosuppression [53]. The evaluation of total IgE levels has significance in stratifying patients with atopic variants of EGID or suggesting further consideration for occult parasitic infections. Skin prick testing to a panel of food and aeroallergens helps to identify sensitizations to specific allergens; indeed, patients with the atopic variant of EGID have evidence of IgE sensitization to a mean of 14 different food groups [54]. A preliminary study has suggested a value for delayed cutaneous hypersensitivity testing (skin patch testing) for specific food antigens, in further identifying allergic variants of EE [34].

The diagnosis of EGID is dependent upon the microscopic evaluation of endoscopic biopsy samples, with careful attention to the quantity, location, and characteristics of the eosinophilic inflammation. Patients with EGID often present with a clear history and positive biopsy results for the disease but have a variety of endoscopic findings [55]. It is not uncommon for endoscopic appearances of the gastrointestinal tract to look normal; thus, microscopic evaluation of biopsy samples is essential. Furthermore, the disease often has patchy involvement, necessitating the analysis of multiple endoscopic biopsies from each intestinal segment [56]. Because no widely accepted diagnostic criteria has been established for EGID, the diagnosis is dependent upon the expertise of the physicians involved in the evaluation of the biopsy samples. While the normal esophagus is devoid of eosinophils, the rest of the gastrointestinal tract contains readily detectable eosinophils [57]. Thus, differentiation of EGID from the normal condition relies on several factors including: (1) eosinophil quantification (and comparisons to normal values at each medical center); (2) the location of eosinophils (eg, their presence in abnormal positions such as the intraepithelial and intestinal crypt regions); (3) associated pathological abnormalities (eg, epithelial hyperplasia as in the case of EE); and (4) the absence of pathological features suggestive of other primary disorders (eg, neutrophilia associated with IBD, or vasculitis associated with Churg-Strauss syndrome). Based on these criteria, patients often suffer from symptoms for an extended period of time (mean of 4 years) before a bona fide diagnosis of EGID is established [58].

Eosinophilic esophagitis

Among all primary gastrointestinal eosinophilic diseases, EE is unique primarily because the esophagus in a healthy individual is completely devoid of eosinophils, unlike other parts of the GI tract [59]. Therefore, any eosinophils in the esophagus may indicate a disease process. In general, esophageal eosinophil numbers in EE are much higher than in GERD. The diagnosis of EE is usually defined as a positive esophageal biopsy showing more than 15 eosinophils per high-power field (HPF). In most cases, esophageal eosinophil numbers in GERD are under seven, and the concurrence of GERD and allergy may have 7 to 20 eosinophils/HPF. However, a recent study by Ngo and colleagues [60] reported three GERD patients with esophageal eosinophil numbers between 21/HPF and 52/HPF who were successfully treated with a proton pump inhibitor. The key difference between EE and GERD is not the absolute numbers of eosinophils in the esophagus; instead, EE patients will have persistent esophageal eosinophilia, even with proton pump inhibitor treatment.

Treatment of eosinophil associated gastrointestinal disorders

Principles of treatment for EE and eosinophilic gastroenteritis are similar. Eliminating the dietary intake of the foods implicated by skin prick or radioallergosorbent (RAST) testing has variable effects, but complete resolution is generally achieved with an amino acid-based elemental diet [61,62]. Once disease remission has been obtained by dietary modification, the specific food groups are slowly reintroduced (at approximately 3-week intervals for each food group) and endoscopy is performed every 3 months to identify sustained remission or disease flare-up. Drugs, such as cromoglycate, montelukast, ketotifen, suplatast tosilate, mycophenolate mofetil (an inosine monophosphate dehydrogenase inhibitor), and "alternative Chinese medicines" have been advocated [26], but are generally not successful, in the authors' experience. In our institution, an appropriate therapeutic approach includes a trial of food elimination, if sensitization is found by food skin testing or RAST. If no sensitization is found, or if specific food avoidance is not feasible, an elemental formula is instituted.

Up to now, the management of EGID, besides elemental diet as mentioned above, has included four parts: systemic and topical steroids, noncorticosteroid therapy, management of other EGID complications (such as iron deficiency and anemia), and the management of therapeutic toxicity [63]. Anti-inflammatory drugs (systemic or topical steroids) are the main therapy in cases where diet restriction is not feasible or has failed to improve the disease. For systemic steroid therapy, a course of 2 to 6 weeks of therapy with relatively low doses seems to work better than a 7-day course of burst glucocorticoids. There are several forms of topical glucocorticoids designed to deliver drugs to specific segments of the gastrointestinal tract (eg, budesonide tablets, such as Entocort, designed to deliver drugs to the ileum and proximal colon). As with asthmatic treatment, topical steroids have a better benefit-to-risk effect compared with systemic steroids. Currently, anti-IL-5 and anti-IgE trials are in progress and some studies have shown promising results [59,64,65]. In severe cases, refractory glucocorticoid therapy, intravenous alimentation or immunosuppressive antimetabolite therapy (azathioprine or 6-mercaptopurine) are alternatives. Finally, even if GERD is not present, neutralization of gastric acidity (with proton pump inhibitors) may improve symptoms and the degree of esophageal and gastric pathology.

Gastrointestinal eosinophilia in hypereosinophilic syndrome

The term HES was introduced by Anderson and Hardy in 1968 to designate patients with marked eosinophilia in the absence of other causes of eosinophilia [66]. They reported three patients, all males between the ages of 34 and 47, who suffered from cardiopulmonary symptoms, fever, diaphoresis, weight loss and marked eosinophilia. Two of the patients died, and at autopsy their hearts were enlarged and showed mural thrombi. Multiple organs are involved in HES, including heart, lung, skin, nervous system, and GI system. Because of the involvement of the GI system, HES may be confused with EGID. However, HES usually involves many other organs with heart, skin, and central nervous system as its major target organs. The treatment for HES is similar to those used for patients with chronic myelogenous leukemia, including prednisone, hydroxyurea, and interferon-α. Chusid and colleagues [67] formulated the diagnostic criteria for HES to include: (1) persistent eosinophilia of at least 1500 cells/mm^2 for a minimum of 6 months; (2) lack of known causes for eosinophilia (eg, parasitic or allergic triggers); and (3) symptoms and signs of organ system involvement. Based on these diagnostic criteria, patients with EGID and blood eosinophil counts greater than 1500/mm^2 meet the diagnostic criteria. However, patients with EGID generally do not have the high risk of life-threatening complications associated with classic HES, such as cardiomyopathy or central nervous system involvement. Notably, considerable heterogeneity among HES patients has been recognized. For example, T-cell clones producing the characteristic Th2 cytokines, IL-4 and IL-5, have been found in patients satisfying the diagnostic criteria for HES [68,69].

Perhaps the most striking advance in our understanding of HES has resulted from treatment of HES patients with the tyrosine kinase inhibitor, imatinib mesylate [70–74]. Imatinib was introduced for the treatment of chronic myelogenous leukemia and has had a remarkable effect in that disease. Treatment of many HES patients with imatinib mesylate causes a dramatic reduction of peripheral blood and bone marrow eosinophils, suggesting that certain HES patients express a novel kinase sensitive to imatinib mesylate. Further investigation of the ability of imatinib mesylate to treat HES patients revealed the existence of an 800 kilobase deletion in chromosome 4, bringing together an upstream DNA sequence homologous to a yeast protein, referred to as FIP1, and designated as like FIP1, or FIP1-L1 and the gene for the cytoplasmic domain of the platelet derived growth factor alpha (PDGFRA) receptor [70,75]. This fusion gene is transcribed and translated, yielding a novel kinase referred to as FIP-L1-PDGFRA; FIP-L1-PDGFRA is exquisitely sensitive to imatinib in vitro, thus explaining the remarkable sensitivity of HES patients to this drug. The FIP-L1-PDGFRA fusion gene cooperates with IL-5 overexpression in a murine model of HES, suggesting that both pathogenic events cooperate in disease etiology [76]. The patients generally responsive to imatinib are those most characteristic of "classic" HES, namely males between the ages of 20 and 50 who present clinically with marked peripheral blood eosinophilia. Recently, these patients have been shown to meet minor criteria for systemic mastocytosis, having elevated levels of serum mast cell tryptase and high numbers of dysplastic mast cells in the bone marrow [77,78]. These patients go on to develop eosinophilic endomyocardial disease with embolization to peripheral organs, including the extremities and the brain, and they strikingly resemble the patients originally designated by Hardy and Anderson [66].

However, it appears that any disease that results in prolonged and marked eosinophilia can be associated with endomyocardial disease. For example, endomyocardial disease has occurred during the course of helminth infections and also in various malignancies associated with marked eosinophilia [79–81]. Thus, patients with marked eosinophilia are at risk for the development of cardiac disease regardless of the underlying etiology of the eosinophilia. Accordingly, routine surveillance of the cardio-respiratory system (eg, echocardiograms and plethysmography) in patients with EGID and peripheral blood eosinophilia is warranted. Based on these concerns, the diagnosis of HES in patients with EGID should always be considered, especially in patients who develop extragastrointestinal manifestations (eg, splenomegaly, or cutaneous, cardiac, or respiratory systems). As such, additional diagnostic testing for HES should be considered, including bone marrow analysis (searching for evidence of myelodysplasia), serum mast cell tryptase and vitamin B_{12} levels (both moderately elevated in classic HES), and genetic analysis for the presence of the FIP1-L1-PDGFRA fusion event [77].

Gastrointestinal eosinophilia from known causes

There are a variety of other known causes of GI eosinophilia, including parasitic infections, other allergic disorders, GERD, IBD, drug reactions, malignancy, Churg-Strauss syndrome, celiac disease, systemic lupus erythematosus, and solid organ transplantation. Among those causes, parasitic infections are the most common cause of gastrointestinal eosinophilia in developing countries. In developed countries, allergic causes have become the dominant cause for gastrointestinal eosinophilia. Among the infectious causes of gastrointestinal eosinophilia, aside from the number one cause of parasitic infections, helicobacter pylori infection has also been reported. Medications causing GI eosinophilia include gold salts, azathioprine, gemfibrozil, enalapril, carbamazepine, clofazimine, and cotrimoxazole. In the Churg-Strauss syndrome and polyarteritis nodosa, characteristic findings include eosinophilic infiltrate involving the small vessels in the intestinal tract and other organs. In IBD, eosinophils usually represent only a small percentage of the infiltrating leukocytes [82,83], but their level has been proposed to be a negative prognostic indicator [83,84].

Summary

Gastrointestinal eosinophilia, as a broad term for abnormal eosinophil accumulation in the GI tract, involves many different disease identities. These diseases include primary eosinophil associated gastrointestinal diseases, gastrointestinal eosinophilia in HES, and all gastrointestinal eosinophilic states associated with known causes. Although each of these diseases has its unique features, it is important to recognize that there is no absolute boundary between them. As an example, HES is a systemic eosinophilic disease, but it may also involve the gastrointestinal tract and not be associated with apparent causes, as in primary gastrointestinal eosinophilia. Similarly, primary EGID has a strong association with allergy, yet it is generally not considered a secondary eosinophilia. Different disease mechanisms likely account for these various states. For example, the eosinophilic esophagitis appears to be primarily driven by IL-5 and eotaxin-3, whereas evidence is emerging that eosinophilic enteritis may be primarily driven by eotaxin-1 [85]. As such, targeted therapy with antieotaxins, eotaxin receptor blockers (eg, CCR3 antagonists), or humanized anti-IL-5 therapeutics are likely to be useful therapy in the future, and early clinical trials have supported their potential utility [64].

Acknowledgments

The authors are grateful to Andrea Lippelman for her help during the writing of this article.

References

[1] Kato M, Kephart GM, Talley NJ, et al. Eosinophil infiltration and degranulation in normal human tissue. Anat Rec 1998;252(3):418–25.

[2] Mishra A, Hogan SP, Lee JJ, et al. Fundamental signals regulate eosinophil homing to the gastrointestinal tract. J Clin Invest 1999;103(12):1719–27.

[3] Rothenberg ME, Mishra A, Brandt EB, et al. Gastrointestinal eosinophils. Immunol Rev 2001;179:139–55.

[4] Straumann A, Kristl J, Conus S, et al. Cytokine expression in healthy and inflamed mucosa: probing the role of eosinophils in the digestive tract. Inflamm Bowel Dis 2005;11(8):720–6.

[5] Gleich GJ, Frigas E, Loegering DA, et al. Cytotoxic properties of the eosinophil major basic protein. J Immunol 1979;123(6):2925–7.

[6] Gleich GJ, Adolphson CR. The eosinophilic leukocyte: structure and function. Adv Immunol 1986;39:177–253.

[7] Slifman NR, Loegering DA, McKean DJ, et al. Ribonuclease activity associated with human eosinophil-derived neurotoxin and eosinophil cationic protein. J Immunol 1986;137(9): 2913–7.

[8] Rosenberg HF, Dyer KD, Tiffany HL, et al. Rapid evolution of a unique family of primate ribonuclease genes. Nat Genet 1995;10(2):219–23.

[9] Young JD, Peterson CG, Venge P, et al. Mechanism of membrane damage mediated by human eosinophil cationic protein. Nature 1986;321(6070):613–6.

[10] Jacoby DB, Gleich GJ, Fryer AD. Human eosinophil major basic protein is an endogenous allosteric antagonist at the inhibitory muscarinic M2 receptor. J Clin Invest 1993;91:1314–8.

[11] Kita H. The eosinophil: a cytokine-producing cell? J Allergy Clin Immunol 1996;97(4): 889–92.

[12] Gharaee-Kermani M, Phan SH. The role of eosinophils in pulmonary fibrosis. Int J Mol Med 1998;1:43–53.

[13] Phipps S, Ying S, Wangoo A, et al. The relationship between allergen-induced tissue eosinophilia and markers of repair and remodeling in human atopic skin. J Immunol 2002;169(8): 4604–12.

[14] Lucey DR, Nicholson WA, Weller PF. Mature human eosinophils have the capacity to express HLA-DR. Proc Natl Acad Sci USA 1989;86(4):1348–51.

[15] Lacy P, Levi-Schaffer F, Mahmudi-Azer S, et al. Intracellular localization of interleukin-6 in eosinophils from atopic asthmatics and effects of interferon gamma. Blood 1998;91(7):2508–16.

[16] Shi HZ, Humbles A, Gerard C, et al. Lymph node trafficking and antigen presentation by endobronchial eosinophils. J Clin Invest 2000;105(7):945–53.

[17] Mattes J, Yang M, Mahalingam S, et al. Intrinsic defect in T cell production of interleukin (IL)-13 in the absence of both IL-5 and eotaxin precludes the development of eosinophilia and airways hyperreactivity in experimental asthma. J Exp Med 2002; 195(11):1433–44.

[18] Lewis RA, Austen KF, Soberman RJ. Leukotrienes and other products of the 5-lipoxygenase pathway. Biochemistry and relation to pathobiology in human diseases. N Engl J Med 1990;323(10):645–55.

[19] Torpier G, Colombel JF, Mathieu-Chandelier C, et al. Eosinophilic gastroenteritis: ultrastructural evidence for a selective release of eosinophil major basic protein. Clin Exp Immunol 1988;74(3):404–8.

[20] Klein NC, Hargrove RL, Sleisenger MH, et al. Eosinophilic gastroenteritis. Medicine 1970; 2:215–25.

[21] Cello JP. Eosinophil gastroenteritis: a complex disease entity. Am J Med 1979;67:1097–114.

[22] Bischoff S, Crowe SE. Food allergy and the gastrointestinal tract. Curr Opin Gastroenterol 2004;20(2):156–61.

[23] Schappi MG, Smith VV, Milla PJ, et al. Eosinophilic myenteric ganglionitis is associated with functional intestinal obstruction. Gut 2003;52(5):752–5.

[24] Sawatzky DA, Kingham PJ, Court E, et al. Eosinophil adhesion to cholinergic nerves via ICAM-1 and VCAM-1 and associated eosinophil degranulation. Am J Physiol Lung Cell Mol Physiol 2002;282(6):L1279–88.

[25] Nie Z, Nelson CS, Jacoby DB, et al. Expression and regulation of intercellular adhesion molecule-1 on airway parasympathetic nerves. J Allergy Clin Immunol 2007;119(6):1415–22.

[26] Noel RJ, Putnam PE, Collins MH, et al. Clinical and immunopathologic effects of swallowed fluticasone for eosinophilic esophagitis. Clin Gastroenterol Hepatol 2004;2(7):568–75.

[27] Noel RJ, Putnam PE, Rothenberg ME. Eosinophilic esophagitis. N Engl J Med 2004;351(9): 940–1.

[28] Caldwell JH, Tennerbaum JI, Bronstein HA. Serum IgE to eosinophilic gastroenteritis. N Engl J Med 1975;292:1388–90.

[29] Scudamore HH, Phillips SF, Swedlund HA, et al. Food allergy manifested by eosinophilia, elevated immunoglobulin E level, and protein-losing enteropathy: the syndrome of allergic gastroenteropathy. J Allergy Clin Immunol 1982;70:129–36.

[30] Furuta GT, Ackerman SJ, Wershil BK. The role of the eosinophil in gastrointestinal diseases. Curr Opin Gastroenterol 1995;11:541–7.

[31] Iacono G, Carroccio A, Cavataiio F, et al. Gastroesophageal reflux and cow's milk allergy in infants: a prospective study. J Allergy Clin Immunol 1996;97:822–7.

[32] Sampson HA. Food allergy. JAMA 1997;278:1888–94.

[33] Walsh SV, Antonioli DA, Goldman H, et al. Allergic esophagitis in children: a clinicopathological entity. Am J Surg Pathol 1999;23(4):390–6.

[34] Spergel J, Rothenberg ME, Fogg M. Eliminating eosinophilic esophagitis. Clin Immunol 2005;115(2):131–2.

[35] Kelly KJ, Lazenby AJ, Rowe PC, et al. Eosinophilic esophagitis attributed to gastroesophageal reflux: improvement with an amino acid-based formula. Gastroenterology 1995;109 (5):1503–12.

[36] Oyaizu N, Uemura Y, Izumi H, et al. Eosinophilic gastroenteritis: immunohistochemical evidence for IgE mast cell-mediated allergy. Acta Pathol Jpn 1985;35:759–66.

[37] Bischoff SC. Mucosal allergy: role of mast cells and eosinophil granulocytes in the gut. Baillieres Clin Gastroenterol 1996;10(3):443–59.

[38] Rothenberg ME, Mishra A, Brandt EB, et al. Gastrointestinal eosinophils in health and disease. Adv Immunol 2001;78:291–328.

[39] Sampson HA. Food allergy. Part 1: immunopathogenesis and clinical disorders. J Allergy Clin Immunol 1999;103(5):717–28.

[40] Fox VL, Nurko S, Furuta GT. Eosinophilic esophagitis: it's not just kid's stuff. Gastrointest Endosc 2002;56(2):260–70.

[41] Bates B. 'Explosion' of eosinophilic esophagitis in children. Pediatr News 2000;34:4.

[42] Croese J, Fairley SK, Masson JW, et al. Clinical and endoscopic features of eosinophilic esophagitis in adults. Gastrointest Endosc 2003;58(4):516–22.

[43] Cury EK, Schraibman V, Faintuch S. Eosinophilic infiltration of the esophagus: gastro-esophageal reflux versus eosinophilic esophagitis in children—discussion on daily practice. J Pediatr Surg 2004;39(2):e4–7.

[44] Attwood SE, Smyrk TC, Demeester TR, et al. Esophageal eosinophilia with dysphagia. A distinct clinicopathologic syndrome. Dig Dis Sci 1993;38(1):109–16.

[45] Cantu P, Velio P, Prada A, et al. Ringed oesophagus and idiopathic eosinophilic oesophagitis in adults: an association in two cases. Dig Liver Dis 2005;37(2):129–34.

[46] Fujiwara H, Morita A, Kobayashi H, et al. Infiltrating eosinophils and eotaxin: their association with idiopathic eosinophilic esophagitis. Ann Allergy Asthma Immunol 2002;89(4): 429–32.

[47] Munitiz V, Martinez de Haro LF, Ortiz A, et al. Primary eosinophilic esophagitis. Dis Esophagus 2003;16(2):165–8.

[48] Lucendo Villarin AJ, Carrion Alonso G, Navarro Sanchez M, et al. Eosinophilic esophagitis in adults, an emerging cause of dysphagia. Description of 9 cases. Rev Esp Enferm Dig 2005; 97(4):229–39.

[49] Straumann A, Simon HU. The physiological and pathophysiological roles of eosinophils in the gastrointestinal tract. Allergy 2004;59(1):15–25.

[50] Ruchelli E, Wenner W, Voytek T, et al. Severity of esophageal eosinophilia predicts response to conventional gastroesophageal reflux therapy. Pediatr Dev Pathol 1999;2(1): 15–8.

[51] Liacouras CA, Ruchelli E. Eosinophilic esophagitis. Curr Opin Pediatr 2004;16:560–6.

[52] Walker NI, Croese J, Clouston AD, et al. Eosinophilic enteritis in northeastern Australia. Pathology, association with Ancylostoma caninum, and implications. Am J Surg Pathol 1995;19(3):328–37.

[53] Al Samman M, Haque S, Long JD. Strongyloidiasis colitis: a case report and review of the literature. J Clin Gastroenterol 1999;28(1):77–80.

[54] Assa'ad AH, Putnam PE, Collins MH, et al. Pediatric patients with eosinophilic esophagitis: an 8-year follow-up. J Allergy Clin Immunol 2007;119(3):731–8.

[55] Straumann A, Spichtin HP, Bucher KA, et al. Eosinophilic esophagitis: red on microscopy, white on endoscopy. Digestion 2004;70(2):109–16.

[56] Lee JH, Rhee PL, Kim JJ, et al. The role of mucosal biopsy in the diagnosis of chronic diarrhea: value of multiple biopsies when colonoscopic finding is normal or nonspecific. Korean J Intern Med 1997;12(2):182–7.

[57] DeBrosse CW, Case JW, Putnam PE, et al. Quantity and Distribution of Eosinophils in the Gastrointestinal Tract of Children. Pediatr Dev Pathol 2006;9:210–8.

[58] Guajardo JR, Plotnick LM, Fende JM, et al. Eosinophil-associated gastrointestinal disorders: a world-wide-web based registry. J Pediatr 2002;141(4):576–81.

[59] Lowichik A, Weinberg AG. A quantitative evaluation of mucosal eosinophils in the pediatric gastrointestinal tract. Mod Pathol 1996;9(2):110–114.

[60] Ngo P, Furuta GT, Antonioli DA, et al. Eosinophils in the esophagus—peptic or allergic eosinophilic esophagitis? Case series of three patients with esophageal eosinophilia. Am J Gastroenterol 2006;101(7):1666–70.

[61] Justinich C, Katz A, Gurbindo C, et al. Elemental diet improves steroid-dependent eosinophilic gastroenteritis and reverses growth failure. J Pediatr Gastroenterol Nutr 1996;23(1): 81–5.

[62] Kelly KJ, Lazenby AJ, Rowe PC, et al. Eosinophilic esophagitis attributed to gastroesophageal reflux: improvement with an amino acid-based formula. Gastroenterology 1995; 109(5):1503–12.

[63] Foroughi S, Prussin C. Clinical management of eosinophilic gastrointestinal disorders. Curr Allergy Asthma Rep 2005;5(4):259–61.

[64] Garrett JK, Jameson SC, Thomson B, et al. Anti-interleukin-5 (mepolizumab) therapy for hypereosinophilic syndromes. J Allergy Clin Immunol 2004;113(1):115–9.

[65] Stein ML, Collins MH, Villanueva JM, et al. Anti-IL-5 (mepolizumab) therapy for eosinophilic esophagitis. J Allergy Clin Immunol 2006;118(6):1312–9.

[66] Anderson RE, Hardy WR. Hypereosinophilia. Ann Intern Med 1968;69(6):1331–2.

[67] Chusid MJ, Dale DC, West BC, et al. The hypereosinophilic syndrome: analysis of fourteen cases with review of the literature. Medicine (Baltimore) 1975;54(1):1–27.

[68] Roufosse F, Cogan E, Goldman M. The hypereosinophilic syndrome revisited. Annu Rev Med 2003;54:169–84.

[69] Simon HU, Plotz SG, Dummer R, et al. Abnormal clones of T cells producing interleukin-5 in idiopathic eosinophilia. N Engl J Med 1999;341(15):1112–20.

[70] Cools J, DeAngelo DJ, Gotlib J, et al. A tyrosine kinase created by fusion of the PDGFRA and FIP1L1 genes as a therapeutic target of imatinib in idiopathic hypereosinophilic syndrome. N Engl J Med 2003;348(13):1201–14.

[71] Cortes J, Ault P, Koller C, et al. Efficacy of imatinib mesylate in the treatment of idiopathic hypereosinophilic syndrome. Blood 2003;101:4717–16.

[72] Schaller JL, Burkland GA. Case report: rapid and complete control of idiopathic hypereosinophilia with imatinib mesylate. Med Gen Med 2001;3(5):9.

[73] Ault P, Cortes J, Koller C, et al. Response of idiopathic hypereosinophilic syndrome to treatment with imatinib mesylate. Leuk Res 2002;26(9):881–4.

[74] Gleich GJ, Leiferman KM, Pardanani A, et al. Treatment of hypereosinophilic syndrome with imatinib mesilate. Lancet 2002;359(9317):1577–8.

[75] Griffin JH, Leung J, Bruner RJ, et al. Discovery of a fusion kinase in EOL-1 cells and idiopathic hypereosinophilic syndrome. Proc Natl Acad Sci U S A 2003;100(13):7830–5.

[76] Yamada Y, Rothenberg ME, Lee AW, et al. The FIP1L1-PDGFR{alpha} fusion gene cooperates with IL-5 to induce murine hypereosinophilic syndrome (HES)/chronic eosinophilic leukemia (CEL)-like disease. Blood 2006;107:4071–9.

[77] Klion AD, Noel P, Akin C, et al. Elevated serum tryptase levels identify a subset of patients with a myeloproliferative variant of idiopathic hypereosinophilic syndrome associated with tissue fibrosis, poor prognosis, and imatinib responsiveness. Blood 2003;101(12):4660–6.

[78] Klion AD, Robyn JA, Akin C, et al. Molecular remission and reversal of myelofibrosis in response to imatinib mesylate treatment in patients with the myeloproliferative variant of hypereosinophilic syndrome. Blood 2003;101:4660–6.

[79] Yoshida T, Naganuma T, Niizawa M, et al. [A case of eosinophilic gastroenteritis accompanied by perimyocarditis, which was strongly suspected]. Nippon Shokakibyo Gakkai Zasshi 1995;92(8):1183–8 [in Japanese].

[80] Hussain A, Brown PJ, Thwaites BC, et al. Eosinophilic endomyocardial disease due to high grade chest wall sarcoma. Thorax 1994;49(10):1040–1.

[81] Andy JJ, Ogunowo PO, Akpan NA, et al. Helminth associated hypereosinophilia and tropical endomyocardial fibrosis (EMF) in Nigeria. Acta Trop 1998;69(2):127–40.

[82] Walsh RE, Gaginella TS. The eosiniophil in inflammatory bowel disease. Scand J Gastroenterol 1991;26:1217–24.

[83] Desreumaux P, Nutten S, Colombel JF. Activated eosinophils in inflammatory bowel disease: do they matter? Am J Gastroenterol 1999;94(12):3396–8.

[84] Nishitani H, Okabayashi M, Satomi M, et al. Infiltration of peroxidase-producing eosinophils into the lamina propria of patients with ulcerative colitis. J Gastroenterol 1998;33(2):189–95.

[85] Blanchard C, Wang N, Rothenberg ME. Eosinophilic esophagitis: pathogenesis, genetics, and therapy. J Allergy Clin Immunol 2006;118(5):1054–9.

showed echocardiographic features of left ventricular free wall thickening, 37% showed an increase in left atrial transverse dimension, and 27% showed an increase in right ventricular transverse dimension [3]. Unsuspected pericardial effusions were found by echocardiography in 32% of these patients [3]. In a Mayo Clinic series of 51 patients who had HES, 49% had cardiac disease by echocardiography. This group with echocardiographic evidence of HES also had higher rates of embolization, clinical heart failure, and cardiac surgery [2].

In recent years, cardiac MRI has emerged as a highly useful noninvasive modality for the diagnosis of cardiac involvement in HES. Cardiac MRI is more sensitive to and specific for the detection of ventricular thrombi than is transthoracic or transesophageal echocardiography (Fig. 3) [31]. Delayed-enhancement gadolinium imaging is capable of detecting myocardial fibrosis and inflammation (Fig. 4) [32]. Cardiac MRI uses inversion-recovery prepared T1-weighted gradient-echo sequencing after the intravenous administration of gadolinium chelate to demonstrate nonviable tissue as delayed enhancement [33]. Delayed enhancement resulting from fibrosis is more intense than delayed enhancement due to inflammation [31]. There are several recent case reports describing cardiac MRI as an adjunct diagnostic modality in HES [24,31,33,34]. One report describes the use of cine-MRI to aid in right ventricular endomyocardectomy in a patient who had HES [35].

Despite steadily improving noninvasive methods to aid in the diagnosis of HES, endomyocardial biopsy remains the diagnostic gold standard (Fig. 5). Serial myocardial biopsies are used to provide information on the clinical course of cardiac disease and the response to treatment. The

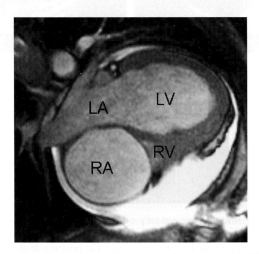

Fig. 3. Cine-MRI in a four-chamber view of the same patient presented in Fig. 1 using a steady-state free precession technique. Note that the right ventricular cavity is nearly obliterated. *Abbreviations:* LA, left atrium; LV, left ventricle; RA, right atrium; RV, right ventricle. (*Courtesy of* Drs. Patricia Bandettini and Andrew Arai, Bethesda, MD.)

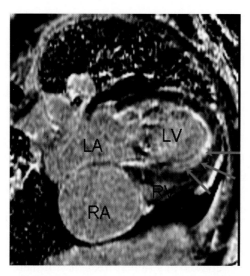

Fig. 4. Delayed hyperenhancement images of the same patient presented in Fig. 1 obtained 20 minutes after administration of gadolinium contrast using an inversion recovery gradient-echo technique validated for imaging myocardial infarction. There is a bright white rim of enhancement lining the left ventricle (*arrows*), which is consistent with endomyocardial fibrosis. *Abbreviations:* LA, left atrium; LV, left ventricle; RA, right atrium; RV, right ventricle. (*Courtesy of* Drs. Patricia Bandettini and Andrew Arai, Bethesda, MA.)

histopathologic features of HES endomyocardial diseases include fibrotic thickening of the endocardium; mural thrombosis; and fibrinoid change, thrombosis, and inflammation of the small intramural coronary vessels. Lastly, infiltration of eosinophils into the myocardium and sometimes endocardium also may be detected [11]. Although endomyocardial biopsy is the gold standard, the high resolution of cardiac MRI permits tissue characterization, which makes this technique a promising, and perhaps, more practical method to follow and potentially diagnose cardiac disease in HES.

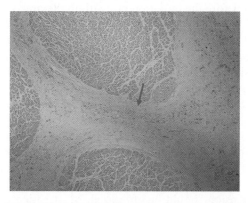

Fig. 5. Histology of fatal endomyocardial fibrosis in the same patient presented in Fig. 1. Arrow denotes areas of intracardiac fibrosis bordered by areas of unaffected myocardium.

Management of hypereosinophilic syndrome heart disease

The initial approach to the cardiac evaluation of a patient who has HES includes a good history and a thorough physical examination looking for evidence of cardiovascular involvement, particularly cardiac decompensation or peripheral thromboembolic events. A baseline electrocardiogram, two-dimensional echocardiogram, and chest radiograph should be obtained. The common findings on electrocardiogram generally are nonspecific and include nonspecific S-T and T wave abnormalities, and, in later stages, evidence of left ventricular hypertrophy. Two-dimensional echocardiography with Doppler flow measurements is essential to evaluate the degree of ventricular hypertrophy, the presence of valvular abnormalities, the presence of mural or apical thrombi, and to estimate ventricular systolic and diastolic function. If initial transthoracic echocardiography is normal, it should be repeated at a minimum of 6-month intervals. If evidence of cardiac disease is found, more frequent echocardiograms may be warranted. The electrocardiogram should be repeated at a similar frequency. If there is evidence of endocardial thickening or difficulty obtaining optimal images, transesophageal echocardiography or cardiac MRI should be performed. If a question of disease involvement or severity still remains, a cardiac biopsy is necessary.

All patients who have evidence of myeloproliferative HES (MHES) or cardiac involvement should be screened by fluorescence in situ hybridization or polymerase chain reaction for the FP mutation, because the tyrosine kinase inhibitor, imatinib, is the treatment of choice for patients with this mutation. Although imatinib therapy is associated with clinical, hematologic, and molecular remission in most patients who have FP-associated CEL, signs and symptoms of congestive heart failure in patients who have endomyocardial fibrosis remain unaffected in most cases [36]. This is likely due to the presence of irreversible structural damage as a result of chronic fibrosis and emphasizes the need for prompt treatment with imatinib in these patients. It is recommended that screening be performed with a baseline serum troponin T level before the initiation of imatinib therapy. Pretreatment with steroids should be initiated before imatinib therapy if the baseline serum troponin T level is elevated or there is evidence of active cardiac disease, because imatinib may be associated with an acute drug-induced cardiomyopathy with resultant clinical decompensation [37–39]. There have been case reports of cardiac toxicity associated with long-term imatinib therapy, although larger clinical databases have not shown similar findings [40,41].

Symptoms of congestive heart failure should be managed with conventional medications, including diuretics, β-adrenergic blockers, angiotensin-converting enzyme inhibitors, angiotensin II receptor blockers, aldosterone antagonists, and digoxin [42]. Control of concomitant comorbid conditions, such as cardiac dysrhythmias, diabetes mellitus, thyroid dysfunction, anemia, and hypertension should be optimized. Most patients who have clinically significant atrioventricular valvular regurgitation no longer need to use prophylactic antibiotic treatment before dental and surgical procedures according to the new American Heart Association guidelines; however, if the patient has a prosthetic heart valve, a history of previous infective endocarditis, or certain congenital heart disorders, antibiotic prophylaxis is still recommended [43].

Surgical intervention secondary to progressive valvular dysfunction may become necessary. The experience with valve replacement in patients who have HES is limited because of the rarity of the disease; however, valve replacement and, less frequently, valve repair in patients who have HES have been described [44,45]. Damaged valves can be replaced with mechanical or bioprosthetic valves. Despite anticoagulation, mechanical valve replacement may have a high incidence of thrombosis, whereas bioprosthetic valves may require more frequent replacement because of deterioration. In 1991, Boustany and colleagues [44] reported a collection of eight cases of mitral valve operations for HES. Since then, six other reports have been published [46]. Mitral valve replacement is the most common surgery performed, although one case of mitral valve annuloplasty for HES has been reported [47]. The use of mechanical valves in this patient group incurs a high risk for thrombosis, despite the use of anticoagulation [48]. In the limited number of patients reported with mechanical valve obstructive thrombosis, reoperation was associated with high mortality [45,48]. Obstruction of mechanical valves may occur rapidly and, in some cases, has been reported to develop within days to months of surgery, despite anticoagulant therapy [49]. Repeat surgery often leads to replacement of the mechanical valve with a bioprosthetic valve.

Because of these considerations, the use of bioprosthetic valves has been advocated, despite the frequent young ages of the patients and apprehension about early valve deterioration. The restrictive cardiomyopathy associated with a small left ventricular cavity is an additional concern and favors the use of a low-profile valve [46]. A report of a young boy who had HES requiring several mitral valve operations described recurrent thrombotic events, despite the use of a bioprosthetic valve and documented therapeutic anticoagulation [49]. Because of these concerns, a heterograft bioprosthesis should be used in conjunction with warfarin therapy. It also is highly recommended that the peripheral eosinophilia be controlled before valve replacement or repair. Most case reports of repeat valve thrombosis were before the use of imatinib treatment and may reflect the effects of persistent uncontrolled eosinophilia.

If the restrictive cardiomyopathy progresses or recurrent valve thrombosis occurs, heart transplantation should be considered. The use of orthotopic heart transplant has been described in only three patients who had HES. All patients are reported to be alive (International Society of Heart and Lung Transplantation Registry 2005) [50]. In the most recent case, a 48-year old man who had HES received an orthotopic heart transplant and—despite treatment with tacrolimus and prednisone—required reintroduction of

Management of thrombotic complications of hypereosinophilic syndrome

In the complete absence of information about whether anticoagulation could prevent the progression of HES cardiac disease from the thrombotic to the fibrotic stage, prophylactic treatment for this indication cannot be recommended; however, patients who have HES with evidence of intracardiac thrombosis by echocardiography or cardiac MRI should be treated with anticoagulant therapy because of reports, limited though they are, that approximately 25% of these patients develop emboli [1,52,53]. On the basis of the published experience with intracardiac thrombosis associated with HES and the much larger experience following myocardial infarction, it is likely that anticoagulation that conforms to the current recommendations for treating thromboembolic disease in other patient populations can significantly reduce, if not eliminate, the risk for emboli in patients who have HES.

A meta-analysis in 1993, for example, concluded that anticoagulation with heparin, but not antiplatelet therapy, can prevent the formation of echocardiographically demonstrated thrombi after myocardial infarction and reduce the risk for embolization [77]. Preventing thrombi is more difficult than preventing emboli, but emboli are the chief source of morbidity. Twenty-two to 56% of patients receiving up to 1000 U/h of unfractionated heparin developed mural thrombi within 11 days after myocardial infarction, but only 0% to 10% of those patients developed clinically apparent emboli [78–83]. Heparin doses exceeding 1000 U/h were more effective. In 1999, a meta-analysis of 31 trials found that the frequency of strokes after myocardial infarction was reduced by 63% in patients who took warfarin with a target INR of 3 to 5 and by 53% in those with an INR of 2 to 3 [84]. In more recent studies, warfarin with an INR of 2.8 to 4.2 and warfarin with an INR of 2 to 2.5 in combination with aspirin, 75 mg/d, were equally protective against strokes and significantly more protective than aspirin, 160 mg/d, alone [85]. In another study, a slightly lower INR (1.5–2.5) in combination with aspirin, 81 mg/d, provided the same level of protection as aspirin, 162 mg/d, alone [86]. Therefore, on the basis of these studies, the threshold INR to prevent cardioemboli seems to be approximately 3.0, although similar results may be achievable with an INR of 2 to 3 supplemented with aspirin. Treatment of thrombosis should begin with an agent that will damp the prothrombotic mechanisms quickly. For arterial thrombosis this means aspirin, with or without a form of heparin, and for venous thrombosis, a form of heparin [87,88]. In a patient who has active thrombosis, warfarin should not be given until heparin is started, because warfarin will not induce therapeutic anticoagulation for several days. If warfarin is given alone, it even may increase coagulability transiently [89,90].

In most patients, the parenteral anticoagulant of choice is a low molecular weight (LMW) heparin because this drug usually requires no monitoring and can be administered to outpatients [91]. Several LMW heparins are marketed. They are similar in efficacy and price. Enoxaparin (Lovenox), dalteparin (Fragmin), and tinzaparin (Innohep) are the most commonly prescribed in the United States and are given subcutaneously every 12 or 24 hours. Because these drugs are excreted by the kidney, they should be used with caution in patients who have renal insufficiency. There is more information about the excretion of enoxaparin than the other LMW heparins. It seems that enoxaparin can be administered safely with creatinine clearances as low as 30 mL/min [92]. The dose is weight-based, even in obese patients, although higher doses of LMW heparin may be required for patients in critical care settings [92,93].

Unlike unfractionated heparin, LMW heparin has minimal, if any, effect on the activated partial thromboplastin time (aPTT) because its anticoagulant activity comes largely from its inhibition of activated factor X (fXa), rather than thrombin; however, if LMW heparin does need monitoring (eg, in a patient with marginal renal function), this is possible with an assay that specifically measures anti-fXa activity in U/mL. Blood for the test should be drawn approximately 4 hours after a subcutaneous dose. Therapeutic anti-fXa levels at that point are 0.5 to 1.2 IU/mL.

Unfractionated heparin is advisable for patients at high risk for bleeding or who are critically ill because its anticoagulant activity can be reversed completely with protamine, and it is only partially dependent upon renal excretion [91]. Although dosing recommendations vary, a commonly used regimen for venous thrombosis is an intravenous bolus of 80 U/kg, followed by 18 u/kg/h by continuous infusion [91]. Traditionally, the dosage has been adjusted 6 hours later to prolong the aPTT to 1.5 to 2.5 times the "control" value; however, this practice often results in subtherapeutic anticoagulation because the sensitivity of the aPTT to heparin varies with different reagents [91]. Also, the meaning of "control" often is unclear. It is recommended that each laboratory establish a therapeutic range of aPTT for heparin based upon calibrations with known amounts of heparin. No therapeutic range is appropriate, however, if the patient's pretreatment aPTT is abnormal. Lupus anticoagulants, which are not rare, can elevate the aPTT to make it especially sensitive to heparin. Such patients will be underanticoagulated significantly if the aPTT is used to adjust their dosage of heparin. Anticoagulation in these patients should be monitored with the anti-fXa assay (therapeutic range, 0.3–0.7 IU/mL, different from that for LMW heparin).

Warfarin should be begun simultaneously with heparin or soon thereafter. Heparin must be continued for at least 5 days and until warfarin has achieved a stable INR between 2 and 3. The transition from heparin to warfarin should not be hurried because unstable anticoagulation at this early stage risks treatment failure.

The downside to antithrombotic treatment, of course, is the risk for bleeding. It has been estimated that 4% to 6% of patients who are treated with standard or LMW heparin for acute deep vein thrombosis develop major bleeding [94–96]. The risk increases with the dosage of anticoagulant and with the presence of comorbid conditions. About 5% of patients taking warfarin have a major bleed each year [85,97–99]; however, the risk for bleeding on warfarin is greatest during the first 3 months of treatment, increases with comorbidities, and increases sharply at INRs greater than 4.5 [96,97,100]. In a study with more than 12,500 patients, the annual risk for major bleeding from antithrombotic dosages of aspirin (≤ 325 mg/d) was 2.7% [101]. Combining aspirin, 100 mg/d, with warfarin at an INR of 3.0 to 4.5 increased the annual risk for major bleeding in patients with artificial heart valves from 10% to 13% [102]. Therefore, the clinical challenge is to balance these bleeding risks with the potential benefits of administering antithrombotic agents.

Patients who have HES can have thromboembolic events unrelated to or only partially related to their hypereosinophilia [71–73]. Therefore, in deciding about the duration of anticoagulation, consideration must be given to whether the initial clinical event followed surgery or occurred during hospitalization or another period of relative immobility [103]. Testing a patient for genetic predispositions (eg, factor V Leiden, prothrombin G20210A) to thrombosis rarely impacts the decision about the duration of anticoagulation [104].

The recommended duration of anticoagulation is based upon the assumption that the risk for recurrent thrombosis or embolism is high until or unless the inciting cause is eliminated. Therefore, in patients who have HES, the duration of anticoagulation should be determined by the activity of the patient's endomyocardial disease. If this is controlled and if echocardiography reveals the absence of thrombus or resolution of thrombus, it is reasonable to discontinue anticoagulation; however, the balance between the risks and benefits of anticoagulation must be reassessed continuously.

Summary

Cardiovascular manifestations of HES are a common cause of morbidity and mortality in an otherwise uncommon disorder. The management of cardiovascular disorders in HES includes normalization of the peripheral eosinophil count; screening for the FP mutation and treating with imatinib if present; optimizing cardiac function by medical and surgical intervention; initiating anticoagulant therapy in patients who have or at risk for thrombotic complications; and considering heart transplantation for patients who have progressive cardiac disease, despite conventional management.

References

[1] Chusid MJ, Dale DC, West BC, et al. The hypereosinophilic syndrome: analysis of fourteen cases with review of the literature. Medicine (Baltimore) 1975;54(1):1–27.
[2] Ommen SR, Seward JB, Tajik AJ. Clinical and echocardiographic features of hypereosinophilic syndromes. Am J Cardiol 2000;86(1):110–3.

[3] Parrillo JE, Borer JS, Henry WL, et al. The cardiovascular manifestations of the hypereosinophilic syndrome. Prospective study of 26 patients, with review of the literature. Am J Med 1979;67(4):572–82.

[4] Loeffler W. Endocarditis parietalis fibroplastica mit Bluteosinophilic. Schweiz Me Wochenschr 1936;66:817.

[5] Ginsberg F, Parrillo JE. Eosinophilic myocarditis. Heart Fail Clin 2005;1(3):419–29.

[6] Cooper LT, Zehr KJ. Biventricular assist device placement and immunosuppression as therapy for necrotizing eosinophilic myocarditis. Nat Clin Pract Cardiovasc Med 2005; 2(10):544–8.

[7] Nutman TB, Miller KD, Mulligan M, et al. Loa loa infection in temporary residents of endemic regions: recognition of a hyperresponsive syndrome with characteristic clinical manifestations. J Infect Dis 1986;154(1):10–8.

[8] Hasley PB, Follansbee WP, Coulehan JL. Cardiac manifestations of Churg-Strauss syndrome: report of a case and review of the literature. Am Heart J 1990;120(4):996–9.

[9] Pela G, Tirabassi G, Pattoneri P, et al. Cardiac involvement in the Churg-Strauss syndrome. Am J Cardiol 2006;97(10):1519–24.

[10] Noth I, Strek ME, Leff AR. Churg-Strauss syndrome. Lancet 2003;361(9357):587–94.

[11] Fauci AS, Harley JB, Roberts WC, et al. NIH conference. The idiopathic hypereosinophilic syndrome. Clinical, pathophysiologic, and therapeutic considerations. Ann Intern Med 1982;97(1):78–92.

[12] Weller PF, Bubley GJ. The idiopathic hypereosinophilic syndrome. Blood 1994;83(10): 2759–79.

[13] Young JD, Peterson CG, Venge P, et al. Mechanism of membrane damage mediated by human eosinophil cationic protein. Nature 1986;321(6070):613–6.

[14] Tai PC, Ackerman SJ, Spry CJ, et al. Deposits of eosinophil granule proteins in cardiac tissues of patients with eosinophilic endomyocardial disease. Lancet 1987;1(8534): 643–7.

[15] Zientek DM, King DL, Dewan SJ, et al. Hypereosinophilic syndrome with rapid progression of cardiac involvement and early echocardiographic abnormalities. Am Heart J 1995; 130(6):1295–8.

[16] Hoffman M, Monroe DM 3rd. A cell-based model of hemostasis. Thromb Haemost 2001; 85(6):958–65.

[17] Ruggeri ZM. Platelet interactions with vessel wall components during thrombogenesis. Blood Cells Mol Dis 2006;36(2):145–7.

[18] Wang JG, Mahmud SA, Thompson JA, et al. The principal eosinophil peroxidase product, HOSCN, is a uniquely potent phagocyte oxidant inducer of endothelial cell tissue factor activity: a potential mechanism for thrombosis in eosinophilic inflammatory states. Blood 2006;107(2):558–65.

[19] Moosbauer C, Morgenstern E, Cuvelier SL, et al. Eosinophils are a major intravascular location for tissue factor storage and exposure. Blood 2007;109(3):995–1002.

[20] Slungaard A, Vercellotti GM, Tran T, et al. Eosinophil cationic granule proteins impair thrombomodulin function. A potential mechanism for thromboembolism in hypereosinophilic heart disease. J Clin Invest 1993;91(4):1721–30.

[21] Venge P, Dahl R, Hallgren R. Enhancement of factor XII dependent reactions by eosinophil cationic protein. Thromb Res 1979;14(4–5):641–9.

[22] Gambacorti Passerini C, Cortellaro M, Cofrancesco E, et al. Possible mechanisms of fibrin deposition in the hypereosinophilic syndrome. Haemostasis 1989;19(1):32–7.

[23] Rohrbach MS, Wheatley CL, Slifman NR, et al. Activation of platelets by eosinophil granule proteins. J Exp Med 1990;172(4):1271–4.

[24] Salanitri GC. Endomyocardial fibrosis and intracardiac thrombus occurring in idiopathic hypereosinophilic syndrome. AJR Am J Roentgenol 2005;184(5):1432–3.

[25] Hendren WG, Jones EL, Smith MD. Aortic and mitral valve replacement in idiopathic hypereosinophilic syndrome. Ann Thorac Surg 1988;46(5):570–1.

[26] Spiegel R, Miron D, Fink D, et al. Eosinophilic pericarditis: a rare complication of idiopathic hypereosinophilic syndrome in a child. Pediatr Cardiol 2004;25(6):690–2.

[27] D'Souza MG, Swistel DG, Castro JL, et al. Hypereosinophilic thrombus causing aortic stenosis and myocardial infarction. Ann Thorac Surg 2003;76(5):1725–6.

[28] Cools J, DeAngelo DJ, Gotlib J, et al. A tyrosine kinase created by fusion of the PDGFRA and FIP1L1 genes as a therapeutic target of imatinib in idiopathic hypereosinophilic syndrome. N Engl J Med 2003;348(13):1201–14.

[29] Subhash HS, Asishkumar M, Jonathan M. Unusual cardiac manifestation of hypereosinophilic syndrome. Postgrad Med J 2002;78(922):490–1.

[30] Shah R, Ananthasubramaniam K. Evaluation of cardiac involvement in hypereosinophilic syndrome: complementary roles of transthoracic, transesophageal, and contrast echocardiography. Echocardiography 2006;23(8):689–91.

[31] Syed IS, Martinez MW, Feng DL, et al. Cardiac magnetic resonance imaging of eosinophilic endomyocardial disease. Int J Cardiol 2007 [epub ahead of print].

[32] Wagner A, Mahrholdt H, Holly TA, et al. Contrast-enhanced MRI and routine single photon emission computed tomography (SPECT) perfusion imaging for detection of subendocardial myocardial infarcts: an imaging study. Lancet 2003;361(9355):374–9.

[33] Plastiras SC, Economopoulos N, Kelekis NL, et al. Magnetic resonance imaging of the heart in a patient with hypereosinophilic syndrome. Am J Med 2006;119(2):130–2.

[34] Puvaneswary M, Joshua F, Ratnarajah S. Idiopathic hypereosinophilic syndrome: magnetic resonance imaging findings in endomyocardial fibrosis. Australas Radiol 2001; 45(4):524–7.

[35] Chandra M, Pettigrew RI, Eley JW, et al. Cine-MRI-aided endomyocardectomy in idiopathic hypereosinophilic syndrome. Ann Thorac Surg 1996;62(6):1856–8.

[36] Klion AD, Robyn J, Akin C, et al. Molecular remission and reversal of myelofibrosis in response to imatinib mesylate treatment in patients with the myeloproliferative variant of hypereosinophilic syndrome. Blood 2004;103(2):473–8.

[37] Klion AD, Bochner BS, Gleich GJ, et al. Approaches to the treatment of hypereosinophilic syndromes: a workshop summary report. J Allergy Clin Immunol 2006;117(6):1292–302.

[38] Pitini V, Arrigo C, Azzarello D, et al. Serum concentration of cardiac troponin T in patients with hypereosinophilic syndrome treated with imatinib is predictive of adverse outcomes. Blood 2003;102(9):3456–7, [author reply: 3457].

[39] Pardanani A, Reeder T, Porrata LF, et al. Imatinib therapy for hypereosinophilic syndrome and other eosinophilic disorders. Blood 2003;101(9):3391–7.

[40] Kerkela R, Grazette L, Yacobi R, et al. Cardiotoxicity of the cancer therapeutic agent imatinib mesylate. Nat Med 2006;12(8):908–16.

[41] Hatfield A, Owen S, Pilot PR. In reply to 'Cardiotoxicity of the cancer therapeutic agent imatinib mesylate'. Nat Med 2007;13(1):13 [author reply: 15–6].

[42] Hunt SA, Abraham WT, Chin MH, et al. ACC/AHA 2005 Guideline update for the diagnosis and management of chronic heart failure in the adult: a report of the American College of Cardiology/American Heart Association Task Force on Practice Guidelines (Writing committee to update the 2001 guidelines for the evaluation and management of heart failure): developed in collaboration with the American College of Chest Physicians and the International Society for Heart and Lung Transplantation: endorsed by the Heart Rhythm Society. Circulation 2005;112(12):e154–235.

[43] Wilson W, Taubert KA, Gewitz M, et al. Prevention of infective endocarditis. Guidelines from the American Heart Association. A guideline from the American Heart Association Rheumatic Fever, Endocarditis, and Kawasaki Disease Committee, Council on Cardiovascular Disease in the Young, and the Council on Clinical Cardiology, Council on Cardiovascular Surgery and Anesthesia, and the Quality of Care and Outcomes Research Interdisciplinary Working Group. Circulation 2007.

[44] Boustany CW Jr, Murphy GW, Hicks GL Jr. Mitral valve replacement in idiopathic hypereosinophilic syndrome. Ann Thorac Surg 1991;51(6):1007–9.

[45] Fuzellier JF, Chapoutot L, Torossian PF. Mitral valve repair in idiopathic hypereosinophilic syndrome. J Heart Valve Dis 2004;13(3):529–31.

[46] Fuzellier JF, Chapoutot L, Torossian PF, et al. Mitral valve replacement in idiopathic eosinophilic endocarditis without peripheral eosinophilia. J Card Surg 2005;20(5):472–4.

[47] Bell JA, Jenkins BS, Webb-Peploe MM. Clinical, haemodynamic, and angiographic findings in Loffler's eosinophilic endocarditis. Br Heart J 1976;38(6):541–8.

[48] Watanabe K, Tournilhac O, Camilleri LF. Recurrent thrombosis of prosthetic mitral valve in idiopathic hypereosinophilic syndrome. J Heart Valve Dis 2002;11(3):447–9.

[49] Radford DJ, Garlick RB, Pohlner PG. Multiple valvar replacements for hypereosinophilic syndrome. Cardiol Young 2002;12(1):67–70.

[50] Korczyk D, Taylor G, McAlistair H, et al. Heart transplantation in a patient with endomyocardial fibrosis due to hypereosinophilic syndrome. Transplantation 2007;83(4): 514–6.

[51] Solley GO, Maldonado JE, Gleich GJ, et al. Endomyocardiopathy with eosinophilia. Mayo Clin Proc 1976;51(11):697–708.

[52] Moore PM, Harley JB, Fauci AS. Neurologic dysfunction in the idiopathic hypereosinophilic syndrome. Ann Intern Med 1985;102(1):109–14.

[53] Spry CJ, Davies J, Tai PC, et al. Clinical features of fifteen patients with the hypereosinophilic syndrome. Q J Med 1983;52(205):1–22.

[54] Ishii T, Koide O, Hosoda Y, et al. Hypereosinophilic multiple thrombosis. A proposal of a new designation of disseminated eosinophilic "collagen disease". Angiology 1977;28(6): 361–75.

[55] Ishii T, Sternby NH, Hosoda Y. Hypereosinophilic multiple thrombosis. Vasa 1978;7(3): 303–8.

[56] Fitzpatrick JE, Johnson C, Simon P, et al. Cutaneous microthrombi: a histologic clue to the diagnosis of hypereosinophilic syndrome. Am J Dermatopathol 1987;9(5):419–22.

[57] Kanno H, Ouchi N, Sato M, et al. Hypereosinophilia with systemic thrombophlebitis. Hum Pathol 2005;36(5):585–9.

[58] Funahashi S, Masaki I, Furuyama T. Hypereosinophilic syndrome accompanying gangrene of the toes with peripheral arterial occlusion—a case report. Angiology 2006;57(2): 231–4.

[59] Elouaer-Blanc L, Zafrani ES, Farcet JP, et al. Hepatic vein obstruction in idiopathic hypereosinophilic syndrome. Arch Intern Med 1985;145(4):751–3.

[60] Valente O, Scarpinella-Bueno MA. Deep venous thrombosis in hypereosinophilic syndrome. Am Fam Physician 1994;50(5):921–2.

[61] Kojima K, Sasaki T. Veno-occlusive disease in hypereosinophilic syndrome. Intern Med 1995;34(12):1194–7.

[62] Mukai HY, Ninomiya H, Mitsuhashi S, et al. Thromboembolism in a patient with transient eosinophilia. Ann Hematol 1996;72(2):93–5.

[63] Zylberberg H, Valla D, Viguie F, et al. Budd-Chiari syndrome associated with 5q deletion and hypereosinophilia. J Clin Gastroenterol 1996;23(1):66–8.

[64] Yamada T, Shinohara K, Katsuki K. A case of idiopathic hypereosinophilic syndrome complicated with disseminated intravascular coagulation. Am J Hematol 1998;59(1):100–1.

[65] Schulman H, Hertzog L, Zirkin H, et al. Cerebral sinovenous thrombosis in the idiopathic hypereosinophilic syndrome in childhood. Pediatr Radiol 1999;29(8):595–7.

[66] Kikuchi K, Minami K, Miyakawa H, et al. Portal vein thrombosis in hypereosinophilic syndrome. Am J Gastroenterol 2002;97(5):1274–5.

[67] Walker M. Idiopathic hypereosinophilia associated with hepatic vein thrombosis. Arch Intern Med 1987;147(12):2220–1.

[68] Uemura K, Nakajima M, Yamauchi N, et al. Sudden death of a patient with primary hypereosinophilia, colon tumours, and pulmonary emboli. J Clin Pathol 2004;57(5):541–3.

[69] Liapis H, Ho AK, Brown D, et al. Thrombotic microangiopathy associated with the hypereosinophilic syndrome. Kidney Int 2005;67(5):1806–11.

[70] Sakuta R, Tomita Y, Ohashi M, et al. Idiopathic hypereosinophilic syndrome complicated by central sinovenous thrombosis. Brain Dev 2007;29(3):182–4.

[71] Narayan S, Ezughah F, Standen GR, et al. Idiopathic hypereosinophilic syndrome associated with cutaneous infarction and deep venous thrombosis. Br J Dermatol 2003;148(4): 817–20.

[72] Gumruk F, Gurgey A, Altay C. A case of hypereosinophilic syndrome associated with factor V Leiden mutation and thrombosis. Br J Haematol 1998;101(1):208–9.

[73] Johnston AM, Woodcock BE. Acute aortic thrombosis despite anticoagulant therapy in idiopathic hypereosinophilic syndrome. J R Soc Med 1998;91(9):492–3.

[74] Harley JB, Fauci AS, Gralnick HR. Noncardiovascular findings associated with heart disease in the idiopathic hypereosinophilic syndrome. Am J Cardiol 1983;52(3):321–4.

[75] Tanaka H, Kawai H, Tatsumi K, et al. Surgical treatment for Loffler's endocarditis with left ventricular thrombus and severe mitral regurgitation: a case report. J Cardiol 2006;47(4): 207–13.

[76] Hanowell ST, Kim YD, Rattan V, et al. Increased heparin requirement with hypereosinophilic syndrome. Anesthesiology 1981;55(4):450–2.

[77] Vaitkus PT, Barnathan ES. Embolic potential, prevention and management of mural thrombus complicating anterior myocardial infarction: a meta-analysis. J Am Coll Cardiol 1993;22(4):1004–9.

[78] Friedman MJ, Carlson K, Marcus FI, et al. Clinical correlations in patients with acute myocardial infarction and left ventricular thrombus detected by two-dimensional echocardiography. Am J Med 1982;72(6):894–8.

[79] Visser CA, Kan G, Lie KI, et al. Left ventricular thrombus following acute myocardial infarction: a prospective serial echocardiographic study of 96 patients. Eur Heart J 1983;4(5): 333–7.

[80] Gueret P, Dubourg O, Ferrier A, et al. Effects of full-dose heparin anticoagulation on the development of left ventricular thrombosis in acute transmural myocardial infarction. J Am Coll Cardiol 1986;8(2):419–26.

[81] Davis MJ, Ireland MA. Effect of early anticoagulation on the frequency of left ventricular thrombi after anterior wall acute myocardial infarction. Am J Cardiol 1986;57(15):1244–7.

[82] Turpie AG, Robinson JG, Doyle DJ, et al. Comparison of high-dose with low-dose subcutaneous heparin to prevent left ventricular mural thrombosis in patients with acute transmural anterior myocardial infarction. N Engl J Med 1989;320(6):352–7.

[83] Nihoyannopoulos P, Smith GC, Maseri A, et al. The natural history of left ventricular thrombus in myocardial infarction: a rationale in support of masterly inactivity. J Am Coll Cardiol 1989;14(4):903–11.

[84] Anand SS, Yusuf S. Oral anticoagulant therapy in patients with coronary artery disease: a meta-analysis. JAMA 1999;282(21):2058–67.

[85] Hurlen M, Abdelnoor M, Smith P, et al. Warfarin, aspirin, or both after myocardial infarction. N Engl J Med 2002;347(13):969–74.

[86] Fiore LD, Ezekowitz MD, Brophy MT, et al. Department of Veterans Affairs Cooperative Studies Program Clinical Trial comparing combined warfarin and aspirin with aspirin alone in survivors of acute myocardial infarction: primary results of the CHAMP study. Circulation 2002;105(5):557–63.

[87] The International Stroke Trial (IST): a randomised trial of aspirin, subcutaneous heparin, both, or neither among 19435 patients with acute ischaemic stroke. International Stroke Trial Collaborative Group. Lancet 1997;349(9065):1569–81.

[88] Buller HR, Agnelli G, Hull RD, et al. Antithrombotic therapy for venous thromboembolic disease: the Seventh ACCP Conference on Antithrombotic and Thrombolytic Therapy. Chest 2004;126(3 Suppl):401S–28S.

[89] Brandjes DP, Heijboer H, Buller HR, et al. Acenocoumarol and heparin compared with acenocoumarol alone in the initial treatment of proximal-vein thrombosis. N Engl J Med 1992;327(21):1485–9.

[90] Deykin D. Warfarin therapy. 1. N Engl J Med 1970;283(13):691–4.
[91] Hirsh J, Raschke R. Heparin and low-molecular-weight heparin: the Seventh ACCP Conference on Antithrombotic and Thrombolytic Therapy. Chest 2004;126(3 Suppl): 188S–203S.
[92] Lim W, Dentali F, Eikelboom JW, et al. Meta-analysis: low-molecular-weight heparin and bleeding in patients with severe renal insufficiency. Ann Intern Med 2006;144(9):673–84.
[93] Priglinger U, Delle Karth G, Geppert A, et al. Prophylactic anticoagulation with enoxaparin: is the subcutaneous route appropriate in the critically ill? Crit Care Med 2003; 31(5):1405–9.
[94] Nieuwenhuis HK, Albada J, Banga JD, et al. Identification of risk factors for bleeding during treatment of acute venous thromboembolism with heparin or low molecular weight heparin. Blood 1991;78(9):2337–43.
[95] Zidane M, Schram MT, Planken EW, et al. Frequency of major hemorrhage in patients treated with unfractionated intravenous heparin for deep venous thrombosis or pulmonary embolism: a study in routine clinical practice. Arch Intern Med 2000;160(15):2369–73.
[96] Landefeld CS, Beyth RJ. Anticoagulant-related bleeding: clinical epidemiology, prediction, and prevention. Am J Med 1993;95(3):315–28.
[97] Palareti G, Leali N, Coccheri S, et al. Bleeding complications of oral anticoagulant treatment: an inception-cohort, prospective collaborative study (ISCOAT). Italian Study on Complications of Oral Anticoagulant Therapy. Lancet 1996;348(9025):423–8.
[98] Beyth RJ, Quinn LM, Landefeld CS. Prospective evaluation of an index for predicting the risk of major bleeding in outpatients treated with warfarin. Am J Med 1998;105(2):91–9.
[99] Buresly K, Eisenberg MJ, Zhang X, et al. Bleeding complications associated with combinations of aspirin, thienopyridine derivatives, and warfarin in elderly patients following acute myocardial infarction. Arch Intern Med 2005;165(7):784–9.
[100] Hylek EM, Singer DE. Risk factors for intracranial hemorrhage in outpatients taking warfarin. Ann Intern Med 1994;120(11):897–902.
[101] Yusuf S, Zhao F, Mehta SR, et al. Effects of clopidogrel in addition to aspirin in patients with acute coronary syndromes without ST-segment elevation. N Engl J Med 2001;345(7): 494–502.
[102] Turpie AG, Gent M, Laupacis A, et al. A comparison of aspirin with placebo in patients treated with warfarin after heart-valve replacement. N Engl J Med 1993;329(8):524–9.
[103] Anderson FA Jr, Spencer FA. Risk factors for venous thromboembolism. Circulation 2003; 107(23 Suppl 1):I9–16.
[104] Kearon C. Duration of therapy for acute venous thromboembolism. Clin Chest Med 2003; 24(1):63–72.

ELSEVIER
SAUNDERS

Immunol Allergy Clin N Am
27 (2007) 477–492

IMMUNOLOGY
AND ALLERGY
CLINICS
OF NORTH AMERICA

Pulmonary Eosinophilic Syndromes

Michael E. Wechsler, MD, MMSc

Pulmonary & Critical Care Division, Harvard Medical School,
Brigham & Women's Hospital, 15 Francis Street, Boston, MA 02115, USA

Although eosinophils are normal constituents of the lungs, several pulmonary eosinophilic syndromes are characterized by an increased number of eosinophils in peripheral blood, in lung tissue, in sputum, in bronchoalveolar lavage (BAL) fluid, or in all of these. These pulmonary eosinophilic syndromes generally are characterized by increased respiratory symptoms, abnormal radiographic appearance, and the potential for systemic manifestations. Because the eosinophil plays such an important role in each of these syndromes, it often is difficult to distinguish between them. Nonetheless, there are important clinical and pathologic differences, and because of differences in prognosis and treatment paradigms, it is important to understand and appreciate the distinguishing features of each of these conditions. This article focuses on the clinical manifestations of these syndromes, ways to distinguish between them, and on the general diagnostic approach to the patient eosinophilia and lung disease.

Classifying pulmonary eosinophilic syndromes and general approach

Eosinophilia is a feature of many different lung diseases. In some conditions, eosinophils are increased in the blood but not in the lung tissue; in other diseases, there may be significant eosinophilia in the lung tissue but not in the peripheral blood. In others, there may be lung eosinophilia without any radiographic evidence of disease. Because eosinophilia is a prominent feature of so many different diseases, the first step in classifying pulmonary eosinophilic syndromes is distinguishing between primary pulmonary eosinophilic lung disorders and those in which eosinophilia is secondary to a specific cause such as a drug reaction, an infection, a malignancy, or another pulmonary condition such as asthma. Box 1 lists primary and secondary pulmonary eosinophilic disorders, the former of which are the main focus of this article.

E-mail address: mwechsler@rics.bwh.harvard.edu

Box 1. Pulmonary eosinophilic syndromes

Primary pulmonary eosinophilic disorders
Acute eosinophilic pneumonia
Chronic eosinophilic pneumonia
Churg-Strauss syndrome
Hypereosinophilic syndrome

Pulmonary disorders of known cause associated with eosinophilia
Asthma and eosinophilic bronchitis
Allergic bronchopulmonary aspergillosis
Bronchocentric granulomatosis
Drug/toxin reaction
Infection
- Parasitic/helminthic disease
  Loffler's syndrome
  Tropical pulmonary eosinophilia
  Ascaris
  Paragonimus
  Strongyloides
  Trichinosis
- Nonparasitic infection
  Tuberculosis
  Coccidioides

Lung diseases associated with eosinophilia
Bronchiolitis obliterans organizing pneumonia
Hypersensitivity pneumonitis
Idiopathic pulmonary fibrosis
Pulmonary Langerhans cell granulomatosis

Malignant neoplasms associated with eosinophilia
Leukemia
Lymphoma
Lung cancer
Adenocarcinoma of various organs
Squamous cell carcinoma of various organs

Systemic disease associated with eosinophilia
Postradiation pneumonitis
Rheumatoid arthritis
Sarcoidosis
Sjögren's syndrome

For each patient, a detailed history is of utmost importance and can help elucidate the origin of the underlying disease. Details regarding onset, timing, and precipitants of specific symptoms can help distinguish one diagnosis from another. History regarding pharmacologic, occupational, and environmental exposures is instructive, and family and travel history is crucial. In addition to details about the sinuses and lungs, it is important to inquire about systemic manifestations and to assess for physical findings of cardiac, gastrointestinal, neurologic, dermatologic, and genitourinary involvement, all of which may give clues to specific diagnoses. Once the details from history and physical examination are teased out, laboratory testing (including measurements of blood eosinophils, cultures, and markers of inflammation), spirometry, and radiographic imaging can help distinguish between different diseases. Often, however, BAL or transbronchial or open lung biopsies are required. In many cases, biopsies or noninvasive diagnostic studies of other organs (eg, echocardiogram, electromyogram) can be helpful.

Acute eosinophilic pneumonia

First described in the 1980s, acute eosinophilic pneumonia is a syndrome characterized by fevers, acute respiratory failure that often requires mechanical ventilation, diffuse pulmonary infiltrates (Fig. 1), and pulmonary eosinophilia in a previously healthy individual (Box 2) [1,2].

Clinical features and etiology

At presentation, acute eosinophilic pneumonia often is mistaken for acute lung injury or acute respiratory distress syndrome until BAL is performed and reveals more than 25% eosinophils. The predominant symptoms of acute eosinophilic pneumonia are cough, dyspnea, malaise, myalgias, night sweats, and pleuritic chest pain. Findings on physical examination include high fevers, basilar rales, and rhonchi on forced expiration. Acute eosinophilic

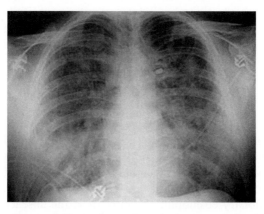

Fig. 1. Diffuse pulmonary infiltrates in a patient who has acute eosinophilic pneumonia.

Box 2. Diagnostic criteria of acute eosinophilic pneumonia

Acute febrile illness with respiratory manifestations of more than
  1 month's duration
Hypoxemic respiratory failure
Diffuse pulmonary infiltrates on chest radiograph
BAL eosinophilia > 25%
Absence of parasitic, fungal, or other infection
Absence of drugs known to cause pulmonary eosinophilia
Quick clinical response to corticosteroids
Failure to relapse after discontinuation of corticosteroids

---

pneumonia most often affects men between ages of 20 and 40 years who have no history of asthma. Although no clear etiology has been identified, several case reports have linked acute eosinophilic pneumonia to recent initiation of tobacco smoking or exposure to other environmental stimuli including dust from indoor renovations [3] or even World Trade Center dust [4].

Laboratory and radiologic features

In addition to a suggestive history, the key to establishing a diagnosis of acute eosinophilic pneumonia is the presence of more than 25% eosinophilia in BAL fluid. Lung biopsies show eosinophilic infiltration with acute and organizing diffuse alveolar damage, but it generally is not necessary to proceed to biopsy to establish a diagnosis [5]. Although patients present with an elevated white blood cell count, in contrast to other pulmonary eosinophilic syndromes, acute eosinophilic pneumonia often is not associated with peripheral eosinophilia on presentation. Peripheral eosinophilia often occurs, however, between 7 and 30 days after disease onset, with mean eosinophil counts of 1700 cells/mm^3 [3]. The erythrocyte sedimentation rate (ESR) and C-reactive protein and IgE levels are high but nonspecific; high-resolution CT is always abnormal with bilateral random patchy, ground-glass, or reticular opacities and small pleural effusions in as many as two thirds of patients [6]. Pleural fluid is characterized by a high pH with marked eosinophilia. Pulmonary function testing is notable for a restrictive defect with a reduced diffusion capacity.

Clinical course and response to therapy

Although some patients improve spontaneously [3], most patients require admission to an ICU and respiratory support with either invasive (intubation) on noninvasive mechanical ventilation. What distinguishes acute eosinophilic pneumonia from other cases of acute lung injury and from some of the other pulmonary eosinophilic syndromes is the absence of organ dysfunction or multisystem organ failure other than respiratory failure. One of the other characteristic features of acute eosinophilic pneumonia is the high degree of corticosteroid responsiveness and the excellent prognosis. Another distinguishing feature of acute eosinophilic pneumonia is the complete clinical and radiographic recovery without recurrence or residual sequelae that occurs in almost all patients within several weeks of initiation of therapy.

Chronic eosinophilic pneumonia

In contrast to acute eosinophilic pneumonia, chronic eosinophilic pneumonia is a more indolent syndrome that is characterized by pulmonary infiltrates and eosinophilia in both the tissue and blood (Box 3) [7]. Most patients are female nonsmokers with a mean age of 45 years, and patients usually do not develop the acute respiratory failure and significant hypoxemia seen in acute eosinophilic pneumonia [5]. As in Churg-Strauss syndrome (CSS), most patients have asthma, and many have a history of allergies. The airflow obstruction tends to worsen with disease activity but responds to corticosteroids.

Clinical and radiographic features

Patients present with a subacute illness over weeks to months, with cough, low-grade fevers, progressive dyspnea, weight loss, wheezing, malaise, night sweats, and a chest radiograph with migratory bilateral, peripheral, or pleural-based opacities. Although this "photographic-negative pulmonary edema" appearance on chest radiograph and chest CT is pathognomonic of chronic eosinophilic pneumonia, fewer than 25% of patients present with this finding (Fig. 2) [8]. Other radiographic findings include atelectasis, pleural effusions, lymphadenopathy, and septal line thickening [9].

Laboratory features

Almost 90% of patients have peripheral eosinophilia with mean eosinophil counts of more than 30% of the total white blood cell count [10]. BAL eosinophilia is also an important distinguishing feature with mean BAL eosinophil counts close to 60%. Both peripheral and BAL eosinophilia are very responsive to treatment with corticosteroids. Other laboratory features of chronic eosinophilic pneumonia include increased ESR, C-reactive protein, platelets,

---

Box 3. Chronic eosinophilic pneumonia

1. Respiratory symptoms of usually more than 2 weeks' duration
2. BAL and/or blood eosinophilia
3. Pulmonary infiltrates (often with a peripheral predominance on chest imaging)
4. Exclusion of any known cause of eosinophilic lung disease.

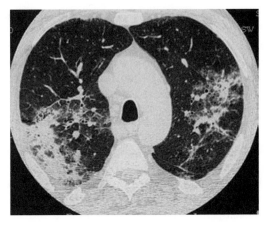

Fig. 2. Peripheral pulmonary infiltrates in a patient who has chronic eosinophilic pneumonia. (*From* Cottin V, Cordier JF. Eosinophilic pneumonias. Allergy 2005;60:844; with permission.)

and IgE. Often lung biopsy is not required to establish a diagnosis but may show accumulation of eosinophils and histiocytes in the lung parenchyma and interstitium, as well as bronchiolitis obliterans organizing pneumonia, but with minimal fibrosis (Fig. 3).

Systemic manifestations and treatment response

Similar to acute eosinophilic pneumonia, nonrespiratory manifestations are uncommon, but arthralgias, neuropathy, and skin and gastrointestinal symptoms have been reported [5]; their presence may suggest CSS or hyper-eosinophilic syndrome (HES). Another similarity is the rapid response to corticosteroids with quick resolution of peripheral and BAL eosinophilia

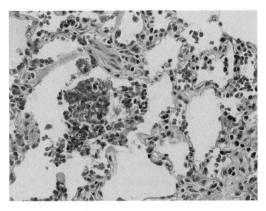

Fig. 3. Accumulation of intra-alveolar eosinophils in chronic eosinophilic pneumonia (hematoxylin and eosin, original magnification ×40). (*Courtesy of* Yadira Sanchez and Sara Vargas, Boston Children's Hospital, Boston, MA.)

and improvement in symptoms. In contrast to acute eosinophilic pneumonia, however, more than 50% of patients relapse, and many require prolonged courses of corticosteroids for months to years [10].

Churg-Strauss syndrome

Also known as "allergic angiitis granulomatosis," CSS is a complex syndrome characterized by eosinophilic vasculitis that may involve multiple organ systems including the lungs, heart, skin, gastrointestinal tract, and nervous system. Although CSS is characterized by peripheral and pulmonary eosinophilia with infiltrates on chest radiograph, the primary features that distinguish CSS from other pulmonary eosinophilic syndromes are the presence of eosinophilic vasculitis in the setting of asthma and the involvement of multiple end organs (a feature it shares with HES). Although perceived to be quite rare, the incidence of this disease seems to have increased in the last few years, particularly in association with various asthma therapies [11].

Diagnostic criteria

Diagnostic criteria have included both clinical and pathologic features (Box 4), but the criteria most commonly used to describe CSS are those adopted by the American College of Rheumatology in 1990 [12]. These criteria include both clinical and pathologic features and define CSS as the presence of four of the following six features: asthma, eosinophilia, neuropathy, pulmonary infiltrates, paranasal sinus abnormality, and presence of eosinophilic vasculitis (Fig. 4).

Clinical features

CSS occurs with equal frequency in men and women and typically occurs in several phases [13]. The prodromal phase is characterized by asthma and allergic rhinitis and usually begins when the individual is in his/her 20s or 30s, typically persisting for many years. The eosinophilic infiltrative phase is characterized by peripheral eosinophilia and eosinophilic tissue infiltration of various organs including the lungs and gastrointestinal tract. The third phase is the vasculitic phase and may be associated with constitutional signs and symptoms including fever, weight loss, malaise, and fatigue. The mean age at time of diagnosis is 48 years with a range of 14 to 74 years; the average length of time between diagnosis of asthma and vasculitis is 9 years [14].

Similar to other pulmonary eosinophilic syndromes, constitutional symptoms are common in CSS and include weight loss of 10 to 20 lb, fevers, and diffuse myalgias and migratory polyarthralgias. Myositis may be present with evidence of vasculitis on muscle biopsies. In contrast to the eosinophilic pneumonias, CSS involves many organ systems including the lungs, skin, nerves, heart, gastrointestinal tract, and kidneys.

Box 4. Criteria used in diagnosis of Churg-Strauss syndrome

Churg and Strauss, 1951
1. Asthma
2. Necrotizing vasculitis of small and medium arteries and veins
3. Eosinophil infiltration around involved vessels and tissues
4. Extravascular granulomas
5. Fibrinoid necrosis of involved tissues

Lanham, 1984
1. Asthma
2. Eosinophilia > 1.5 × 107
3. Systemic vasculitis involving two or more organs

American College of Rheumatology, 1990
1. Asthma
2. Eosinophilia > 10%
3. Neuropathy
4. Pulmonary infiltrates
5. Paranasal sinus abnormality
6. Extravascular eosinophil infiltration on biopsy

Chapel Hill, 1994
1. Asthma
2. Eosinophilia
3. Eosinophil-rich granulomatous inflammation involving the respiratory tract
4. Necrotizing vasculitis affecting small- to medium-sized vessels

---

Data from Wechsler ME, Pauwels R, Drazen JD. Leukotriene modifiers and Churg-Strauss syndrome: adverse effect or response to corticosteroid withdrawal? Drug Saf 1999;21:241–51.

Respiratory. Almost all patients who have CSS have asthma that arises in adulthood with a mean age of onset of 35 years. It often occurs in individuals who have no family history of atopy. The asthma is usually severe; oral corticosteroids often are required to control symptoms but may lead to suppression of vasculitic symptoms. Although the severity of asthma may increase as the underlying disease progresses, asthma symptoms may abate in some instances as the vasculitis becomes manifest. Common symptoms include cough, dyspnea, sinusitis, and allergic rhinitis; alveolar hemorrhage and hemoptysis also may occur.

Neurologic. More than three fourths of patients who have CSS have neurologic manifestations [14]. Mononeuritis multiplex often involves the

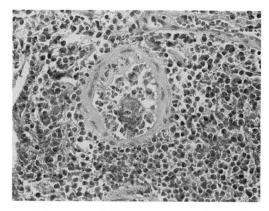

Fig. 4. Eosinophilic vasculitis in the lung of a patient who has Churg-Strauss syndrome. (*Courtesy of* Yadira Sanchez and Sara Vargas, Boston Children's Hospital, Boston, MA.)

peroneal nerve but also can affect the ulnar, radial, internal popliteal, and, occasionally, cranial nerves. Polyneuropathy often develops in the absence of treatment and may be symmetric or asymmetric. Cerebral hemorrhage and infarction can be important causes of death in these patients. Despite treatment, neurologic sequelae are common.

Dermatologic. Approximately half of patients who have CSS develop dermatologic manifestations. These manifestations include palpable purpura, skin nodules, urticarial rashes, and livedo.

Cardiovascular. The heart is a primary target organ in CSS, and heart involvement often portends a worse prognosis [13]. Granulomas, vasculitis, and widespread myocardial damage may be found on biopsy or at autopsy. Cardiomyopathy and heart failure may be seen in up to half of all patients but often are at least partially reversible. Acute pericarditis, constrictive pericarditis, myocardial infarction, and other electrocardiographic changes may occur.

Gastrointestinal. Eosinophilic infiltration of the gastrointestinal tract may result in abdominal pain, diarrhea, gastrointestinal bleeding, and colitis. Ischemic bowel, pancreatitis, and cholecystitis also have been reported in association with CSS and usually portend a worse prognosis [15].

Renal. Renal involvement is more common than once thought. Approximately 25% of patients have some degree of renal involvement that may include proteinuria, glomerulonephritis, renal insufficiency, and, rarely, renal infarct. Systemic hypertension also is common.

Laboratory abnormalities

Eosinophilia greater than 10% is one of the defining features of this illness and may be as high as 75% of the peripheral white blood cell count. It is present at the time of diagnosis in more than 80% of subjects but may respond quickly (often within 24 hours) to initiation of systemic corticosteroid therapy. Even in the absence of systemic eosinophilia, tissue eosinophilia may be present.

Although not specific to CSS, antineutrophil cytoplasmic antibodies (ANCA), mostly with a perinuclear staining pattern, are present in up to two thirds of patients [16]. Nonspecific laboratory abnormalities that may be present in patients who have CSS include a marked elevation in ESR, a normochromic normocytic anemia, an elevated IgE, hypergammaglobulinemia, and positive rheumatoid factor and antinuclear antibodies. BAL often reveals significant eosinophilia, but this sign may be seen in the other eosinophilic lung diseases. Pulmonary function testing often reveals an obstructive defect similar to asthma.

Radiographic features

Chest radiographic abnormalities are extremely common in CSS and consist of bilateral, nonsegmental, patchy infiltrates that often migrate and may be interstitial or alveolar in appearance. Reticulonodular and nodular disease without cavitation can be seen, as can pleural effusions and hilar adenopathy. The most common CT findings include bilateral ground-glass opacity and airspace consolidation that is predominantly subpleural [17]. Other CT findings include bronchial wall thickening, hyperinflation, interlobular septal thickening, lymph node enlargement, and pericardial and pleural effusions. Angiography may be used diagnostically and may show signs of vasculitis in the coronary, central nervous system, and peripheral vasculature.

Etiology and pathologic features of Churg-Strauss syndrome

Like other pulmonary eosinophilic syndromes, the exact etiology of CSS is unknown. CSS probably represents an autoimmune process because of the prominence of allergic features and the presence of immune complexes, heightened T-cell immunity, and altered humoral immunity, as evidenced by elevated levels of serum IgE and rheumatoid factor. The presence of ANCA in about half of patents also suggests an immune-mediated mechanism. Although the exact role of ANCA in CSS and other vasculitides remains unclear, the binding of ANCA to vascular walls is thought to contribute to vascular inflammation and injury as well as to chemotaxis of inflammatory cells. CSS has been associated with various asthma therapies, including leukotriene modifiers [18,19] and inhaled corticosteroids [20], but no causal link has been established. It seems either that the syndrome occurs coincidentally to the use of these medications or that these medications facilitate systemic steroid withdrawal that unmasks the syndrome.

Pathologically, CSS is characterized by tissue infiltration by eosinophils, extravascular granulomas, and necrotizing vasculitis, which may occur in isolation or may coexist and commonly are found in the lungs, heart, skin, muscle, liver, spleen, and kidneys. The eosinophilic vasculitis predominantly affects small and medium-sized arteries and veins and may include fibrinoid necrosis and thrombosis. Granulomas are not seen in many patients but when present are peri- or extravascular and are characterized by degenerated eosinophils with necrotic collagen at the center, surrounded by epithelioid cells and giant cells.

Treatment and prognosis of Churg-Strauss syndrome

Most patients diagnosed as having CSS have been diagnosed previously as having asthma, rhinitis, and sinusitis and have received treatment for these disorders with inhaled or systemic corticosteroids. In patients who have CSS but who are perceived to have severe asthma, these therapies may delay the diagnosis of CSS by masking the signs of vasculitis. Corticosteroids dramatically alter the course of CSS: up to 50% of those who are untreated die within 3 months of diagnosis [21], but in treated patients the 6-year survival rate exceeds 70% [14]. Common causes of death include heart failure, cerebral hemorrhage, renal failure, and gastrointestinal bleeding. Recent data suggest that clinical remission may be obtained in more than 90% of patients treated. Approximately 25% of those patients may relapse, often because of corticosteroid tapering; a rising eosinophil count heralds the relapse [14]. Myocardial, gastrointestinal, and renal involvement most often portends a poor prognosis. In such cases, treatment with higher doses of corticosteroids or the addition of cytotoxic agents such as cyclophosphamide often is warranted. Although survival does not differ between those treated or not treated with cyclophosphamide, treatment is associated with a reduced incidence of relapse and an improved clinical response to treatment [15]. Other therapies that have been used successfully in the management of CSS include azathioprine, methotrexate, mycophenolate, intravenous gamma globulin, and interferon alpha. Plasma exchange has not been shown to provide any additional benefit [14].

Hypereosinophilic syndrome

A detailed overview of the main HES (those not primarily involving the lung) is given elsewhere in this volume. Briefly, HES constitutea a heterogeneous group of disease entities manifest by persistent eosinophilia in excess of 1500 eosinophils/mm^3 in association with end-organ damage or dysfunction, in the absence of secondary causes of eosinophilia [22]. In addition to familial, undefined, and overlap syndromes with incomplete criteria, the predominant HES subtypes are the myeloproliferative and lymphocytic variants (Box 5). The myeloproliferative variant may be divided into three subgroups: (1) chronic eosinophilic leukemia with demonstrable cytogenetic

Box 5. Hypereosinophilic syndromes

Myeloproliferative variants
Etiology unknown
PDGFRA-associated HES
Chronic eosinophilic leukemia

Lymphocytic variants
Familial
Undefined
  • Benign
  • Complex
  • Episodic

Overlap/organ-restricted eosinophilic disorders (including eosinophilic pneumonia)

Associated conditions (including CSS)

abnormalities and/or blasts on peripheral smear; (2) the PDGFRA-associated HES attributed to a constitutively activated tyrosine kinase fusion protein (Fip1L1-PDGFRα) caused by a chromosomal deletion on 4q12; and (3) the FIP1-negative variant associated with eosinophilia and at least four of the following: dysplastic peripheral eosinophils, increased serum B_{12}, increased tryptase, anemia, thrombocytopenia, splenomegaly, bone marrow cellularity in excess of 80%, spindle-shaped mast cells, and myelofibrosis. In the lymphocytic variant, hypereosinophilia seems to occur in response to the production of eosinophilopoietic cytokines, particularly interleukin-5, by clonal populations of phenotypically abnormal, activated T lymphocytes [23]. In these patients T-cell receptor rearrangement analysis often demonstrates T-cell clonality, and serum IgE and thymus- and activation-regulated chemokine levels are elevated.

Extrapulmonary manifestations of hypereosinophilic syndrome
    More common in men than in women, HES occurs between the ages of 20 and 50 years and is characterized by significant extrapulmonary involvement, including infiltration of the heart, gastrointestinal tract, kidney, liver, joints, and skin. Cardiac involvement includes myocarditis and/or endomyocardial fibrosis, as well as a restrictive cardiomyopathy [23].

Pulmonary manifestations of hypereosinophilic syndrome
    As in other pulmonary eosinophilic syndromes, patients who have HES manifest high levels of blood, BAL, and tissue eosinophilia. Lung involvement occurs in 40% of these patients and is characterized by cough, dyspnea, and pulmonary infiltrates [5]. Although it often is difficult to discern

the pulmonary infiltrates and effusions seen on chest radiography from pulmonary edema resulting from cardiac involvement, findings on CT scan include interstitial infiltrates, ground-glass opacities, and small nodules. HES typically is not associated with ANCA.

Course and response to therapy

Unlike the other pulmonary eosinophilic syndromes, less than half of patients who have HES respond to corticosteroids as first-line therapy. Treatment options include hydroxyurea, cyclosporine, and interferon, but imatinib has emerged as an important therapeutic option for patients who have the myeloproliferative variant. Anti-interleukin-5 therapy with mepolizumab also holds promise for these patients and is being investigated currently.

Diagnosis and differential diagnosis of pulmonary eosinophilic syndromes

The key to managing the pulmonary eosinophilic syndromes is establishing a firm diagnosis. The first step in this process is excluding secondary causes of pulmonary eosinophilia, as listed in Box 1. One must exclude one of the many medications or toxins that have been associated with eosinophilic lung diseases. One must rule out parasitic involvement caused by infestation by nematodes such as *Ascaris* and *Strongyloides* and other parasites that can cause tropical eosinophilia or Loffler's syndrome. One must exclude *Aspergillus* colonization that may be associated with allergic bronchopulmonary aspergillosis, as well as infection with other micro-organisms. Finally, one must take a careful history and perform a detailed evaluation to exclude malignancies, other systemic conditions such as sarcoidosis, and other lung diseases such as pulmonary fibrosis and bronchiolitis obliterans, each of which may present with eosinophilia.

Because all of the pulmonary eosinophilic syndromes are characterized by blood and BAL eosinophilia as well as pulmonary infiltrates, it can be difficult to differentiate between them. Indeed, it often is speculated that all these conditions are related and on a continuum, with some unknown mechanism responsible for targeting eosinophils and their toxins to specific organs, such as the lung. Nonetheless, one can often establish a diagnosis by using a combination of clinical, laboratory, pathologic, and radiographic criteria (Table 1).

For instance, isolated pulmonary involvement with peripheral eosinophilia is associated with either acute or chronic eosinophilic pneumonias, depending on the relative acuity of symptoms. Generally, the presence of ANCA or vasculitis and eosinophilia in an individual who has airway obstruction is sufficient for a diagnosis of CSS. Patients who have HES have eosinophilia with multiorgan involvement and may present in a manner similar to CSS; however, these entities are not associated with vasculitis and often do not have asthma as a primary disease feature. Bronchoscopy with

Table 1
Distinguishing features of various eosinophilic lung diseases

Feature	Acute eosinophilic pneumonia	Chronic eosinophilic pneumonia	Churg-Strauss syndrome	Hypereosinophilic syndrome
Onset	Acute (days)	Indolent (weeks/months)	Indolent (months/years)	Indolent (months/years)
Imaging	Diffuse	Peripheral	Patchy	Patchy
Fulminant respiratory failure	++	−	−	−
Asthma/allergy history	−	+	++	−
Smoking history	+	−	−	−
Vasculitis	−	−	++	−
Antineutrophil cytoplasmic antibody	−	−	+	−
Cardiac involvement	−	±	+	++
Neurologic	−	±	++	++
Requirement for therapies other than corticosteroids	−	−	+	++

Abbreviations: −, rarely occurs; +/−, occasionally occurs; +, commonly occurs; ++, occurs most of the time.

BAL should be considered in cases of lung disease with eosinophilia. If the BAL is unrevealing, consideration should be given to obtaining lung tissue by means of a transbronchial or open-lung biopsy, depending on the clinical and radiographic findings. Video-assisted thoracoscopic surgery (VATS) can substitute for a thoracotomy to provide tissue. If disease is more parenchymal and peripheral, a transbronchial biopsy is less likely to be revealing, and VATS or a limited thoracotomy should be considered.

Although a biopsy specimen often can help tease out differences, noninvasive surrogates including CT scan, electromyogram, nerve conduction studies, or other blood tests often can be used to establish a diagnosis. Once the proper diagnosis is established, one can treat the specific disease entity appropriately. Work-up of the patient who has eosinophilia and lung disease thus should include the following laboratory studies: complete blood cell count with differential, ESR, C-reactive protein, ANCA, vitamin B_{12}, immunoglobulins including IgE, electrolytes and liver enzymes, tryptase, urinalysis, stool assessment for ova and parasites, and strong consideration of bone marrow analysis. All organ systems should be evaluated including consideration of the following: dilated eye examination, EKG, echocardiogram, pulmonary function studies, detailed skin, vascular, and neurologic examinations, and consideration of imaging of specific organs such as the lungs, heart, kidney, and gastrointestinal tract.

Summary

Pulmonary eosinophilic syndromes are a heterogeneous group of disorders that are associated with peripheral blood and/or tissue eosinophilia. It is critical to make a quick diagnosis and to treat aggressively with corticosteroids and other therapies to prevent long-term sequelae. Establishing a diagnosis is facilitated by the use of noninvasive and invasive markers and by judicious use of CT scans and other tests.

References

[1] Badesch DB, King TE, Schwarz MI. Acute eosinophilic pneumonia: a hypersensitivity phenomenon. Am Rev Respir Dis 1989;139:249–52.

[2] Allen JN, Pacht ER, Gadek JE, et al. Acute eosinophilic pneumonia as a reversible cause of noninfectious respiratory failure. N Engl J Med 1989;321:569–74.

[3] Philit F, Etienne-Mastroianni B, Parrot A, et al. Idiopathic acute eosinophilic pneumonia: a study of 22 patients. The Groupe d'Etudes et de Recherche sur les Maladies Orphelines Pulmonaires (GERMO'P). Am J Respir Crit Care Med 2002;166:1235–9.

[4] Rom WN, Weiden M, Garcia R, et al. Acute eosinophilic pneumonia in a New York City firefighter exposed to World Trade Center dust. Am J Respir Crit Care Med 2002;166: 797–800.

[5] Cottin V, Cordier JF. Eosinophilic pneumonias. Allergy 2005;60:841–57.

[6] Cheon JE, Lee KS, Jung GS, et al. Acute eosinophilic pneumonia: radiographic and CT findings in six patients. Am J Roentgenol 1996;167:1195–9.

[7] Carrington CB, Addington WW, Goff AM, et al. Chronic eosinophilic pneumonia. N Engl J Med 1969;280:787–98.

[8] Jederlinic PJ, Sicilian L, Gaensler EA. Chronic eosinophilic pneumonia. A report of 19 cases and a review of the literature. Medicine (Baltimore) 1988;67:154–62.

[9] Arakawa H, Kurihara Y, Niimi H, et al. Bronchiolitis obliterans with organizing pneumonia versus chronic eosinophilic pneumonia: high-resolution CT findings in 81 patients. Am J Roentgenol 2001;176:1053–8.

[10] Marchand E, Reynaud-Gaubert M, Lauque D, et al. Idiopathic chronic eosinophilic pneumonia. A clinical and follow-up study of 62 cases. The Groupe 'Etudes et de Recherche sur les Maladies Orphelines Pulmonaires (GERMO'P). Medicine (Baltimore) 1998;77: 299–312.

[11] Wechsler ME, Pauwels R, Drazen JD. Leukotriene modifiers and Churg-Strauss syndrome: adverse effect or response to corticosteroid withdrawal? Drug Saf 1999;21:241–51.

[12] Masi AT, Hunder GG, Lie JT, et al. The American College of Rheumatology 1990 criteria for the classification of Churg-Strauss syndrome (allergic granulomatosis and angiitis). Arthritis Rheum 1990;33(8):1094–100.

[13] Lanham JG, Elkon KB, Pusey CD, et al. Systemic vasculitis with asthma and eosinophilia: a clinical approach to the Churg-Strauss syndrome. Medicine 1983;63:65–81.

[14] Guillevin L, Cohen P, Gayraud M, et al. Churg-Strauss syndrome: clinical study and long-term follow-up of 96 patients. Medicine 1999;78:26–37.

[15] Conron M, Beynon HLC. Churg-Strauss syndrome. Thorax 2000;55:870–7.

[16] Hagen EC, Daha MR, Hermans J, et al. The diagnostic value of standardized assays for antineutrophil cytoplasmic antibodies in idiopathic systemic vasculitis. Kidney Int 1998;53: 743–53.

[17] Choi YH, Im JG, Han BK, et al. Thoracic manifestations of Churg-Strauss syndrome. Chest 2000;117:117–24.

[18] Wechsler ME, Garpestad E, Flier SR, et al. Pulmonary infiltrates, eosinophilia, and cardio-myopathy following corticosteroid withdrawal in patients with asthma receiving zafirlukast. JAMA 1998;279:455–7.

[19] Wechsler ME, Finn D, Gunawardena D, et al. Churg-Strauss syndrome in patients receiving montelukast as treatment for asthma. Chest 2000;117:708–13.

[20] Le Gall C, Pham S, Vignes S, et al. Inhaled corticosteroids and Churg-Strauss syndrome: a report of five cases. Eur Respir J 2000;15(5):978–81.

[21] Allen JN, Davis WB. Eosinophilic lung diseases. Am J Respir Crit Care Med 1994;150: 1423–38.

[22] Klion AD, Bochner BS, Gleich GJ, et al. Approaches to the treatment of hypereosinophilic syndromes: a workshop summary report. J Allergy Clin Immunol 2006;117:1292–302.

[23] Klion AD. Recent advances in the diagnosis and treatment of hypereosinophilic syndromes. Hematology 2005;209–14.

ELSEVIER
SAUNDERS

Immunol Allergy Clin N Am
27 (2007) 493–518

IMMUNOLOGY
AND ALLERGY
CLINICS
OF NORTH AMERICA

Treatment of Hypereosinophilic Syndromes with Prednisone, Hydroxyurea, and Interferon

Joseph H. Butterfield, MD[a,b,*]

[a]Division of Allergic Diseases, Mayo Clinic, 200 First Street SW, Rochester, MN 55905, USA
[b]Mayo Clinic College of Medicine, 200 First Street SW, Rochester, MN 55905, USA

The subclassification of hypereosinophilic syndromes (HES) continues to improve as the molecular basis for these serious ailments becomes better understood. It is only natural to anticipate that treatment options for patients with HES will evolve as well. This has, indeed, been the case with the introduction of imatinib mesylate and anti-interleukin (IL)-5 monoclonal antibodies, such as mepolizumab. Yet, for many patients with hypereosinophilia, prednisone, hydroxyurea, and interferon alpha 2b (IFN-α) provide a rational and cost-effective approach to treatment.

Experience with these medications is extensive. Even for IFN-α, the most recent of these agents, clinical experience with its use in the treatment of HES now extends to over 15 years. Additionally, judicious dosing with combinations of these medications will frequently allow excellent control of eosinophilia, while avoiding side effects attendant with high doses of any one of them used as a single agent. Finally, with time, the doses necessary for control of eosinophilia often decreases, thereby reducing the possibility of side effects and lowering the cost of treatment.

There has never been a double-blind crossover study of the effectiveness of any of the current treatments used for HES. The use of glucocorticoids (GC) as treatment options for HES evolved from their known anti-inflammatory effects, discovered [1,2] and applied [3,4] in the mid 20th century. Although clinical observations dating back to the early 20th century documented a marked eosinopenia in various clinical emergencies [5,6], another 50 years passed before the role of the adrenal cortex in these processes was appreciated. The diurnal variation in eosinophil numbers [7–9] was

---

* Division of Allergic Diseases, Mayo Clinic, 200 First Street SW, Rochester, MN 55905.
E-mail address: butterfield.joseph@mayo.edu

recognized as a phenomenon that was in antiphase with serum cortisol concentrations [10], and was absent in human beings with severe untreated adrenal cortical insufficiency [8]. The Thorn test for adrenal cortical insufficiency was based on the failure of hypoadrenal patients to develop eosinopenia following corticotropin (ACTH) administration [11,12].

Glucocorticoid treatment of hypereosinophilic syndromes

In vitro studies

Eosinophils and glucocorticoid receptors

Eosinophils possess approximately 11 thousand high-affinity (Kd = 15.3 ± 0.6 nM dexamethasone) GC receptor sites per cell [13], indicating that receptor-ligand interactions on eosinophils can occur at physiologic concentrations of GC. Eosinophils from patients with HES, however, are heterogeneous in their GC receptor expression and GC binding sites may, in fact, be undetectable on HES eosinophils [14].

Glucocorticoid effect on eosinophils and eosinophilopoiesis

The eosinopenia that develops and reaches a nadir 4 hours after cortisone administration to normal volunteers [15,16] cannot be explained by either a "lytic" effect on eosinophils [17] or by sequestration of eosinophils in the reticuloendothelial system [18,19]. To examine this effect further, researchers have examined the effect of GC on eosinophil colony-forming cells (EO-CFC). Yet in vitro studies of GC on eosinophil colony growth have yielded a mixed picture of their effects and mechanism of action. These studies have used various GC model systems, readouts, and sources of EO-CFC (bone marrow and peripheral blood from normal volunteers, atopic patients, and HES patients) as well as CD34+ cells. Several studies have shown no effect of GC on eosinophil division and colony formation, even at nonphysiologic concentrations of GC [20,21], whereas others have demonstrated colony inhibition by a direct [22] effect on EO-CFC or by an indirect effect via accessory cells [23]. These results have done little to clarify the mechanism of the clinical effect of GC to cause eosinopenia, and suggest that eosinophil colony formation may not be an adequate model for examining the effect of GCs on eosinophilopoiesis.

In vitro effect of glucocorticoids on the production and action of eosinophil-active cytokines

In many reports GC have been shown to inhibit the effect of eosinophil-active cytokines derived from various cellular sources.

Eosinophil colony-stimulating factor. In an early work, Raghavachar and colleagues [24] showed that addition of hydrocortisone to T-cell clones from an HES patient inhibited production of eosinophil colony-stimulating factor in a double-layer agar culture system.

Granulocyte-macrophage colony-stimulating factor. Various GC inhibit the eosinophil survival-promoting activity of granulocyte-macrophage colony-stimulating factor (GM-CSF), through a direct effect on the eosinophils [25] and by inhibiting production of GM-CSF [26].

Interleukin-5. IL-5, the predominant cytokine produced by HES-derived T-cells [27] enhances eosinophil survival, chemotaxis, and activation [28,29]. In addition, in some HES patients, abnormal clones of CD3$^-$CD4$^+$ or CD3$^+$CD4$^-$CD8$^-$ T-cells that produce IL-5 are present [30]. Dexamethasone acts at the level of gene transcription, as well as by posttranscriptional mechanisms, to inhibit IL-5 synthesis and release. Expression of the IL-5 gene in human peripheral blood mononuclear cells is inhibited by dexamethasone in doses as low as 10^{-9}M [31].

Effects on eosinophil apoptosis and survival

IL-5's enhancement of eosinophil survival can be inhibited by dexamethasone and methylprednisolone, but not by hydrocortisone [32]. Incubation of normodense eosinophils with increasing concentrations of GM-CSF, IL-3, or IL-5 abolishes this effect [33]. The problems with applying in vitro studies to clinical practice are no better illustrated than by examination of the effect of GC on eosinophil apoptosis. The results of several studies are summarized in Table 1, and show that depending on the source of eosinophils (HES patients, normal volunteers, asymptomatic atopic patients, or cord blood-derived eosinophils) and in vitro culture conditions, an increase, decrease, or no effect on apoptosis may be found [34–39]. For a comprehensive

Table 1
Results of eosinophil apoptosis studies

Eosinophil source	GC used	Effect on apoptosis	Reference
Normal volunteers, Asymptomatic atopics	Dexamethasone	Increased	[37]
Normal volunteers	Mometasone	Increased	[38]
Eosinophils from HES patients[a]	Dexamethasone	Heterogeneous responses (−16.8%-inhibition of apoptosis to +87.8%)	[35]
Healthy Subjects	Dexamethasone	Increased $P = .002$	[35]
Cord Blood CD-34(+'ve) cells + cytokines	Dexamethasone	Decrease apoptosis in day 7 cultures $P < .02$ No significant change in day 14 cultures Increased apoptosis in day 21 and day 28 cultures $P < .02$	[34]
Eosinophils from HES patients	Dexamethasone	Increased	[36]

[a] In vitro effect did not correlate with clinical effect of steroids.

review of GC-induced apoptotic effects on human eosinophils, see Druilhe and colleagues [40].

Clinical experience with corticotropin and glucocorticoids
in hypereosinophilic syndromes

The circulating eosinophil population in HES is comprised of cells with a prolonged half-life [41]. In early studies, hydrocortisone infusion to two subjects with marked eosinophilia caused an exponential decrease of circulating cells in one patient and a linear decrease in the second, suggesting that in hypereosinophilic states the kinetics of eosinophil production and loss from the circulation may vary markedly [42]. Corticotropin (20 mg–50 mg four times daily) administered to eosinophilic ($1000/mm^3$–$15,000/mm^3$) patients was shown to decrease peripheral eosinophil levels but had no effect on medullary eosinophil numbers [43]. This finding was substantiated in several subsequent studies in which GC administration caused disparate results in the peripheral blood (eosinopenia) and bone marrow (increase or no change) [35,44,45].

Corticotropin and GC were used early-on in attempts to control "eosinophilic leukemia" and "disseminated eosinophilic collagen disease." The term "hypereosinophilic syndromes" was not used before 1968. As reflected below, the early clinical reports suffer from a lack of uniformity in the clinical terminology and criteria used to delineate eosinophilic syndromes, and by the variability of the dose, duration, and type of GC used.

The decade of the 1940s saw the discovery of the potent anti-inflammatory effect of corticotropin and cortisone [3,46] and the realization that adrenal cortical activity caused eosinopenia [11]. The decade of the 1950s was dominated by reports of the use of corticotropin for eosinophilia. In 1953 Rothstein and colleagues [47] first reported the benefit of corticotropin in eosinophilic leukemia. This case was followed by others, describing reduction—often temporary—in eosinophil numbers, and symptomatic improvement from corticotropin use [48,49]. During the decade of the 1960s reports of GC use began to supplant those of corticotropin for eosinophilic disorders. These reports were notable for wide ranges of dosages and treatment durations. Treatment of "eosinophilic leukemia" [50–53], "fibroplastic parietal endocarditis with eosinophilia" [54,55], "collagen disease with eosinophilia" [56], and "disseminated eosinophilic collagen disease" [57] with GC gave results that were not always successful or long lasting.

Hardy and Anderson in 1968 [58] distinguished "hypereosinophilic syndromes" from eosinophilic leukemia. Nonetheless, for many years, diverse terminology persisted. The duration of treatment, dosages of GC used, and effectiveness in these conditions were far from uniform perhaps, in part, reflecting the nonstandardization of cases described [59–64]. Finally, in 1975 Chusid and colleagues [65] published the criteria that since have served as the basis for defining the HES, thereby establishing a level playing field for comparing treatment responses. Of the 13 reports of "physiologic to massive doses of prednisone, dexamethasone, and cortisone" and 5 reports of corticotropin cited in the literature to that time, little permanent change in total eosinophilic counts or clinical symptoms was found [65]. Within a few years, a study by Parrillo and colleagues [66] of 26 subjects fulfilling the criteria for HES reported that prednisone (60 mg/day for 1–2 weeks) gave a good (38%) or partial (31%) response, and that responders could be maintained with burst or every-other-day regimens. Their patients had a significant improvement in 3-year survival when compared with historical controls, among whom the median survival time was 12 months.

Characteristics of glucocorticoid nonresponders and glucocorticoid responders

Not all HES patients respond equally well to GC. From Parrilo's [66] report, approximately 30% of HES patients did not respond to GC. Patients with elevated levels of serum B_{12} [67], folate deficiency, basophilia greater than 3%, bone marrow chromosomal abnormalities, and low leukocyte alkaline phosphatase scores did not respond well to GC. Subsequent reports suggest that the lack of response to GC correlates with the absence of detectable GC receptor expression in HES patients [14]. In one case, disappearance of GC binding correlated with the appearance of leukemic markers [14].

Characteristics of patients who responded well to GC included increased serum IgE levels (2338 ± 684 international units or IU/mL for responders versus 51 ± 27 IU/mL for nonresponders) and clinical findings of episodic severe angioedema, a profound and prolonged eosinopenic response 4 to 12 hours after challenge with prednisone 60 mg, and lack of hepatosplenomegaly [65,68,69]. In one patient a change from prednisone to the combination of methylprednisolone plus troleandomycin was effective, whereas prednisolone alone or the combination of prednisone and hydroxyurea was not [70].

Treatment recommendations for the use of GC for HES in adults include an initial dose of 1 mg/kg or 60 mg/day of prednisone. A substantial fall in the total eosinophil count to this initial dose presages an overall favorable response to GC. After 1 to 2 weeks patients can be converted to 60 mg every other day and can be reassessed for clinical symptoms and response of involved organs after 3 months [71]. Favorable clinical, hematologic, and organ system response can be followed by a gradual reduction of the prednisone dosage. Patients not responding to prednisone are candidates for addition of cytotoxic agents.

Clinical control of organ system manifestations of hypereosinophilic syndromes with glucocorticoids

A major goal of treating HES is to control or reverse organ damage caused by infiltration and degranulation of eosinophils. Although GC have been reportedly effective in the global response of reducing eosinophilia and prolonging life in HES, individual reports of specific organ system responses to GC are surprisingly rare. Success or failure with the use of GC in HES-related organ damage must be tempered with a realization that when these agents are begun early in the course of illness the chance for clinical benefit is greatly enhanced, whereas when patients present with severe end-organ damage from ongoing HES or the duration of GC treatment is short, the chance for reversing clinical deterioration is small, even if the eosinophilia can be brought under control.

Response of neurologic manifestations of hypereosinophilic syndromes to glucocorticoids

Hypereosinophilia has been associated not only with peripheral neuropathy, but also with features of encephalopathy, as well as focal central nervous system symptoms or death from emboli or hemorrhage [72,73]. There are several reports of prednisone-induced improvement in peripheral neuropathy, which can be a presenting feature of HES [74,75]. Early GC therapy has been effective in reversing clinical features of acute encephalopathy in HES [76,77]. Pulse intravenous high dose methylprednisolone, 1 gm/day for 5days, has also been successfully employed to treat encephalopathic features of HES [78].

Response of cardiovascular features of hypereosinophilic syndromes to glucocorticoids

Cardiovascular manifestations of HES span a range of anatomic and clinical problems, each of which can be considered separately when one assesses the response to GC. The presence of asymptomatic endocardial lesions may precede overt cardiac disease by substantial periods of time [79].

Clinical signs from cardiac dysfunction in HES include dyspnea, chest pain and signs of congestive heart failure, pulmonary edema [80], murmur of mitral regurgitation, cardiomegaly, and T-wave inversions [81]. Prednisolone 40 mg/day to 60 mg/day has been used, along with bed rest and diuretics, to treat acute episodes of heart failure in patients with early heart disease, and maintenance on a lower dose, 10 mg/day, appeared to prevent progression of cardiac findings [82]. HES patients treated with imatinib mesylate may develop acute myocyte degeneration and acute ventricular dysfunction. It is uncertain why certain HES patients develop this acute complication and others do not, however GC can be used to prevent or treat acute left ventricular dysfunction in this circumstance [83,84]. Treatment with GC (prednisolone or prednisone 40 mg/day–60 mg/day) has resulted in clinical and biopsy-proven improvement of active eosinophilic endomyocarditis, disappearance of eosinophilic infiltration and eosinophil cationic protein deposition, improved congestive heart failure and left ventricular ejection fraction [85–87], resolution of EKG changes of posterior myocardial infarction, and normalization of creatine phosphokinase values [88].

Valvular involvement in HES includes tricuspid, mitral, and aortic valve regurgitation caused by endocardial inflammation, and fibrosis affecting papillary muscles and chordae tendineae producing papillary muscle dysfunction [81]. It has become clear that even with successful prosthetic valve replacement, recurrent valve obstruction can occur if the eosinophilia goes unchecked [89,90].

Vascular events and disseminated intravascular coagulation

Once large vessel arterial occlusion has occurred in HES, treatment with GC will not result in re-establishment of vessel patency, even if there is a dramatic eosinopenic response [91]. Combined treatment with urokinase and GC has been successful in a case of HES-associated pulmonary thromboembolism [92]. Control of HES-associated disseminated intravascular coagulation has necessitated the use of both GC and low molecular weight heparin [93] or the combination of GC and cyclosporine [94].

Response of dermatologic involvement to glucocorticoids

Skin findings in HES are primarily erythematous pruritic papules and nodules, urticaria and angioedema, petechiae, and hemorrhage [65,95]. Prednisolone-responsive dermal lesions (facial and extremity edema, urticaria) may be the sole manifestation of hypereosinophilia [96]. Incapacitating mucosal ulcers, which may affect the oropharynx, gastrointestinal tract, and genitalia [97,98] have been associated with severe cases of HES, and are resistant to treatment with GC [99]. Skin involvement, associated with the expression of eotaxin by lesional dermal endothelial cells and elevated serum IL-5 levels, has responded well to prednisolone [100]. Betamethasone-responsive bullous changes with profound swelling [101], and deflazacort-responsive solar urticaria [102], are other examples of GC-responsive, selective skin involvement in HES.

Response of gastrointestinal tract involvement to glucocorticoids

Sclerosing cholangitis, with or without associated colitis, is a recognized, though rare, example of gastrointestinal involvement by HES [103,104]. Prednisone has generally been effective in controlling the eosinophilia and clinical symptoms in these patients [103,105,106], as well as cholestatic liver disease associated with HES [107], "hepatobiliary masses," and obstructive jaundice [108].

Hydroxyurea treatment of hypereosinophilic syndromes

For HES patients with poor prognostic signs, such as very high leukocyte counts, congestive heart failure, splenomegaly, or the presence of myeloblasts in the peripheral blood [66], therapy with prednisone alone often may not be sufficient to control HES. In these cases, and for HES patients unresponsive to other agents, addition of hydroxyurea to their regimens is often of great benefit.

Hydroxyurea is well absorbed after oral administration. Following transport by diffusion into cells, hydroxyurea is converted to a free radical nitroxide, which causes inactivation of ribonucleotide reductase, inhibition of DNA synthesis, and synchronization of the surviving cell population [109]. Early studies of colony-formation kinetics of bone marrow cells from normal volunteers using hydroxyurea suicide showed that eosinophil colonies develop more slowly than granulocyte colonies from a population of small cells that have a lower rate of hydroxyurea suicide [110].

Hydroxyurea has been most beneficial in the treatment of HES, not as a single agent, where its use can cause cytopenias necessitating its cessation [111], but when added to other agents in a combined treatment program. As early as the mid 1970s the utility of adding hydroxyurea was reported for eosinophilic leukemia [112]. In 1976 Solley and colleagues [113] reported the benefit of giving hydroxyurea (500 mg four times a day) to a patient with eosinophilic endomyocardiopathy unresponsive prednisone. This was followed by lowering of total leukocyte count, and the percentage of eosinophils and resolution of hepatosplenomegaly.

The first large scale study to report the benefit of adding hydroxyurea to the treatment of patients who were GC failures was by Parrillo and colleagues [66] in 1978. In this study, six of eight HES subjects with at least one poor prognostic sign and evidence of cardiac involvement (seven of eight had failed treatment with prednisolone) responded to addition of hydroxyurea, and the remaining two subjects experienced a partial response. Based on this study, hydroxyurea 1 g/day to 2 g/day was recommended for use in GC unresponsive patients to lower the total leukocyte count 5,000 cells/mm^3 to 10,000 cells/mm^3, with subsequent re-evaluation of clinical status at regular intervals. Occasional patients may respond to doses of hydroxyurea below 1 g/day, especially when hydroxyurea is used in combination with other agents (see below); however, doses above 2 g/day should generally be avoided because of the risk of cytopenias. Depending on the patient's clinical status and the urgency to reduce the total eosinophil count, it is reasonable to begin treatment with 0.5 g/day to 1.0 g/day of hydroxyurea. Thereafter gradual advancement of the daily dose by 0.5 g every 2 to 4 weeks can be guided by the response of the total eosinophil count and clinical symptoms.

The combination of hydroxyurea and prednisone can result in clinical improvement of cardiac fibrosis [114], cerebellar involvement (documented by resolution of hyperintense lesions on MRI scan) [115], and for HES-associated mucosal lesions [99]. Beyond its use with prednisone, hydroxyurea combined with INF-α has been a useful regimen for control of myeloproliferative HES [116,117] and eosinophilic leukemia with a t(2;5) (p23;q35) translocation [118]. Sequential addition of hydroxyurea to INF-α has allowed control of the disease when initial therapy with interferon was not successful [119]. In a case of GC-resistant HES associated with aberrant T-cells and greatly increased levels of IL-2 and IL-15, addition of hydroxyurea caused control of eosinophilia, disappearance of the aberrant T-cells, and normalization of IL-2 and IL-15 values after 2 months. In this patient, serum levels of the primary eosinophil-active cytokines IL-3, IL-5, and GM-CSF were normal throughout the clinical course [120].

In the author's own experience with HES-associated recalcitrant coronary artery spasm, addition of hydroxyurea 500 mg/day to 1000 mg/day to a partially successful program of prednisone and imatinib mesylate gave excellent control of eosinophilia and resolution of clinical symptoms [121].

Interferons in the treatment of hypereosinophilic syndromes

It has now been over 15 years since the first case reports appeared describing the clinical benefit that the biologic response modifier IFN-α exhibited for HES patients resistant to prednisone and hydroxyurea [122,123]. During the intervening years the value of IFN-α in the treatment of HES has been substantiated in numerous clinical reports.

IFN-α has proven effective in HES resistant individually to prednisone [124–127] and hydroxyurea [122,124,125,128], to treatment with the combination of hydroxyurea and prednisone [122–124,129–132], and to less commonly used agents and drug combinations, including prednisone in combination with cyclophosphamide and hydroxyurea [124], vincristine/ prednisone/hydroxyurea [133], methylprednisolone/busulfan [126], etoposide [125,134], 2-chlorodeoxyadenosine [126], melphalan [130], prednisone/ cyclosporine [134], and vincristine [135]. As mentioned above [116–119], in combination with hydroxyurea, IFN-α can be a potent regimen to control HES including HES-associated mucosal lesions [136].

In vitro effects of interferon-α

Interferon-α reduces circulating levels of eosinophil granule proteins

The clinically beneficial effects of IFN-α derive from its effects on eosinophil proliferation, migration, activation, and survival. A functional receptor for IFN-α is present on eosinophils taken from patients with various eosinophilic disorders, though there is a wide variation of 20% to 86% in the percentage of positive cells [137]. Release of eosinophil derived neurotoxin and eosinophil cationic protein, by eosinophils activated with IgA or IgE immune complexes, is inhibited by preincubation with IFN-α [137]. Statistically, significant reductions in another eosinophil granule protein, major basic protein, have been documented in HES patients undergoing treatment with IFN-α [134]. Because eosinophil granule proteins have been found to have detrimental effects on various tissues, including Purkinje cells and cardiac cells [138,139], these combined results suggest that one of the beneficial effects of IFN-α is to reduce toxic levels of eosinophil granule proteins in the circulation and possibly in tissues.

Interferon-α inhibits eosinophilopoiesi

In vitro studies showed that IFN-α, IFN-β, and IFN-γ were each able to suppress bone marrow colony formation by a direct effect on colony-forming cells, an effect that was not dependent on the presence of monocytes, T lymphocytes, or B lymphocytes. However, this effect was not specific for eosinophil colonies [140]. The ability of IFN-α to directly inhibit eosinophil colony growth by nonadherent, non-T bone marrow cells stimulated with either IL-5 or GM-CSF suggests a direct inhibition of eosinophilopoiesis [141]. Furthermore, because eosinophils themselves produce IL-5 [142], interruption of this autocrine loop by blocking eosinophil proliferation may serve to reduce eosinophil numbers, activation, and survival in HES.

Interferon-α regulates eosinophil active cytokine production

One mechanism by which IFN-α can regulate cytokine production is by promoting development of the T-helper lymphocyte Th_1 subset of clonal $CD4^+$ T cells that secrete IL-2 and IFN-γ [143–146]. IFN-γ inhibits differentiation and tissue migration of eosinophils from IL-3 and IL-5-stimulated umbilical cord mononuclear cells (UCMNC) [147]. Both IFN-α and IFN-γ decrease viability and increase apoptosis of UCMNC-derived eosinophils, with IFN-α being a more effective apoptotic agent [148]. The combination of tissue necrosis factor alpha (TNF-α) and IFN-γ can induce differentiation of the eosinophil line EoL-1 into a noneosinophil monocyte/macrophage lineage [149]. This suggests that potentially immature eosinophils may be diverted to noneosinophil differentiation by the presence of these cytokines at the appropriate time.

Gene expression of IL-5, GM-CSF, TNF-α, and IL-13 in peripheral blood mononuclear cells stimulated by mitogen is inhibited by IFN-α [150]. Because IL-13 and TNF-α, through their induction of circulating adhesion molecules VCAM and ICAM-1 on endothelium, allow eosinophils with integrin counter-receptors leukocyte adhesion molecules VLA-4 and LFA-1 to transmigrate to sites of activation, the inhibition of gene expression of these cytokines may add to the benefit of IFN-α in HES by preventing eosinophil infiltration into and damage at sites of inflammation [151,152].

In several other systems studied, including allergen-induced proliferation of T-cell clones and their production of IL-5 and GM-CSF [150], IL-5 production by mitogen-stimulated lymphocytes [150,153], and IL-5, TNF-α, and GM-CSF production by human cord blood-derived mast cells [154], the ability of IFN-α to inhibit cytokines critical to the proliferation, activation, and survival of eosinophils has been confirmed. The clinical relevance of these in vitro observations is reflected in a report of IFN-α induced clinical and cytogenetic remission in an HES patient with elevated IL-5 levels and chromosomal abnormalities of chromosome 5, the site of genes for IL-5, IL-3, and GM-CSF [125].

Several investigators have reported the presence of IL-5 producing $CD3^+CD4^-CD8^-$, and $CD3^-CD4^+$ abnormal T-cell clones [30,155–157]. HES with these abnormal T-cells is termed "lymphocytic or L-HES." In vitro clonal T-helper lymphocyte Th_2 $CD3^-CD4^+$ cells have a high rate of spontaneous apoptosis when compared with $CD3^+CD4^+$ T-cells from normal volunteers. The finding that IFN-α protects against spontaneous $CD3^-CD4^+$ apoptosis but not Fas ligand-induced apoptosis has raised the question as to the safety of using IFN-α in these patients [158]. In one of the patients reported with a predominance of $CD3^-CD4^+$ cells, treatment with IFN-α was associated with expansion of this circulating clone, development of peripheral T-cell lymphoma, and recurrence of hypereosinophilia [158]. Further study must determine the significance of this finding compared with the ability of IFN-α to reduce IL-5 production by clonal T-cells, and to control hypereosinophilia and elevated soluble IL-2 receptor levels in some lymphoma patients [159]. The association of clonal T-cell proliferation with eosinophilia is well recognized [160–162]; however there has been no recognized increase in the occurrence of lymphoma in HES patients receiving IFN-α. Currently, the recommended treatment for patients with L-HES is prednisone alone [163] or in combination with hydroxyurea [164].

Clinical spectrum of interferon-α effectiveness in hypereosinophilic syndromes

Treatment of hypereosinophilic syndromes with chromosomal abnormalities

There are numerous examples of successful cytogenetic remission of HES patients, with chromosomal abnormalities, by the use of IFN-α. These successes include one HES patient with trisomy 8 and elevated serum IL-2 receptor levels, who responded to treatment with IFN-α and hydroxyurea with cytogenetic remission and decreased IL-2 receptor values [165], and one patient with nullisomy Y treated only with IFN-α, who had a reduction to 15% of cells with this abnormality [126].

Because the gene coding for IL-3, IL-5, and GM-CSF reside on the long arm of chromosome 5 [166], the effect of IFN-α in HES patients with cytogenetic abnormalities involving chromosome 5 is of special interest. Case reports document IFN-α induced cytogenetic and clinical remission in one patient with a 46, XY, t(5;9)(q32;q33) abnormality [110] treated with IFN-α and hydroxyurea, and in two other patients treated with IFN-α alone: one patient with a complex chromosomal translocation—46, XY, t(3;9;5)(q25;q34;q33)—and elevated IL-5 levels [125], and one patient with a t(1;5) abnormality with complete hematologic and major cytogenetic response (17 of 20 normal metaphases) [167].

Other reported cytogenetic successes entail combined use of IFN-α with other agents: (1) resolution of a chromosome 10 abnormality in a patient with cardiovascular involvement treated with prednisone, hydroxyurea, and

IFN-α [168]; (2) resolution of a t(5;12)(q33;p13) translocation in a patient treated with IFN-α plus cytosine arabinoside for 13 months, followed by hydroxyurea and vincristine [169]; (3) long lasting cytogenetic response and resolution of eosinophilia in a 48-year-old female having a myeloproliferative disorder with marked eosinophilia and a 46, XX t(4;7)(q11;p13) karyotype. For this last patient, IFN-α was added to an unsuccessful program of prednisone and hydroxyurea and the combination proved efficacious [132].

Organ system responses to interferon-α

Effective control of hypereosinophilia by IFN-α is accompanied by resolution or improvement of organ system dysfunction, including hepatomegaly [122], splenomegaly [110,123,130,167], and hepatosplenomegaly [124]. Nowhere is this better illustrated than by divergent results observed following valve replacement surgery in HES. Resistance to the effects of IFN-α has been associated with cardiorespiratory failure following valve replacement [170], whereas control of eosinophilia after valve replacement is followed by continued satisfactory valve performance and resolution or prevention of cardiovascular complications [129,168]. Examples of beneficial cardiac and cardiopulmonary outcomes, following control of eosinophilia following IFN-α, include improvement of cardiovascular function and congestive heart failure [124,125], reversal of electrocardiogram changes [122], partial resolution of a left ventricular obliterative mass [131], resolution of pulmonary infiltrates [127], reduction in restrictive lung defect [122], and control of asthma symptoms [171]. IFN-α was the first therapy found to be effective for incapacitating mucosal ulcers [99,130,134], a herald of a subset of HES with poor prognosis [97]. Pruritic papules, nodules and plaques associated with HES have also responded to IFN-α [127,172].

Interferon-γ

IFN-γ, which has received scant clinical attention in the treatment of HES, is equal to IFN-α in its ability to suppress multipotential hematopoietic progenitors in vitro, and exceeds the inhibitory effect of IFN-α on colony growth by the colony forming units granulocyte-macrophage (CFU-GM) [140]. In limited clinical usage, IFN-γ reduced peripheral eosinophilia in a hypereosinophilic, aspirin-sensitive, nonatopic patient when used at a dose of 50 μg/m^2 3 days per week for 4 weeks [173].

Effective doses, duration of therapy, pegylated interferon-α,
and safety profile

HES patients respond equally well to IFN-α 2B and IFN-α 2A [132], which differ by only one amino acid [174]. IFN-α, administered by subcutaneous injection, is available as a powder for reconstitution, as a solution for injection, and as a solution in prefilled multidose pens. The range of doses reportedly effective for HES is quite broad, from 0.5 to 3×10^6 U every other day [171] to 6.25×10^6 U per day [169], with numerous intermediary doses reportedly beneficial [124,129,131,134]. Commonly, a starting dose of 3×10^6 U Mondays, Wednesdays, and Fridays is used. With prolonged use, no apparent resistance to the eosinopenic effect of IFN-α has been observed [124,134,136,169,171]. Subsequent reports have also demonstrated that, once control of eosinophilia has been achieved, the dose of IFN-α necessary to maintain remission is frequently substantially lower than that needed to initially bring the eosinophilia under control [127,135,171]. Sustained remissions after discontinuation of IFN-α have been reported [127,130,175], though rebound eosinophilia has also occurred [134,171]. Re-treatment with IFN-α of rebound eosinophilia, occurring 6 months after discontinuance of IFN-α, was successful [126].

PEG-intron is a long-acting preparation of IFN-α in which polyethylene glycol (PEG), molecular weight 12,000, is linked through histidine-34 on IFN-α. PEG-intron maintains its biologic effects, yet can be given once per week [176]. Because the need for long-term, repeated dosing with IFN-α, frequently 3 to 7 days per week for extended periods of time may be uncomfortable and daunting to patients, investigators have begun to substitute PEG-intron in HES patients receiving IFN-α who have controlled eosinophil counts and are stable clinically. Similar to dosing with IFN-α, investigators have found that dosing with PEG-intron could be reduced gradually with time [177]. Fig. 1 shows the clinical course of an HES patient whose eosinophilia was initially treated with prednisone. Subsequently IFN-α was instituted as a steroid-sparing agent and prednisone was tapered, reduced, and discontinued. Because of a stable course on IFN-α at 3×10^6 U three times per week, PEG-intron was given, beginning at a dose of 80 mcg/week, a dose based on her body mass. Subsequently, dosage reductions to 64 mcg/week, and then to 48 mcg/week were possible. PEG-intron may therefore be useful in maintaining stable HES patients with reduced frequency of injections and discomfort.

The frequency of nonlimiting side effects, such as flu-like symptoms, gastrointestinal system disorders, musculoskeletal system disorders, and nervous system and psychiatric disorders reported with IFN-α treatment for HES do not differ substantially from the frequency of those side effects when IFN-α is used to treat other conditions. As noted above, the dose of IFN-α can often be reduced. Reported side effects necessitating dose reduction include exacerbation of autoimmune disorders, including autoimmune thyroiditis, psoriasis, and ulcerative colitis in patients with hematological disorders receiving 6 to 25×10^6 U/week [178].

Although not specific for HES patients, neuropsychiatric side effects of depression and suicide ideation are common reasons for discontinuing IFN-α [179]. Psychosis, including delusions of parasite infestation in one HES patient, has occurred with IFN-α use [180]. Other reports include: aggravation

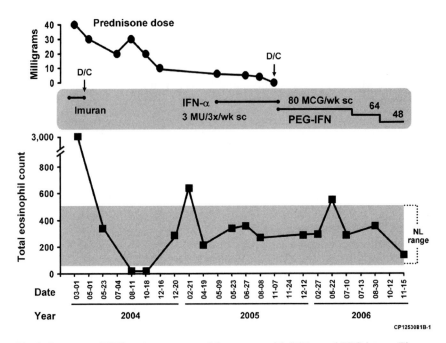

Fig. 1. Response of HES patient to sequential treatment with INF-α and PEG-intron. The patient's eosinophilia could not be controlled with less than 20 mg of prednisone per day. Addition of INF-α, 2b 3 million units three times per week, allowed tapering and discontinuation of prednisone. Because of a very stable clinical course, a trial of PEG-intron was given at an initial dose of 80 μg per week, while INF-α 2b was discontinued. Her eosinophil counts and clinical condition remained in good control and PEG-intron was subsequently tapered as indicated.

of urticaria and pruritus after 2 weeks of treatment in a 14-month-old child with a clonal abnormality [46,XX, add(8)(p23)] [181], necessitating discontinuation of IFN-α; one case of reversible renal insufficiency and nephrotic syndrome-range proteinuria following one year's treatment with IFN-α and hydroxyurea [182]; and a second case report of reversible nephrotoxicity that occurred in an HES patient already receiving IFN-α when recombinant human granulocyte colony-stimulating factor (rh-G-CSF) was added to his program. For the latter patient, cessation of rh-G-CSF, but not cessation of IFN-α, was followed by improved renal function [133]. Fetal development has been normal in a pregnant woman with HES given IFN-α [183], and the wife of a man given IFN-α also had a normal pregnancy and healthy infant [134].

Failure of interferon-α to control eosinophilia

There are several reasons why IFN-α may not control eosinophilia. Eosinophils are heterogeneous in IFN-α receptor expression [137]; however the clinical relevance of this variability has not been conclusively documented. Other considerations include inadequate dose, intolerance of side effects, and premature cessation of treatment. Antibodies to IFN-α have not been documented in HES patients. The failure of IFN-α has been associated with clinical organ dysfunction [170,184,185], and has occurred in the presence of trisomy 8 [128,185], and other chromosomal abnormalities [181], or granulocytic sarcomas [134,181]. Temporary benefit without lasting control of eosinophilia has also occurred [186–188].

Childhood hypereosinophilia

Childhood HES, is rare, and warrants separate mention. Childhood HES may precede, follow, or accompany acute lymphoblastic leukemia [189–193], which requires treatment with chemotherapeutic agents in addition to GC. Children with HES experience many of the same types of organ dysfunction as do adults with HES, and produce eosinophil-active cytokines as do adult patients [194]. In a review of 18 published cases of childhood HES in 1987 a majority, 15, had involvement of the cardiovascular system as the major cause of morbidity and mortality [195]. Cardiovascular symptoms, such as heart failure [195,196], and pleural and pericardial effusions [197] may respond dramatically to treatment solely with GC; however peripheral arterial occlusion [198] and progression of restrictive cardiomyopathy to dilated cardiomyopathy, despite prednisone-induced hematologic remission, has occurred [199].

GC treatment alone is unlikely to be effective when the initial leukocyte count nears or exceeds 100,000/mm^3 [200,201]. Dermatologic and gastrointestinal involvement in childhood HES respond well to treatment with GC [106,202], including a child with the FIP1L1-PDGFRA rearrangement who presented with intense pruritus [202].

Various doses of GC have been reported effective in the treatment of children. Prolonged, low dose prednisone can be an effective option in some childhood cases of HES [203]; moreover, the eventual ability to discontinue GC therapy after variable amounts of time is noted in several reports [197,203–205]. Control of HES with methylprednisolone (20 mg/kg/day) in two siblings unresponsive to conventional doses (2 mg/kg/day) was associated with phenotypic changes in eosinophils that included increase in Fas (CD95) and decrease in CD11b and CD18 in one sibling [206].

Complications of severe hypereosinophilia include right ventricular thrombosis [207], prosthetic mitral valve obstruction [208], and acute pericarditis necessitating pericardiocentesis [209]. It is occasionally possible to discontinue GC [209] even after these complications, while prolonged multidrug therapy with oral GC, hydroxyurea, and warfarin has been necessary for other patients [207].

Reports of childhood HES treated with hydroxyurea or IFN-α are not numerous. Addition of hydroxyurea, 20 mg/kg/day, to an unsuccessful treatment program of prednisone resulted normalization of the total

Table 2
The cost of treating hypereosinophilic syndromes

Drug	Dosing regimen	Cost/day	Cost/month (30 days)
Prednisone 5–10 mg	1 tablet once daily	$2.63–$2.65	$78.90–$79.50
Prednisone 20 mg	1 tablet once daily	$2.68	$80.40
Prednisone 60 mg	1 tablet once daily	$2.83	$84.90
Hydroxyurea 500 mg	1 capsule every other day	$2.90	$43.50
Hydroxyurea 1000 mg	2 capsules (1000 mg) daily	$3.20	$96.00
Hydroxyurea 1500 mg	3 capsules (1500 mg) daily	$3.50	$105.00
Interferon alpha 2b	3 MU[a] 3x/week	$97.88	$1,174.56
Interferon alpha 2b	3 MU 7x/week	$97.88	$2,936.40
Interferon alpha 2b	5 MU 3x/week	$131.81	$1,581.72
Interferon alpha 2b	5 MU 7x/week	$131.81	$3,954.30
PEG-intron	80 mcg once a week	$354.10	$1,416.40

Source: Mayo Clinic pharmacy. Patient's cost calculated as acquisition cost plus 25% markup plus pharmacy fee.
[a] Million units.

eosinophil count in an 11-year-old boy who presented with pericardial effusion [210]. Hydroxyurea 2.7 g/m^2 was briefly used in an 8-year-old boy with HES, but was discontinued in lieu of vincristine [200]. Chronic hydroxyurea therapy, 50 mg/kg/day has been effective in controlling myelodysplastic syndrome with t(5;12)(q31; p12-p13) with eosinophilia in an 8-year-old girl [211]. IFN-α, 5 MU/m^2/day, successfully controlled hypereosinophilia in a 5-month-old boy after the failure of GC [212].

Cost of treatment

Of first importance in the treatment of HES are the effectiveness and tolerability of the medications used. However, a little-discussed but important consideration in the treatment of HES is the long-term financial cost of therapy. Listed in Table 2 are the monthly direct patient costs of treatment of HES with varying doses of prednisone, hydroxyurea, IFN-α, and PEG-intron. From this table several points are worth emphasizing. Low-dose prednisone alone or in combination with hydroxyurea can be an economical approach to controlling HES. IFN-α is a much more expensive therapeutic option. If PEG-intron, which can be administered once per week, is effective, the cost of treatment is comparable or less than that of IFN-α, which frequently must be administered three or more times per week.

References

[1] Germuth FG Jr, Ottinger B. Effect of 12-hydroxy-11-dehydrocorticosterone (compound E) and of ACTH on arthus reaction and antibody formation in the rabbit. Proc Soc Exp Biol Med 1950;4:815–23.
[2] Dougherty TF, Schneebeli GL. Role of cortisone in regulation of inflammation. Proc Soc Exp Biol Med 1950;74:854–9.

[3] Hench PS, Kendall EC, Slocumb CH, et al. The effect of a hormone of the adrenal cortex (17-hydroxy-11-dehydrocorticosterone: compound E) and of pituitary adrenocorticotrophic hormone on rheumatoid arthritis; preliminary report. Proc Staff Meet Mayo Clin 1949;24: 181–97.

[4] Shick RM, Baggenstoss AH, Polley HF. The effects of cortisone and ACTH on periarteritis nodosa and cranial arteritis. Preliminary report. Proc Staff Meet Mayo Clin 1950;25: 135–44.

[5] Zappert J. Ueber das Vorkommen der eosinophilen Zellen in menschlichen blute. Z Klin Med 1893;23:227–308.

[6] Staubli C. Die klininische bedeutung der eosinophilie. Ergeb Inn Med Kinderheilkd 1910;6: 192–220.

[7] Doe RP, Flink EB, Goodsell MG. Relationship of diurnal variation in 17-hydroxycorticosteroid levels in blood and urine to eosinophils and electrolyte excretion. J Clin Endocrinol Metab 1956;16:196–206.

[8] Visscher MB, Halberg F. Daily rhythms in the number of circulating eosinophils and some related phenomena. Ann N Y Acad Sci 1955;59:834–49.

[9] Arnoldsson H, Helander E. Some aspects on the problem of eosinophilia. Errors of method, diurnal rhythm and eosinophilia in allergy. Acta Allergol 1958;12:96–112.

[10] Kaine HD, Seltzer HS, Conn JW. Mechanism of diurnal eosinophil rhythm in man. J Lab Clin Med 1955;45:247–52.

[11] Thorn GW, Forsham PH, Prunty FTG, et al. A test for adrenal cortical insufficiency. The response to pituitary adrenocorticotrophic hormone. J Am Med Assoc 1948;137: 1005–9.

[12] Prunty FTG. Techniques for the evaluation of adrenal cortical function by the use of adrenocorticotrophin: a review. J Clin Pathol 1950;3:87–105.

[13] Peterson AP, Altman LC, Hill JS, et al. Glucocorticoid receptors in normal human eosinophils: comparison with neutrophils. J Allergy Clin Immunol 1981;68:212–7.

[14] Prin L, Lefebvre PP, Gruart V, et al. Heterogeneity of human eosinophil glucocorticoid receptor expression in hypereosinophilic patients: absence of detectable receptor correlates with resistance to corticotherapy. Clin Exp Immunol 1989;78:383–9.

[15] Best WR, Samter M. Variation and error in eosinophil counts of blood and bone marrow. Blood 1951;6:61–74.

[16] Kellgren JH, Janus O. The eosinopenic response to cortisol and ACTH in normal subjects. Br Med J 1951;2:1183–7.

[17] Esseltier AF, Jeanneret P, Kopp E, et al. Evidence against destruction of eosinophils by glucocorticoids as shown by in vitro experiments. Endocrinology 1954;54:477–9.

[18] Sevitt S. The spleen and blood eosinopenia. J Clin Pathol 1955;8:42–6.

[19] Esseltier AF, Jeanneret RL, Morandi L. The mechanism of glucocorticoid eosinopenia. Contribution to the physiology of eosinophile granulocytes. Blood 1954;9:531–49.

[20] Krippaehne ML, Osgood EE. Studies of the influences of cortisone and hydrocortisone on human leukocytes in culture and in eosinophilic leukemia. Acta Haematol 1955;13: 145–52.

[21] Suda T, Miura Y, Ijima H, et al. The effect of hydrocortisone on human granulopoiesis in vitro with cytochemical analysis of colonies. Exp Hematol 1983;11:114–21.

[22] Bjornson BH, Harvey JM, Rose L. Differential effect of hydrocortisone on eosinophil and neutrophil proliferation. J Clin Invest 1985;76:924–9.

[23] Slovick FT, Abboud CN, Brennan JK, et al. Modulation of in vitro eosinophil progenitors by hydrocortisone: role of accessory cells and interleukins. Blood 1985;66:1072–9.

[24] Raghavachar A, Fleischer S, Frickhofen N, et al. T-lymphocyte control of human eosinophilic granulopoiesis: clonal analysis in an idiopathic hypereosinophilic syndrome. J Immunol 1987;139:3753–8.

[25] Lamas AM, Leon OG, Schleimer RP. Glucocorticoids inhibit eosinophil responses to granulocyte-macrophage colony-stimulating factor. J Immunol 1991;147:254–9.

[26] Daffern PJ, Jagels MA, Saad JJ, et al. Upper airway epithelial cells support eosinophil survival in vitro through production of GM-CSF and prostaglandin E2: regulation by glucocorticoids and TNF-alpha. Allergy Asthma Proc 1999;20:243–53.

[27] Schrezenmeier H, Thome SD, Tewald F, et al. Interleukin-5 is the predominant eosinophilopoietin produced by cloned T lymphocytes in hypereosinophilic syndrome. Exp Hematol 1993;21:358–65.

[28] Yamaguchi Y, Hayashi Y, Sugama Y, et al. Highly purified murine interleukin 5 (IL-5) stimulates eosinophil function and prolongs in vitro survival. IL-5 as an eosinophil chemotactic factor. J Exp Med 1988;167:1737–42.

[29] Wang JM, Rambaldi A, Biondi A, et al. Recombinant human interleukin 5 is a selective eosinophil chemoattractant. Eur J Immunol 1989;19:701–5.

[30] Simon H-U, Plotz SG, Dummer R, et al. Abnormal clones of T cells producing interleukin-5 in idiopathic eosinophilia. N Engl J Med 1999;341:1112–20.

[31] Rolfe FG, Hughes JM, Armour CL, et al. Inhibition of interleukin-5 gene expression by dexamethasone. Immunology 1992;77:494–9.

[32] Hallsworth MP, Litchfield TM, Lee TH. Glucocorticoids inhibit granulocyte-macrophage colony-stimulating factor-1 and interleukin-5 enhanced in vitro survival of human eosinophils. Immunology 1992;75:382–5.

[33] Wallen N, Kita H, Weiler D, et al. Glucocorticoids inhibit cytokine-mediated eosinophil survival. J Immunol 1991;147:3490–5.

[34] Bloom JW, Chacko J, Lohman IC, et al. Differential control of eosinophil survival by glucocorticoids. Apoptosis 2004;9:97–104.

[35] Debierre-Grockiego F, Fuentes V, Prin L, et al. Differential effect of dexamethasone on cell death and STAT5 activation during in vitro eosinophilopoiesis. Br J Haematol 2003;123: 933–41.

[36] Debierre-Grockiego F, Leduc I, Prin L, et al. Dexamethasone inhibits apoptosis of eosinophils isolated from hypereosinophilic patients. Immunobiology 2001;204: 517–23.

[37] Letuve S, Druilhe A, Grandsaigne M, et al. Critical role of mitochondria, but not caspases during glucocorticosteroid-induced human eosinophil apoptosis. Am J Respir Cell Mol Biol 2002;26:565–71.

[38] Meagher LC, Cousin JM, Seckl JR, et al. Opposing effects of glucocorticoids on the rate of apoptosis in neutrophilic and eosinophilic granulocytes. J Immunol 1996;156: 4422–8.

[39] Zhang X, Moilanen E, Adcock IM, et al. Divergent effect of mometasone on human eosinophil and neutrophil apoptosis. Life Sci 2002;71:1523–34.

[40] Druilhe A, Letuve S, Pretolani M. Glucocorticoid-induced apoptosis in human eosinophils: mechanisms of action. Apoptosis 2003;8:481–5.

[41] Dale DC, Hubert RT, Fauci A. Eosinophil kinetics in the hypereosinophilic syndrome. J Lab Clin Med 1976;87:487–95.

[42] Hudson B, Doig A. Observations on the nature of hormone-induced eosinopenia. Australas Ann Med 1957;6:228–37.

[43] Essellier AF, Wagner WF. Das verhalten der eosinophilen in blut und knochenmark auf verbreichung von adrenocorticotrophin. Klin Wochenschr 1952;30:705–9.

[44] Root SW, Andrews GA. Effect of ACTH on the eosinophil count in peripheral blood and bone marrow. Am J Med Sci 1953;226:304–9.

[45] Rosenthal RL, Wald N, Yager A, et al. Effects of cortisone and ACTH therapy on eosinophils of the bone marrow and blood. Proc Soc Exp Biol Med 1950;75:740–1.

[46] Hench PS, Kendall EC, Slocumb CH, et al. Effects of cortisone acetate and pituitary ACTH on rheumatoid arthritis, rheumatic fever and certain other conditions. Arch Med Interna 1950;85:545–666.

[47] Rothstein I, Spring M, Berley BS. Effect of ACTH in a case of eosinophilic leukemia. N Y State J Med 1953;53:1461–3.

[48] Engfeldt B, Zetterstrom R. Disseminated eosinophilic collagen disease; a clinical and pathological study of a clinical entity related to Loffler's syndrome. Acta Med Scand 1956;153: 337–53.

[49] Fadell EJ, Crone RI, Leonard ME, et al. Eosinophilic leukemia. Arch Intern Med 1957;99: 819–23.

[50] Chen HP, Smith HS. Eosinophilic leukemia. Ann Intern Med 1960;52:1343–52.

[51] Bentley HP, Reardon AE, Knoedler JP, et al. Eosinophilic leukemia. Report of a case, with review and classification. Am J Med 1961;30:310–22.

[52] Thomas JR. Eosinophilic leukemia presenting with erythrocytosis. Blood 1963;22: 639–45.

[53] Bruenwald H, Kiossoglou KA, Mitus WJ, et al. Philadelphia chromosome in eosinophilic leukemia. Am J Med 1965;39:1003–10.

[54] Brink AJ, Weber HW. Fibroplastic parietal endocarditis with eosinophilia. Loffler's endocarditis. Am J Med 1963;34:52–70.

[55] Roberts WC, Liegler DG, Carbone PP. Endomyocardial disease and eosinophilia. A clinical and pathologic spectrum. Am J Med 1969;46:28–42.

[56] Karle H, Videbaek A. Eosinophilic leukaemia or a collagen disease with eosinophilia. Dan Med Bull 1966;13:41–5.

[57] Pierce LE, Hosseinian AH, Constantine AB. Disseminated eosinophilic collagen disease. Blood 1967;29:540–9.

[58] Hardy WR, Anderson RE. The hypereosinophilic syndromes. Ann Intern Med 1968;68: 1220–9.

[59] Benvenisti DA, Ultman JE. Eosinophilic leukemia: report of 5 cases and review of the literature. Ann Intern Med 1969;71:731–45.

[60] Fledelius H. Extreme persistent eosinophilia with high serum B12 values. A report of two cases. Acta Med Scand 1970;187(3):235–40.

[61] Sheperd AJ, Walsh CH, Archer RK, et al. Eosinophilia, splenomegaly and cardiac disease. Br J Haematol 1971;2:233–9.

[62] Manko MA, Cooper JH, Myers RN. Disseminated hypereosinophilic disease. Am J Gastroenterol 1972;5:318–25.

[63] Yam LT, Li CY, Necheles TF, et al. Pseudoeosinophilia, eosinophilic endocarditis and eosinophilic leukemia. Am J Med 1972;53:193–202.

[64] Flannery EP, Dillon DE, Freeman MV, et al. Eosinophilic leukemia with fibrosing endocarditis and short Y chromosome. Ann Intern Med 1972;77:223–8.

[65] Chusid MJ, Dale DC, West BC, et al. The hypereosinophilic syndrome: analysis of fourteen cases with review of the literature. Medicine (Baltimore) 1975;54:1–27.

[66] Parrillo JE, Fauci AS, Wolff SM. Therapy of the hypereosinophilic syndrome. Ann Intern Med 1978;89:167–72.

[67] Flaum MA, Schooley RT, Fauci AS, et al. A clinicopathologic correlation of the idiopathic hypereosinophilic syndrome. I. Hematologic manifestations. Blood 1981;58:1012–20.

[68] Parrillo JE, Lawley TJ, Frank MM, et al. Immunologic reactivity in the hypereosinophilic syndrome. J Allergy Clin Immunol 1979;64:113–21.

[69] Bush RK, Geller M, Busse WW, et al. Response to corticosteroids in the hypereosinophilic syndrome. Association with increased serum IgE levels. Arch Intern Med 1978; 138:1244–6.

[70] Edwards D, Wald JA, Dobozin BS, et al. Troleandomycin and methylprednisolone for treatment of the hypereosinophilic syndrome [letter to the editor]. N Engl J Med 1987; 317:573–4.

[71] Schooley RT, Parrillo JE, Wolff SM, et al. Management of the idiopathic hypereosinophilic syndrome. In: Mahmoud AAF, Austen KF, editors. The eosinophil in health and disease. New York: Grune & Stratton; 1980. p. 323–43.

[72] Moore PM, Harley JB, Fauci AS. Neurologic dysfunction in the idiopathic hypereosinophilic syndrome. Ann Intern Med 1985;102:109–14.

[73] Kocaturk H, Yilmaz M. Idiopathic hypereosinophilic syndrome associated with multiple intracardiac thrombi. Echocardiography 2005;22:675–6.

[74] Bell D, Mackay IG, Pentland B. Hypereosinophilic syndrome presenting as peripheral neuropathy. Postgrad Med J 1985;61:429–32.

[75] Prick JJW, Gabreels-Festen AAWM, Korten JJ, et al. Neurological manifestations of the hypereosinophilic syndrome (HES). Clin Neurol Neurosurg 1988;90:269–73.

[76] Moreau Th, Derex L, Confavreux Ch. Acute encephalopathy and idiopathic hypereosinophilic syndrome: clinical and MRI response to early steroid treatment. Eur J Neurol 1997;4: 618–21.

[77] Fernandez-Miranda C, Ruiz L, Dominguez J, et al. Reversible encephalopathy as first manifestation of hypereosinophilic syndrome. Eur J Intern Med 1996;7:41–2.

[78] Lebbink J, Laterre EC. Idiopathic hypereosinophilic syndrome revealed by central nervous system dysfunction. Acta Neurol Belg 1996;96:137–40.

[79] Borer JS, Henry WL, Epstein SE. Echocardiographic observations in patients with systemic infiltrative disease involving the heart. Am J Cardiol 1977;39:184–8.

[80] Londhey VA, Nadkar MY, Kini SH, et al. Idiopathic hypereosinophilic syndrome manifesting as pulmonary oedema. J Assoc Physicians India 2003;51:414–5.

[81] Parrillo JE, Borer JS, Henry WL, et al. The cardiovascular manifestations of the hypereosinophilic syndrome. Prospective study of 26 patients, with review of the literature. Am J Med 1979;67:572–82.

[82] Davies J, Spry CJF, Sapsford R, et al. Cardiovascular features of 11 patients with eosinophilic endomyocardial disease. Quarterly Journal of Medicine, New Series LII 1983;205: 23–9.

[83] Pardanani A, Reeder T, Porrata LF, et al. Imatinib therapy for hypereosinophilic syndrome and other eosinophilic disorders. Blood 2003;101:3391–7.

[84] Pitini V, Arrigo C, Azzarello D, et al. Serum concentration of cardiac troponin T in patients with hypereosinophilic syndrome treated with imatinib is predictive of adverse outcomes [letter to the editor]. Blood 2003;102:3456–7.

[85] Harley JB, Fauci AS, Gralnick HR. Noncardiovascular findings associated with heart disease in the idiopathic hypereosinophilic syndrome. Am J Cardiol 1983;32:321–4.

[86] Huntgeburth M, Lindner M, Fries JWU, et al. Hypereosinophilic syndrome associated with acute necrotizing myocarditis and cardiomyopathy. Z Kardiol 2005;94:761–6.

[87] Hayashi S-I, Isobe M, Okubo Y, et al. Improvement of eosinophilic heart disease after steroid therapy: successful demonstration by endomyocardial biopsied specimens. Heart Vessels 1999;14:104–8.

[88] Maruyoshi H, Nakatani S, Yasumura Y, et al. Loffler's endocarditis associated with unusual ECG change mimicking posterior myocardial infarction. Heart Vessels 2003;18: 43–6.

[89] Arsiwala S, Peek G, Davies M, et al. Hypereosinophilic syndrome: cause of prosthetic valve obstruction. J Thorac Cardiovasc Surg 1995;110:545–6.

[90] Frustaci A, Abdulla AK, Possati G, et al. Persisting hypereosinophilia and myocardial activity in the fibrotic stage of endomyocardial disease. Chest 1989;96:674–5.

[91] Ponsky TA, Brody F, Giordano J, et al. Brachial artery occlusion secondary to hypereosinophilic syndrome. J Vasc Surg 2005;42:796–9.

[92] Ohashi H, Itoh M, Goto Y, et al. Pulmonary thromboembolism in a patient with idiopathic hypereosinophilic syndrome. Japanese Journal of Rheumatology 1997;7:115–21.

[93] Yeung T, Lau S, Wong K. An unusual case of hypereosinophilic syndrome and disseminated intravascular coagulation. Chin Med J 2005;118:1582–4.

[94] Lee JS, Lee H-K, Lee SS, et al. A case of idiopathic hypereosinophilic syndrome complicated with pulmonary thromboembolism and disseminated intravascular coagulation. Tuberculosis and Respiratory Diseases 2004;57:573–8.

[95] Kazmierowski JA, Chusid MJ, Parrillo JE, et al. Dermatologic manifestations of the hypereosinophilic syndrome. Arch Dermatol 1978;114:531–5.

[96] Barna M, Kemeny L, Dobozy A. Skin lesions as the only manifestation of the hypereosinophilic syndrome. Br J Dermatol 1997;136:646–7.

[97] Leiferman KM, O'Duffy JD, Perry HO, et al. Recurrent incapacitating mucosal ulcerations. A prodrome of the hypereosinophilia syndrome. JAMA 1982;247:1018–20.

[98] Aksahoshi M, Hoshino S, Teramura M, et al. Recurrent oral and genital ulcers as the prodrome of the hypereosinophilic syndrome: report of a probable case. Nippon Naika Gakkai Zasshi 1987;76:421–4.

[99] Barouky R, Bencharif L, Badet F, et al. Mucosal ulcerations revealing primitive hypereosinophilic syndrome. Eur J Dermatol 2003;13:207–8.

[100] Tsunemi Y, Idezuki T, Nakamura K, et al. Dermal endothelial cells express eotaxin in hypereosinophilic syndrome. J Am Acad Dermatol 2003;49:918–21.

[101] Offidani A, Bernardini MI, Simonetti O, et al. Hypereosinophilic dermatosis: skin lesions as the only manifestation of the idiopathic hypereosinophilic syndrome? Br J Dermatol 2000; 143:675–7.

[102] Aragone MG, Nigro A, Parodi A, et al. Solar urticaria as the presenting sign of hypereosinophilic syndrome. Int J Dermatol 1999;38:234.

[103] Delevaux I, Andrie M, Chipponi J, et al. A rare manifestation of idiopathic hypereosinophilic syndrome: sclerosing cholangitis. Dig Dis Sci 2002;47:148–51.

[104] Scheurlen M, Mork H, Weber P. Hypereosinophilic syndrome resembling chronic inflammatory bowel disease with primary sclerosing cholangitis. J Clin Gastroenterol 1992;14: 59–63.

[105] Amin MA, Hamid MA, Saba S. Hypereosinophilic syndrome presenting with eosinophilic colitis, enteritis and cystitis. Chin J Dig Dis 2005;6:206–8.

[106] Ichikawa N, Taniguchi A, Akama H, et al. Sclerosing cholangitis associated with hypereosinophilic syndrome. Intern Med 1997;36:561–4.

[107] Valente AI, Pinto HC, Ramalho F, et al. Idiopathic hypereosinophilic syndrome presenting as cholestatic liver disease. Eur J Gastroenterol Hepatol 1997;9:815–7.

[108] Reyes M, Abraham C, Abedi M, et al. Hypereosinophilic syndrome with hepatobiliary masses and obstructive jaundice. Ann Allergy Asthma Immunol 2005;94: 25–8.

[109] Yarbro JW. Mechanism of action of hydroxyurea. Semin Oncol 1992;19:1–10.

[110] Dresch C, Faille A, Poirer O, et al. Hydroxyurea suicide study of the kinetic heterogeneity of colony forming cells in human bone marrow. Exp Hematol 1979;7:337–44.

[111] Malbrain MLNG, Vanden Bergh H, Zachee P. Further evidence for the clonal nature of the idiopathic hypereosinophilic syndrome: complete haematological and cytogenetic remission induced by interferon-alpha in a case with a unique chromosomal abnormality. Br J Haematol 1996;92:176–83.

[112] Chusid MJ, Dale DC. Eosinophilic leukemia. Remission with vincristine and hydroxyurea. Am J Med 1975;59:297–300.

[113] Solley GO, Maldonado JE, Gleich GJ, et al. Endomyocardiopathy with eosinophilia. Mayo Clin Proc 1976;51:697–708.

[114] Lombardi C, Rusconi C, Faggiano P, et al. Successful reduction of endomyocardial fibrosis in a patient with idiopathic hypereosinophilic syndrome: a case report. Angiology 1995;46: 345–51.

[115] Diaz F, Collazos J. Reversible cerebellar involvement in the idiopathic hypereosinophilic syndrome. Postgrad Med J 1999;75:477–9.

[116] Coutant G, Bletry O, Prin L, et al. Traitement des syndromes hypereosinophiliques a expression myeloproliferative par l'association hydroxyurea-interferon alpha. Annales de Medicine Interne 1993;144:243–50.

[117] Bletry O, Papo T. Les interferons. Interferons alpha et gamma: indications dans es maladies systemiques. Annales de Medicine Interne 1993;144:557–62.

[118] Sato H, Danbara M, Tamura M, et al. Eosinophilic leukaemia with a t(2;5) (p23;q35) translocation. Br J Haematol 1994;87:404–6.

[119] Demiroglu H, Dundar S. Combination of interferon-alpha and hydroxyurea in the treatment of idiopathic hypereosinophilic syndrome. Br J Haematol 1997;97:927–40.

[120] Means-Markwell M, Burgess T, de Keratry D, et al. Eosinophilia with aberrant T cells and elevated serum levels of interleukin-2 and interleukin-15. N Engl J Med 2000;342: 1568–71.

[121] Butterfield JH, Sharkey SW. Control of hypereosinophilic syndrome-associated recalcitrant coronary artery spasm by combined treatment with prednisone, imatinib mesylate and hydroxyurea. Experimental and Clinical Cardiology 2006;11:25–8.

[122] Murphy PT, Fenelly DF, Stuart M, et al. Alfa-interferon in a case of hypereosinophilic syndrome. Br J Haematol 1990;75:619–20.

[123] Zielinski RM, Lawrence WD. Interferon-α for the hypereosinophilic syndrome. Ann Intern Med 1990;113:716–8.

[124] Fruehauf S, Fiehn C, Haas R, et al. Sustained remission of idiopathic hypereosinophilic syndrome following α-Interferon therapy. Acta Haematol 1993;89:91–3.

[125] Yamada O, Kitahara K, Imamura K, et al. Clinical and cytogenetic remission induced by interferon-α in a patient with chronic eosinophilic leukemia associated with a unique t(3;9;5) translocation. Am J Hematol 1998;58:137–41.

[126] Ceretelli S, Capochiani E, Petrini M. Interferon-α in the idiopathic hypereosinophilic syndrome: consideration of five cases. Ann Hematol 1998;77:161–4.

[127] Yoon TY, Ahn G-B, Chang S-H. Complete remission of hypereosinophilic syndrome after interferon-α therapy: report of a case and literature review. J Dermatol 2000;27: 110–5.

[128] Kobayashi M, Katayama T, Ochiai S, et al. Interferon-a therapy for the myeloproliferative variants of hypereosinophilic syndrome. Japan Journal of Clinical Hematology 1993;34: 367–72.

[129] Bockenstedt PL, Santinga JT, Bolling SF. α-Interferon treatment for idiopathic hypereosinophilic syndrome. Am J Hematol 1994;45:248–51.

[130] Acaba L, Mangual A, Garcia EV. Excellent response to interferon therapy in a patient with hypereosinophilic syndrome and elevated serum immunoglobulin E levels. Bol Asoc Med P R 2000;92:59–62.

[131] Baratta L, Afeltra A, Delfino M, et al. Favorable response to high-dose interferon-alpha in idiopathic hypereosinophilic syndrome with restrictive cardiomyopathy. Case report and literature review. Angiology 2002;53:465–70.

[132] Schoffski P, Ganser A, Pascheberg U, et al. Complete haematological and cytogenetic response to interferon alpha-2a of a myeloproliferative disorder with eosinophilia associated with a unique t(3;7) aberration. Ann Hematol 2000;79:95–8.

[133] Hansen PB, Johnsen HE, Hippe E. Hypereosinophilic syndrome treated with α-interferon and granulocyte colony-stimulating factor but complicated by nephrotoxicity. Am J Hematol 1993;43:66–8.

[134] Butterfield JH, Gleich GJ. Interferon-α treatment of six patients with the idiopathic hypereosinophilic syndrome. Ann Intern Med 1994;121:648–53.

[135] Busch FW, Schmidt H, Steinke B. Alpha-Interferon for the hypereosinophilic syndrome. Ann Intern Med 1991;114:338–9.

[136] Esteve K, Cervamtes F, Bosch F, et al. Tratamiento con interferon alfa del sindrome hipereosinofilico idiopatico resistente a la terapeutica convencional. Medicina Cliniica 1996;106: 30–2.

[137] Aldebert D, Lamkhioued B, Desaint C, et al. Eosinophils express a functional receptor for interferon α: inhibitory role of interferon α on the release of mediators. Blood 1996;87: 2354–60.

[138] Durack DT, Ackerman SJ, Loegering DA, et al. Purification of human eosinophil-derived neurotoxin. Proc Natl Acad Sci U S A 1981;78:5165–9.

[139] Kishimoto C, Spry CJ, Tai PC, et al. The in vivo cardiotoxic effect of eosinophilic cationic protein in an animal preparation. Jpn Circ J 1986;50:1264–7.

[140] Broxmeyer HE, Lu L, Platzer E, et al. Comparative analysis of the influences of human gamma, alpha and beta interferons on human multipotential (CFU-GEMM), erythroid (BFU-E) and granulocyte-macrophage (CFU-GM) progenitor cells. J Immunol 1983; 131:1300–5.

[141] Kioke T, Nakamura Y, Enokihara H. Interferon-α inhibits interleukin-5 and granulocyte-macrophage colony stimulating factor production by lymphocytes and suppresses eosinophil colony formation from bone marrow progenitor cells. Dokkyo Journal of Medical Sciences 1998;25:45–52.

[142] Desreumaux P, Janin A, Dubucquoi S, et al. Synthesis of interleukin-5 by activated eosinophils in patients with eosinophilic heart diseases. Blood 1993;82:1553–60.

[143] Paul WE, Seder RA. Lymphocyte responses and cytokines. Cell 1994;76:241–51.

[144] Gutterman JU. Cytokine therapeutics: lessons from interferon α. Proc Natl Acad Sci U S A 1994;91:1198–205.

[145] Parronchi P, De Carli M, Manetti R, et al. IL-4 and IFN (α and γ) exert opposite regulatory effects on the development of cytolytic potential by Th1 or Th2 human T cell clones. J Immunol 1992;149:2977–83.

[146] Schandene L, Cogan E, Crusiaux A, et al. Interferon-α upregulates both interleukin-10 and interferon-γ production by human CD4$^+$ T cells [letter to the editor]. Blood 1997;89: 1110–1.

[147] Ochiai K, Iwamoto I, Takahashi H, et al. Effect of IL-4 and interferon-gamma (IFN-gamma) on IL-3 and IL-5-induced eosinophil differentiation from human cord blood mononuclear cells. Clin Exp Immunol 1995;99:124–8.

[148] Morita M, Lamkhioued B, Gounni AS, et al. Induction by interferons of human eosinophil apoptosis and regulation by interleukin-3, granulocyte/macrophage-colony stimulating factor and interleukin-5. Eur Cytokine Netw 1996;7:725–32.

[149] Nakajuma T, Yamashita N, Matsui H, et al. Induction of differentiation into monocyte/ macrophage cell lineage of a human eosinophilic leukaemia cell line EoL-1 by simultaneous stimulation with tumor necrosis factor-α and interferon-γ. Br J Haematol 1995; 89:258–65.

[150] Krishnaswamy G, Smith JK, Srikanth S, et al. Lymphoblastoid interferon-α inhibits T cell proliferation and expression of eosinophil-activating cytokines. J Interferon Cytokine Res 1996;16:819–27.

[151] Bochner BS, Klunk DA, Sterbinsky SA, et al. IL-13 selectively induces vascular cell adhesion molecule-1 expression in human endothelial cells. J Immunol 1995;154:799–803.

[152] Resnick MB, Weller PF. Mechanisms of eosinophil recruitment. Am J Respir Cell Mol Biol 1993;8:349–55.

[153] Enokihara H, Nakamura Y, Nagashima S, et al. Regulation of interleukin-5 production by interleukin-4, interferon-alpha, transforming growth factor β and interleukin-6. Int Arch Allergy Immunol 1994;104:44–5.

[154] Krishnaswamy G, Hall K, Youngberg G, et al. Regulation of eosinophil-active cytokine production from human cord blood-derived mast cells. J Interferon Cytokine Res 2002; 22:379–88.

[155] Kitano K, Ichikawa N, Mahbub B, et al. Eosinophilia associated with proliferation of CD(3+)4-(8-) alpha beta+ T cells with chromosome 16 anomalies. Br J Haematol 1996; 92:315–7.

[156] Simon HU, Yousefi S, Dommann-Scherrer CC, et al. Expansion of cytokine-producing CD4$^-$ CD8$^-$ T cells associated with abnormal Fas expression and hypereosinophilia. J Exp Med 1996;183:1071–82.

[157] Cogan E, Schandene L, Crusiaux A, et al. Clonal proliferation of type 2 helper T cells in a man with the hypereosinophilic syndrome. N Engl J Med 1994;330:535–8.

[158] Schandene L, Roufosse F, de Lavarfeille A, et al. Interferon α prevents spontaneous apoptosis of clonal Th2 cells associated with chronic hypereosinophilia. Blood 2000;96: 4285–92.

[159] Prin L, Plumas J, Gruart V, et al. Elevated serum levels of soluble interleukin-2 receptor: a marker of disease activity in the hypereosinophilic syndrome. Blood 1991;78:2626–32.

[160] Kitano K, Ichikawa N, Shimodaira S, et al. Eosinophilia associated with clonal T-cell proliferation. Leuk Lymphoma 1997;27:335–42.

[161] Keidan AJ, Castovsky C, De Castro JT, et al. Hypereosinophilic syndrome preceding T cell lymphoblastic lymphoma. Clin Lab Haematol 1985;7:83–8.

[162] Kim CJ, Park SH, Chi JG. Idiopathic hypereosinophilic syndrome terminating as disseminated T-cell lymphoma. Cancer 1991;67:1064–9.

[163] Klion AD, Bochner BS, Gleich GJ, et al. Approaches to the treatment of hypereosinophilic syndromes: a workshop summary report. J Allergy Clin Immunol 2006;117:1292–302.

[164] Sugimoto K, Tamayose K, Sasaki M, et al. More than 13 years of hypereosinophilil associated with clonal $CD3^-CD4^+$ lymphocytosis of Th2/Th0 type. Int J Hematol 2002;75: 281–4.

[165] Quiquandon I, Claisse JF, Capiod JC, et al. α-Interferon and hypereosinophilic syndrome with trisomy 8: karyotypic remission. Blood 1995;85:2284–5.

[166] van Leuween BH, Martinson ME, Webb GC, et al. Molecular organization of the cytokine gene cluster involving the human IL-3, IL-4, IL-5, and GM-CSF genes, on human chromosome 5. Blood 1989;73:1142–8.

[167] Luciano L, Catalano L, Sarrantonio C, et al. αIFN-induced hematologic and cytogenetic remission in chronic eosinophilic leukemia with t(1;5). Haematologica 1999;84:651–3.

[168] Watanabe K, Tournilhad O, Camilleri LF. Recurrent thrombosis of prosthetic mitral valve in idiopathic hypereosinophilic syndrome. J Heart Valve Dis 2002;11(3):447–9.

[169] Granjo E, Lima M, Lopes JM, et al. Chronic eosinophilic leukaemia presenting with erythroderma, mild eosinophilia and hyper-IgE: clinical, immunological and cytogenetic features and therapeutic approach. Acta Haematologica 2002;107:108–12.

[170] van den Anker-Lugtenburg PJ, van't Veer MB. Alpha-interferon in a case of hypereosinophilic syndrome. Br J Haematol 1991;77:258.

[171] Canonica GW, Passalacqua G, Pronzato C, et al. Effective long-term α-interferon treatment for hypereosinophilic syndrome. J Allergy Clin Immunol 1995;96:131–55.

[172] DeYampert NM, Beck LA. Eosinophilia and multiple erythematous indurated plaques. Arch Dermatol 1997;133:1579–84.

[173] Milewski M, Libura M, Undas A, et al. Interferon gamma abolishes aspirin-induced bronchoconstriction in a hypereosinophilic non-atopic patient [abstract 2125]. Eur Respir J 1995;8(Suppl 19):432S.

[174] Vilcek J, Feldman M. The sequences of IFN-alfa-2a and IFN-alfa-2b differ by one amino acid. Historical review: cytokines as therapeutics and targets of therapeutics. Trends Pharmacol Sci 2004;25(4):201–9.

[175] Dicato M, Ries F, Duhem C. Long lasting remission of hypereosinophilic syndrome (HES) after alpha-interferon (IFN) treatment. Blood 1994;84(10 Suppl 1):631A.

[176] Grace M, Youngster S, Gitlin G, et al. Structural and biologic characterization of pegylated recombinant IFN-α2b. J Interferon Cytokine Res 2001;21:1103–15.

[177] Butterfield JH. PEG-Interferon after Interferon alfa-2b for hypereosinophilic syndrome. J Allergy Clin Immunol 2007;119:S222.

[178] Gisslinger H, Eichinger S, Gilly B, et al. Exacerbation of autoimmunity during therapy with recombinant interferon alpha for hematological disorders. Ann Hematol 1992;65(Suppl): A8.

[179] Raison CL, Demetrashivili M, Capuron L, et al. Neuropsychiatric adverse effects of interferon-alpha: recognition and management. CNS Drugs 2005;19:105–23.

[180] Hendrick A. Case report psychosis during interferon in eosinophilic leukaemia. Clin lab Haematol 1994;16:295–6.

[181] Kook H, Cho D, Noh H-Y, et al. Chronic eosinophilic leukemia with unique chromosomal abnormality, add(8)(p23), in a 14-month girl: treatment with imatinib mesilate [abstract 4931]. Blood 2002;100(11):344–5.

[182] Nassar GM, Pedro P, Remmers RE, et al. Reversible renal failure in a patient with the hypereosinophilic syndrome during therapy with alpha interferon. Am J Kidney Dis 1998;31:121–6.

[183] Kanthawatana S, Irani AM, Schwartz LB. Recombinant Interferon-alpha (IFNα) and pregnancy in a patient with hypereosinophilic syndrome. J Allergy Clin Immunol 1998; 101(1):S20–S2S.

[184] Blanquer A, Lopez A, Tarin F, et al. Alpha interferon for hypereosinophilic syndrome. Am J Hematol 1994;47(4):332–3.

[185] George BO, Abdelaal MA, Gang MT, et al. Idiopathic hypereosinophilic syndrome: a report of four cases in Arabs, and a review of the literature. Afr J Med Sci 2001; 30:241–9.

[186] Papo T, Piette J-C, Hermine O. Treatment of the hypereosinophilic syndrome with interferon-α. Ann Intern Med 1995;123:155–6.

[187] Chockalingam A, Jalil A, Shadduck RK, et al. Case Report. Allogeneic peripheral blood stem cell transplantation for hypereosinophilic syndrome with severe cardiac dysfunction. Bone Marrow Transplant 1999;23:1093–4.

[188] Xicoy B, Batlle M, Grau J, et al. Transient demyelinating neurologic lesions in a patient with idiopathic hypereosinophilic syndrome [letter to the editor]. Am J Hematol 2002;69: 153–4.

[189] Katz HT, Haque SJ, Hsieh FH. Pediatric hypereosinophilic syndrome (HES) differs from adult HES. J Pediatr 2005;146:134–6.

[190] Tan AM, Downie PJ, Ekert H. Hypereosinophilia syndrome with pneumonia in acute lymphoblastic leukemia. Aust Paediatr J 1987;23:359–61.

[191] Blatt J, Pjoujansky R, Horn M, et al. Idiopathic hypereosinophilic syndrome terminating in acute lymphoblastic leukemia. Pediatr Hematol Oncol 1992;9:151–5.

[192] Narayanan G, Hussain BM, Chandralekha B, et al. Hypereosinophilic syndrome in acute lymphoblastic leukemia: case report and literature review. Acta Oncol 2000;39:241–3.

[193] Hill A, Metry D. Urticarial lesions in a child with acute lymphoblastic leukemia and eosinophilia. Pediatr Dermatol 2003;20:502–5.

[194] Takamizawa M, Iwata T, Watanabe K, et al. Elevated production of interleukin-4 and interleukin-5 by T cells in a child with idiopathic hypereosinophilic syndrome. J Allergy Clin Immunol 1994;93:1076–8.

[195] Alfaham MA, Ferguson SD, Sihra B, et al. The idiopathic hypereosinophilic syndrome. Arch Dis Child 1987;62:601–13.

[196] Ito T, Harada K, Takada G. An infant with hypereosinophilic syndrome and heart failure markedly responded to prednisolone: serial changes of left ventricular wall thickening and left ventricular diastolic dysfunction observed by echocardiography. Heart Vessels 1998;13: 302–5.

[197] Kao CC, Ou LS, Lin SJ, et al. Childhood idiopathic hypereosinophilic syndrome: report of a case. Asian Pac J Allergy Immunol 2002;20(2):121–6.

[198] Funahashi S, Masaki I, Furuyama T. Hypereosinophilic syndrome accompanying gangrene of the toes with peripheral arterial occlusion: A case report. Angiology 2006;57: 231–4.

[199] Subhash HS, George P, Sowmya G, et al. Progressive dilated cardiomyopathy in a patient with hypereosinophilic syndrome despite prednisone induced hematological remission. J Assoc Physicians India 2001;49:944–5.

[200] Marshall GM, White L. Effective therapy for a severe case of the idiopathic hypereosinophilic syndrome. Am J Pediatr Hematol Oncol 1989;11:178–83.

[201] Horenstein MS, Humes R, Epstein ML, et al. Loffler's endocarditis presenting in 2 children as fever with eosinophilia. Pediatrics 2002;110:1014–8.

[202] Rives S, Alcorta I, Toll T, et al. Idiopathic hypereosinophilic syndrome in children: report of a 7-year-old boy with FIP1L1-PDGFRA rearrangement. J Pediatr Hematol Oncol 2005; 27:663–5.

[203] Rizzari C, Cantu-Rajnoldi A, Masera G. Efficacy of prolonged low-dose steroid treatment in a child with idiopathic hypereosinophilic syndrome: a case report. Pediatr Hematol Oncol 1995;12:209–12.

[204] Venkatesh C, Mahender E, Janani S, et al. Hypereosinophilic syndrome. Indian J Pediatr 2006;73:237–9.

[205] Bakhshi S, Hamre M, Mohamed AN, et al. t(5;9)(q11;134): a novel familial translocation involving abelson oncogene and association with hypereosinophilia. J Pediatr Hematol Oncol 2003;25:82–4.

[206] Uckan D, Hicsonmez G, Tunc B, et al. The analysis of eosinophil and lymphocyte phenotype following single dose of high-dose methylprednisolone in two siblings with marked hyypereosinohilia. Clin Lab Haematol 2001;23:33–7.

[207] Roy R, Ladusans E, Keenen R. Acute hypereosinophilia associated with right ventricular thrombosis. Eur J Pediatr 2005;164:448–50.

[208] Hii MW, Firkin FC, MacIsaac AI, et al. Obstructive prosthetic mitral valve thrombosis in idiopathic hypereosinophilic syndrome: a case report and review of the literature. J Heart Valve Dis 2006;15:721–5.

[209] Spiegel R, Miron D, Fink D, et al. Eosinophilic pericarditis: a rare complication of idiopathic hypereosinophilic syndrome in a child. Pediatr Cardiol 2004;25:690–2.

[210] Jain AK, Dubey AP, Sudha S. Idiopathic hypereosinophilic syndrome-unusual presentation. Indian Pediatr 2004;41:79–82.

[211] Pellier I, Le Moine P, Rialland X, et al. Myelodysplastic syndrome with t(5;12)(q31; p12-p13) and eosinophilia: a pediatric case with review of literature. J Pediatr Hemat Oncol 1996;18:285–8.

[212] Leblond P, Lepers S, Thebaud E, et al. Idiopathic hypereosinophilic syndrome: a case report in an infant. Arch Pediatr 2004;11:219–22.

ELSEVIER
SAUNDERS

Immunol Allergy Clin N Am
27 (2007) 519–527

IMMUNOLOGY
AND ALLERGY
CLINICS
OF NORTH AMERICA

Novel Approaches to Therapy of Hypereosinophilic Syndromes

Hans-Uwe Simon, MD, PhD[a],*, Jan Cools, PhD[b]

[a]Department of Pharmacology, University of Bern,
Friedbuehlstrasse 49, CH-3010 Bern, Switzerland
[b]Department of Molecular and Developmental Genetics, K.U. Leuven,
VIB, Herestraat 49-box 602, B-3000 Leuven, Belgium

The hypereosinophilic syndromes (HES) are a heterogeneous group of disorders that are characterized by the presence of marked blood and tissue eosinophilia resulting in a variety of clinical manifestations. Three criteria, established by Chusid and colleagues [1], define HES: (1) sustained blood eosinophilia of greater than 1500/mL for longer than 6 months; (2) apparent etiologies for eosinophilia must be absent; and (3) patients must have signs of organ involvement. Known causes of eosinophilia include parasitic helminth infections, HIV, allergic disorders, and malignancies. There has been recent progress in our understanding of the pathogenesis of at least some HES subgroups. For instance, T-cell clones expressing interleukin (IL)-5 have been identified as a cause of HES in some patients [2–5]. In other patients, mutations in hematopoietic stem cells largely contribute to the development of HES [6,7]. Currently, such patients are still considered as suffering from HES, although the cause of eosinophilia can be explained.

Corticosteroids are the first-line treatment for most patients, but the most appropriate dose and the duration of therapy have not been evaluated. Usually, patients are treated with a high dosage (>40 mg of prednisone equivalent) initially, and the dosage is reduced gradually. Using this approach, most, but not all, patients who have HES respond. Patients receiving long-term treatment have increased risks for developing opportunistic infections (eg, *Pneumocystis* species–induced pneumonia) and bone loss.

Work in the laboratory of the authors is supported by grants from the Swiss National Science Foundation (grant no. 310000-107526); the Stanley Thomas Johnson Foundation, Bern, Switzerland; the OPO-Foundation, Zurich, Switzerland; grant G.0287.07 of the 'FWO-Vlaanderen;' and grant SCIE2006-34 of the Foundation against Cancer, foundation of public interest.

* Corresponding author.
E-mail address: hus@pki.unibe.ch (H-U. Simon).

doi:10.1016/j.iac.2007.07.003

Corticosteroid-mediated adverse effects often become limiting, and the use of alternative therapies must be considered. Cytotoxic therapies might be used in corticosteroid-refractory HES. For instance, hydroxyurea has been applied successfully at dosages of 1 to 3 g/d [8]; however, these treatments are associated with unwanted hematologic and gastrointestinal effects. Recently, therapeutic progress has been made, particularly in those patients in whom our understanding of the pathogenesis of the disease has improved. This article summarizes these new pharmacologic approaches to the therapy of HES.

Interferon-α

Low-dose (1–3 million U/d) interferon-α has been reported to control HES for prolonged periods of time [9]. In contrast to corticosteroids, eosinophil numbers do not decline rapidly, but a reduction can be expected within 2 to 4 weeks. The antieosinophil effect of interferon-α might be the consequence of its effect on the T helper 1 (Th1)-T helper 2 (Th2) balance [10]; however, interferon-α receptors also are present on eosinophils [11], suggesting that clinical benefits also can be due to the direct effects on eosinophils. It is unclear when eosinophils activate the interferon-α receptor gene during maturation, but it is likely that it occurs late, during terminal differentiation, as observed in neutrophils [12]. Therefore, the effects of interferon-α in patients with mutations in hematopoietic stem cells associated with HES might be limited.

Because interferon-α, even at low doses, has multiple unwanted systemic effects (Box 1), it often is used only in corticosteroid-refractory HES [10]. Interferon-α has been reported to break corticosteroid resistance [10] or, at the least, to act synergistically with corticosteroids in treatment outcomes [9]. Interferon-α has been lifesaving for patients with intractable HES that was resistant to corticosteroids. Interferon-α also has been reported to act synergistically with low-dose hydroxyurea [9].

Anti–interleukin-5 monoclonal antibody

Eosinophil development from hematopoietic stem cells is regulated mainly by IL-5 and, to a lesser extent, IL-3 and granulocyte/macrophage colony-stimulating factor (GM-CSF) [13]. Because IL-5 seems to contribute to the pathogenesis of some HES subgroups [14], it represents a logical therapeutic target for these diseases. Preliminary open-label studies in the treatment of HES with anti–IL-5 monoclonal antibody (mAb) from two companies were encouraging; the treatment reduced blood eosinophil numbers into the normal range within 48 hours [15,16]; however, tissue eosinophilia was reduced by only 50% [15]. Nevertheless, clinical improvement was seen in patients who had HES in association with anti–IL-5 mAb therapy, and the drug was tolerated well.

Box 1. Adverse effects of antieosinophil therapies

Low-dose interferon-α
Flulike symptoms
Nausea
Lack of appetite
Depression
Fatigue
Elevated liver transaminases
Myelosuppression

Imatinib
Nausea
Diarrhea
Rash
Edema
Muscle cramps
Elevated liver transaminases
Myelosuppression
Acute cardiac decompensation?

Mepolizumab
Upper respiratory tract infection
Myalgia

Alemtuzumab
Flulike symptoms (first day only)
Infections
Myelosuppression

Following these initial reports, a randomized, double-blind, placebo-controlled study was conducted with an anti–IL-5 mAb (mepolizumab). Eighty-five patients who had HES without evidence of a Fip1-like 1 (FIP1L1)-platelet-derived growth factor receptor α (PDGFRA) gene fusion (see later discussion) were randomized [17]. This study demonstrated a significant corticosteroid-sparing effect of mepolizumab, which suggests that corticosteroid-mediated morbidity can be reduced by this antibody therapy. Notably, approximately 50% of the mepolizumab-treated patients no longer required any corticosteroids. Therefore, mepolizumab represents the first drug specifically targeting eosinophils that showed clinical usefulness in an eosinophil-based disorder.

Mepolizumab only partially depleted eosinophils from tissues in patients suffering from bronchial asthma [18], eosinophilic dermatitis [15], or eosinophilic esophagitis (A. Straumann and H-U. Simon, unpublished data). The reduction of eosinophil numbers in inflamed tissues is rarely more than

50%, a finding that is independent of the underlying disease. In all of these clinical studies, the dose of mepolizumab was 750 mg, which resulted in a rapid decline of blood eosinophil numbers to normal levels. We recently conducted a mepolizumab study in patients who had eosinophilic esophagitis that confirmed these findings. Increasing the dose to 1500 mg did not lead to increased reductions of eosinophil numbers within the epidermal layer of the esophagus (A. Straumann and H.-U. Simon, unpublished data). Because eosinophils are not depleted from inflamed tissues, it remains to be shown whether mepolizumab is able to prevent, or at least to reduce, end-organ pathology associated with HES.

Mepolizumab seems to be tolerated well [17]. The incidence of adverse effects in mepolizumab-treated patients was in the same range as with placebo, with two exceptions. In the randomized, double-blind, placebo-controlled study of mepolizumab treatment for HES, 21% of the mepolizumab-treated patients developed respiratory infections compared with 10% in the placebo group. In addition, myalgia occurred more frequently with mepolizumab (19% compared with 7% with placebo; see Box 1); however, the latter adverse event also might have been due to the reduction of the corticosteroid dose.

Imatinib

Imatinib, a tyrosine kinase inhibitor, is an effective drug in PDGFRA-associated HES. In this HES subgroup, a gene fusion occurs between FIP1L1 and PDGFRA as the result of an 800-kilobase interstitial deletion on chromosome 4q12 [6,19]. The gene fusion has been identified in eosinophils as well as in multiple other hematopoietic lineages, including neutrophils, monocytes, lymphocytes, and mast cells, suggesting that PDGFRA-associated HES is actually an eosinophilic leukemia that arises from a mutation in a pluripotent hematopoietic stem cell. The imatinib response rate in these patients is nearly 100%, with only a few cases of acquired drug resistance due to a T674I mutation in PDGFRA [6,20]. The reduction in blood eosinophils is seen within 1 week of initiation of therapy. Generally, clinical improvement is seen within 1 month. Low-dose (100 mg/d) imatinib is usually sufficient to control eosinophilia and symptoms. Side effects of imatinib therapy generally are mild and rarely lead to discontinuation of therapy (see Box 1) [21].

The use of imatinib in patients who have HES, in which PDGFRA does not play a role, is controversial. Imatinib does not seem to be useful in treating patients in whom cytokine-producing T cells are the underlying cause of HES; however, it was reported that some FIP1L1/PDGFRA-negative patients who had HES responded to imatinib [6,22]. This raises the possibility that such patients have a rearrangement, mutation, or at least overexpression of a gene encoding a tyrosine kinase. It is likely that most, if not all, patients who have HES and are responsive to imatinib actually suffer from eosinophilic leukemia or chronic myeloid leukemia associated with eosinophilia [7,23].

Other tyrosine kinase inhibitors

Despite the fact that imatinib treatment results in rapid, complete, and durable responses in FIP1L1-PDGFRA positive patients, some of the patients may relapse during imatinib therapy. Four patients have been described who developed resistance to imatinib; in all patients, the resistance was due to a T674I mutation within the kinase domain of FIP1L1-PDGFRA [6,20,24,25]. Despite the fact that FIP1L1-PDGFRA is extremely sensitive to imatinib, the FIP1L1-PDGFRA (T674I) mutant is highly resistant to imatinib, and increasing the dosage of imatinib cannot overcome resistance [6].

PKC412 [26], nilotinib (AMN107) [27,28], and sorafenib (BAY43-9006, Nexavar) [29] are small-molecule kinase inhibitors, with a different structure than imatinib, which show activity against PDGFRA and are under clinical development. The staurosporine derivative PKC412 originally was identified as an inhibitor of protein kinase C (PKC); it subsequently was shown to inhibit tyrosine kinases as well, including KDR, KIT, FLT3, and PDGFR [30]. PKC412 has shown activity in mast cell leukemia with the D816V KIT mutation [31] and is being tested in clinical trials for the treatment of acute myeloid leukemia with the FLT3 mutation [32]. Using in vitro and in vivo models, it was shown that PKC412 inhibits FIP1L1-PDGFRA and the imatinib resistant T674I mutant [26].

Nilotinib (AMN107) was rationally designed as a novel BCR-ABL inhibitor based on modeling of the binding of imatinib to the ABL kinase domain. Similar to imatinib, nilotinib interferes with tyrosine kinase activity by binding to the ATP-binding pocket when the kinase is in an inactive conformation. Nilotinib, however, inhibits proliferation of BCR-ABL transformed cells with a higher potency than does imatinib. In addition, nilotinib is active against several imatinib-resistant BCR-ABL mutants [33]. Nilotinib also inhibits the proliferation of cell lines transformed by activated KIT and PDGFR. Based on these observations, nilotinib also was tested for its activity against FIP1L1-PDGFRA and ETS variant gene 6 (ETV6)-PDGFRB and was found to inhibit these activated kinases at low nanomolar concentrations [28]. In addition, nilotinib showed at least some activity against the imatinib-resistant FIP1L1-PDGFRA (T674I) mutant [27].

Sorafenib (BAY43-9006, Nexavar) was developed as a BRAF inhibitor and was approved recently by the US Food and Drug Administration for the treatment of renal cell carcinoma [34]. More detailed analysis of the specificity of sorafenib revealed that it also had potent activity against RET and PDGFR family kinases. This was confirmed by in vitro studies using cell lines expressing activated FLT3, ETV6-PDGFRB, and FIP1L1-PDGFRA [29,35]. Sorafenib also showed potent activity against the imatinib-resistant FIP1L1-PDGFRA (T674I) mutant [29], which was confirmed recently in vivo by treatment of a FIP1L1-PDGFRA (T674I)-positive chronic eosinophilic leukemia patient with sorafenib (E. Lierman, J. Cools, and P. Vandenberghe, unpublished data).

These inhibitors might be suitable for patients who do not tolerate imatinib or have developed imatinib resistance as a result of the T674I mutation in PDGFRA. It remains to be investigated whether some of these inhibitors could be combined to prevent the development of resistance, especially in patients who have chronic eosinophilic leukemia in blast crisis.

Anti-CD52 monoclonal antibody

CD52 is a glycosyl-phosphotidol-inositol-linked glycoprotein expressed by leukocytes, including T and B cells, as well as eosinophils. An anti-CD52 mAb (alemtuzumab) has been developed that is being used increasingly for the prevention or treatment of acute allograft rejection in organ transplant recipients [36] and in the treatment of chronic lymphocytic leukemia [37]. Alemtuzumab was used in the treatment of two patients who had HES [38,39]. One patient suffered from a clonal T-cell disease associated with HES. The primary cellular target of this antibody in HES remains to be determined. Alemtuzumab treatment increases the risk for opportunistic infections (see Box 1) [40].

Bone marrow transplantation

Attempts to treat HES with allogeneic hematopoietic stem cell transplantation have been reported since 1988 [41–49]. Because HES are a heterogeneous group of uncommon disorders, these reports only represent cases or small series of patients. Clearly, in such a situation, it is difficult to establish a transplantation standard. Because of the high treatment-associated mortality, stem cell transplantation is reserved for patients suffering from aggressive HES that are resistant to drug treatment. In the case of imatinib failure in PDGFRA-associated HES, allogeneic hematopoietic stem cell transplantation represents a confirmed curative option [50].

Summary

There has been recent progress in the understanding of the pathogenesis of HES. This has led to the distinction of subgroups in which the underlying cause has been identified. Consequently, promising new treatment options became available. For instance, the prognosis of PDGFRA-associated HES is poor because of cardiac complications. Imatinib dramatically improves the clinical situation of these patients within 1 month, and it is hoped that it also will improve their long-term survival. The cytokine-driven forms of HES are considered to have a better prognosis, and the availability of mepolizumab might reduce corticosteroid-mediated adverse effects; however, it is unlikely that mepolizumab is able to delete T-cell clones, which have been identified as IL-5–producing cells in some patients. Because such clonal T cells may transform into a T-cell lymphoma, the current therapeutic options for these patients are not satisfying. Moreover, it is unclear whether mepolizumab is useful to reduce HES-associated symptoms and prevent end-organ damage. There are some concerns in this respect, because the antibody seems to deplete eosinophils from affected organs only partially.

Besides the progress in HES therapy, there is some progress regarding measurement of treatment responses. For instance, the presence or absence of the abnormal fusion protein in PDGFRA-associated HES [19] or immunophenotypically abnormal T-cell clones [4,5] allows monitoring of therapeutic effects. In other cases, however, eosinophil numbers and clinical presentations remain the only parameters that are used. No other marker, including eosinophil-derived basic proteins, has been validated. Moreover, no marker is available that predicts eosinophil-mediated tissue damage.

References

[1] Chusid MJ, Dale CD, West BC, et al. The hypereosinophilic syndrome: analysis of fourteen cases with review of the literature. Medicine (Baltimore) 1997;54:1–27.

[2] Cogan E, Schandene L, Crusiaux A, et al. Brief report: clonal proliferation of type 2 helper T cells in a man with the hypereosinophilic syndrome. N Engl J Med 1994;330: 535–8.

[3] Simon HU, Yousefi S, Dommann-Scherrer CC, et al. Expansion of cytokine-producing CD4-CD8- T cells associated with abnormal Fas expression and hypereosinophilia. J Exp Med 1996;183:1071–82.

[4] Simon HU, Plötz SG, Dummer R, et al. Abnormal clones of T cells producing interleukin-5 in idiopathic eosinophilia. N Engl J Med 1999;341:1112–20.

[5] Simon HU, Plötz SG, Simon D, et al. Clinical and immunological features of patients with interleukin-5-producing T cell clones and eosinophilia. Int Arch Allergy Immunol 2001;124: 242–5.

[6] Cools J, DeAngelo DJ, Gotlib J, et al. A tyrosine kinase created by fusion of the PDGFRA and FIP1L1 genes as a therapeutic target of imatinib in idiopathic hypereosinophilic syndrome. N Engl J Med 2003;348:1201–14.

[7] Fletcher S, Bain B. Diagnosis and treatment of hypereosinophilic syndromes. Curr Opin Hematol 2007;14:37–42.

[8] Parrillo JE, Fauci AS, Wolff SM. Therapy of the hypereosinophilic syndrome. Ann Intern Med 1978;89:167–72.

[9] Butterfield JH. Interferon treatment for hypereosinophilic syndromes and systemic mastocytosis. Acta Haematol 2005;114:26–40.

[10] Simon HU, Seelbach H, Ehmann R, et al. Clinical and immunological effects of low-dose IFN-alpha treatment in patients with corticosteroid-resistant asthma. Allergy 2003;58: 1250–5.

[11] Aldebert D, Lamkhioued B, Desaint C, et al. Eosinophils express a functional receptor for interferon alpha: inhibitory role of interferon alpha on the release of mediators. Blood 1996; 87:2354–60.

[12] Martinelli S, Urosevic M, Daryadel A, et al. Induction of genes mediating interferon-dependent extracellular trap formation during neutrophil differentiation. J Biol Chem 2004;279: 44123–32.

[13] Rothenberg ME, Hogan SP. The eosinophil. Annu Rev Immunol 2006;24:147–74.

[14] Klion AD, Bochner BS, Gleich GJ, et al. Approaches to the treatment of hypereosinophilic syndromes: a workshop summary report. J Allergy Clin Immunol 2006;117:1292–302.

[15] Plötz SG, Simon HU, Darsow U, et al. Use of an anti-interleukin-5 antibody in the hypereosinophilic syndrome with eosinophilic dermatitis. N Engl J Med 2003;349:2334–9.

[16] Klion AD, Law MA, Noel P, et al. Safety and efficacy of the monoclonal anti-interleukin 5 antibody, SCH55700, in the treatment of patients with the hypereosinophilic syndrome. Blood 2004;103:2939–41.

[17] Rothenberg M, Klion A, Roufosse F, et al. Corticosteroid reduction and clinical control in patients with hypereosinophilic syndrome treated with mepolizumab, an anti-interleukin-5 monoclonal antibody. Submitted for publication.

[18] Flood-Page PT, Menzies-Gow AN, Kay AB, et al. Eosinophil's role remains uncertain as anti-IL-5 only partially depletes numbers in asthmatic airways. Am J Respir Crit Care Med 2003;167:199–204.

[19] Klion AD, Robyn J, Akin C, et al. Molecular remission and reversal of myelofibrosis in response to imatinib mesylate treatment in patients with the myeloproliferative variant of hypereosinophilic syndrome. Blood 2004;103:473–8.

[20] von Bubnoff N, Sandherr M, Schlimok G, et al. Myeloid blast crisis evolving during imatinib treatment of an FIP1L1-PDGFR alpha-positive chronic myeloproliferative disease with prominent eosinophilia. Leukemia 2005;19:286–7.

[21] Hensley ML, Ford JM. Imatinib treatment: specific issues related to safety, fertility, and pregnancy. Semin Hematol 2003;40(2 Suppl 2):21–5.

[22] La Starza R, Specchia G, Cuneo A, et al. The hypereosinophilic syndrome: fluorescence in situ hybridization detects the del(4)(q12)-FIP1L1/PDGFRA but not genomic rearrangements of other tyrosine kinases. Haematologica 2005;90:596–601.

[23] Simon D, Simon HU. Eosinophilic disorders. J Allergy Clin Immunol 2007;119:1291–300.

[24] Griffin JH, Leung J, Bruner RJ, et al. Discovery of a fusion kinase in EOL-1 cells and idiopathic hypereosinophilic syndrome. Proc Natl Acad Sci U S A 2003;100:7830–5.

[25] Ohnishi H, Kandabashi K, Maeda Y, et al. Chronic eosinophilic leukaemia with FIP1L1-PDGFRA fusion and T674I mutation that evolved from Langerhans cell histiocytosis with eosinophilia after chemotherapy. Br J Haematol 2006;134:547–9.

[26] Cools J, Stover EH, Boulton CL, et al. PKC412 overcomes resistance to imatinib in a murine model of FIP1L1-PDGFRalpha-induced myeloproliferative disease. Cancer Cell 2003;3: 459–69.

[27] von Bubnoff N, Gorantla SP, Thöne S, et al. The FIP1L1-PDGFRA T674I mutation can be inhibited by the tyrosine kinase inhibitor AMN107 (nilotinib). Blood 2006;107:4970–1.

[28] Stover EH, Chen J, Lee BH, et al. The small molecule tyrosine kinase inhibitor AMN107 inhibits TEL-PDGFRbeta and FIP1L1-PDGFRalpha in vitro and in vivo. Blood 2005; 106:3206–13.

[29] Lierman E, Folens C, Stover EH, et al. Sorafenib is a potent inhibitor of FIP1L1-PDGFRa and the imatinib-resistant FIP1L1-PDGFRa T674I mutant. Blood 2006;108:1374–6.

[30] Fabbro D, Ruetz S, Bodis S, et al. PKC412–a protein kinase inhibitor with a broad therapeutic potential. Anticancer Drug Des 2000;15:17–28.

[31] Gotlib J, Berubé C, Growney JD, et al. Activity of the tyrosine kinase inhibitor PKC412 in a patient with mast cell leukemia with the D816V KIT mutation. Blood 2005;106:2865–70.

[32] Stone RM, DeAngelo DJ, Klimek V, et al. Patients with acute myeloid leukemia and an activating mutation in FLT3 respond to a small-molecule FLT3 tyrosine kinase inhibitor, PKC412. Blood 2005;105:54–60.

[33] Weisberg E, Manley PW, Breitenstein W, et al. Characterization of AMN107, a selective inhibitor of native and mutant Bcr-Abl. Cancer Cell 2005;7:129–41.

[34] Escudier B, Eisen T, Stadler WM, et al. Sorafenib in advanced clear-cell renal-cell carcinoma. N Engl J Med 2007;356:125–34.

[35] Lierman E, Lahortiga I, Van Miegroet H, et al. The ability of sorafenib to inhibit oncogenic PDGFRbeta and FLT3 mutants and overcome resistance to other small molecule inhibitors. Haematologica 2007;92:27–34.

[36] Thai NL, Khan A, Tom K, et al. Alemtuzumab induction and tacrolimus monotherapy in pancreas transplantation: one- and two-year outcomes. Transplantation 2006;82:1621–4.

[37] Karlsson C, Hansson L, Celsing F, et al. Treatment of severe refractory autoimmune hemolytic anemia in B-cell chronic lymphocytic leukemia with alemtuzumab (humanized CD52 monoclonal antibody). Leukemia 2007;21:511–4.

[38] Sefcick A, Sowter D, DasGupta E, et al. Alemtuzumab therapy for refractory idiopathic hypereosinophilic syndrome. Br J Haematol 2004;124:558–9.

[39] Pitini V, Teti D, Arrigo C, et al. Alemtuzumab therapy for refractory idiopathic hypereosinophilic syndrome with abnormal T cells: a case report. Br J Haematol 2004;127:477.

[40] Peleg AY, Husain S, Kwak EJ, et al. Opportunistic infections in 547 organ transplant recipients receiving alemtuzumab, a humanized monoclonal CD52 antibody. Clin Infect Dis 2007;44:204–12.

[41] Archimbaud E, Guyotat D, Guillaume C, et al. Hypereosinophilic syndrome with multiple organ dysfunction treated by allogeneic bone marrow transplantation. Am J Hematol 1988; 27:302–3.

[42] Sigmund DA, Flessa HC. Hypereosinophilic syndrome: successful allogeneic bone marrow transplantation. Bone Marrow Transplant 1995;15:647–8.

[43] Fukushima T, Kuriyama K, Ito H, et al. Successful bone marrow transplantation for idiopathic hypereosinophilic syndrome. Br J Haematol 1995;90:213–5.

[44] Esteva-Lorenzo FJ, Meehan KR, Spitzer TR, et al. Allogeneic bone marrow transplantation in a patient with hypereosinophilic syndrome. Am J Hematol 1996;51:164–5.

[45] Sadoun A, Lacotte L, Delwail V, et al. Allogeneic bone marrow transplantation for hypereosinophilic syndrome with advanced myelofibrosis. Bone Marrow Transplant 1997;19: 741–3.

[46] Basara N, Markova J, Schmetzer B, et al. Chronic eosinophilic leukaemia: successful treatment with an unrelated bone marrow transplantation. Leuk Lymphoma 1998;32:189–93.

[47] Vazquez L, Caballero D, Canizo CD, et al. Allogeneic peripheral blood cell transplantation for hypereosinophilic syndrome with myelofibrosis. Bone Marrow Transplant 2000;25: 217–8.

[48] Ueno NT, Anagnostopoulos A, Rondon G, et al. Successful non-myeloablative allogeneic transplantation for treatment of idiopathic hypereosinophilic syndrome. Br J Haematol 2002;119:131–4.

[49] Cooper MA, Akard LP, Thompson JM, et al. Hypereosinophilic syndrome: long-term remission following allogeneic stem cell transplant in spite of transient eosinophilia post-transplant. Am J Hematol 2005;78:33–6.

[50] Halaburda K, Prejzner W, Szatkowski D, et al. Allogeneic bone marrow transplantation for hypereosinophilic syndrome: long-term follow-up with eradication of FIP1L1-PDGFRA fusion transcript. Bone Marrow Transplant 2006;38:319–20.

ELSEVIER
SAUNDERS

Immunol Allergy Clin N Am
27 (2007) 529–549

IMMUNOLOGY
AND ALLERGY
CLINICS
OF NORTH AMERICA

Evaluation and Differential Diagnosis of Marked, Persistent Eosinophilia

Thomas B. Nutman, MD

*Laboratory of Parasitic Diseases, National Institute of Allergy and Infectious Diseases,
National Institutes of Health, Building 4, Room B1-03, 4 Center Drive,
Bethesda, MD 20892-0425, USA*

Elevations in the levels of peripheral blood and tissue eosinophils can occur in a wide variety of disease processes that include infectious, allergic, neoplastic, primary hematologic disorders, and other, often less well-defined entities [1–3]. Worldwide, multicellular helminth (worm) parasites are most commonly associated with significant eosinophilia, followed in frequency by drug hypersensitivity and atopic diseases. Hypereosinophilic syndromes (HES), in contrast, are a set of relatively rare, heterogeneous disorders characterized by persistent eosinophilia (defined as $> 1500/\mu L$ for 6 months) and organ involvement/dysfunction in which other clinical entities have been excluded [4]. The approach to defining these non-HES causes of persistently elevated eosinophil levels is the focus of this review.

Biology of the eosinophil and eosinophilia

Eosinophils are bone marrow–derived leukocytes whose development and terminal differentiation are under the control of several cytokines (interleukin [IL]-3, granulocyte macrophage colony-stimulating factor [GM-CSF], and IL-5), with IL-5 being the cytokine that is primarily responsible for eosinophilopoiesis. Eosinophilia, defined as more than 450 eosinophils/μL (or 500/μL in some studies), is normally measured by sampling peripheral blood, although eosinophils are predominantly found in peripheral tissues [5] (and particularly in those tissues with a mucosal-environmental interface such as the respiratory, gastrointestinal, and lower genitourinary tracts). Physiologically, eosinophil levels in the peripheral blood have a diurnal variation with a peak in the morning, a time at which endogenous steroids are the lowest [6]. Pyogenic inflammation causes eosinopenia, a process that can mask the presence of

E-mail address: tnutman@niaid.nih.gov

0889-8561/07/$ - see front matter. Published by Elsevier Inc.
doi:10.1016/j.iac.2007.07.008

eosinophilia or eosinophil-mediated inflammation. Hypoadrenalism is associated with eosinophilia because of low levels of endogenous glucocorticoids. Eosinophil levels can also be lowered by exogenous administration of medications, including corticosteroids, estrogen, and epinephrine [7,8].

Eosinophils, particularly in disease states associated with hypereosinophilia, can have a variety of phenotypic and functional changes felt to reflect cellular activation. In these situations, the eosinophil on a peripheral smear can appear vacuolated with alterations in granule size, and, on flow cytometric analysis, the eosinophil has characteristic changes in surface molecule expression [9]. By electron microscopy, eosinophils demonstrate piecemeal degranulation [10] when activated.

Hypereosinophilic conditions

Based on more recent classifications of HES that include idiopathic hypereosinophilic syndrome (IHES), platelet-derived growth factor receptor α (PDGFRA)–associated HES, the lymphocytic variant HES (L-HES), familial hypereosinophilia, Churg-Strauss syndrome (CSS), and eosinophil-associated gastrointestinal disease (EGID), HES have been classified as heterogeneous group of uncommon disorders characterized by marked eosinophilia in the peripheral blood, tissues, or both, often without an identifiable cause (see the article by Sheihk and Weller in this issue) [2,4]. It is against this backdrop that an approach to the differential diagnosis of those non-HES (with identifiable causes) associated with persistent, marked eosinophilia (> 1500 eosinophils/μL) and/or evidence of organ dysfunction is discussed. Because there are comprehensive reviews of eosinophilia in general [1,11,12], the focus herein is on those disorders that could be confused with HES.

Infectious diseases

A wide variety of infectious agents, almost exclusively helminth (worm) parasites, elicit eosinophilia [3,11,13]; only a relatively few, however, elicit a sustained, marked increase in eosinophil levels (Box 1) [14]. The pattern and degree of eosinophilia in parasitic infections is determined by the development, migration, and distribution of the parasite within the host as well as by the host's immune response. In general, it is useful to remember that parasites tend to elicit marked eosinophilia when they or their products come into contact with immune effector cells in tissues, particularly during migration. When barriers are erected between the parasite and host or when the parasite no longer invades tissue, the stimulus for eosinophilia is usually absent. Therefore, eosinophilia is highest among parasites with a phase of development that involves migration through tissue (eg, trichinosis, ascariasis, gnathostomiasis, filarial parasites), but a sustained eosinophilic response is not seen among parasites that are wholly intraluminal (eg, adult tapeworms) or contained in a cystic structure (eg, hydatid cysts) unless there

---

Box 1. Conditions associated with marked peripheral blood eosinophilia

Infectious diseases
  Parasitic infections primarily with helminths (see Table 1)
  Certain fungal infections (Allergic bronchopulmonary
    aspergillosis, coccidiomycosis)
  Infestations—scabies, myiasis

Allergic or atopic diseases
  Drug hypersensitivity or medication-associated eosinophilias
  Atopic diseases

Hematologic and neoplastic disorders
  Hypereosinophilic syndromes (HES) including chronic
    eosinophilic leukemia
  Leukemia (acute myelogenous leukemias most commonly,
    B-cell ALL)
  Lymphomas (particularly Hodgkin's, T- and B-cell lymphomas)
  Tumor associated
  Adenocarcinomas
  Squamous carcinomas
  Large-cell lung carcinomas
  Transitional cell carcinoma of the bladder
  Systemic mastocytosis

Immunologic
  Primary immunodeficiency diseases (HyperIgE syndrome,
    Omenn syndrome)
  Graft-versus-host-disease

Endocrinologic disorders
  Hypoadrenalism

Other
  Irradiation
  Atheroembolic disorders
  Sarcoidosis

---

is disruption of the integrity of the cyst wall with leakage of cyst contents and exposure to the immune system [11,13]. Those parasites most likely to induce marked eosinophilia are noted in Table 1. Evaluation of helminth etiologies for marked eosinophilia should be guided not only by the clinical findings, but most often by geographic histories of potential exposures to infections. Approaches to the diagnosis of these infections are suggested in Table 1, provided there is an appropriate exposure history.

Table 1
Helminth infections associated with marked and/or persistent eosinophilia

Parasitic disease Organism(s)	Development and duration of eosinophilia		Main anatomical site(s)	Diagnosis
	Acute	Persistent		
Angiostrongyloidiasis				
Angiostrongylus cantonensis	+		CNS	Larvae in CSF
Angiostrongylus costiricensis	+		GI	Biopsy
Ascariasis	+		GI	Eggs in stool
Clonorchiasis	+	+	Hepatobiliary	Eggs in stool, serology
Fascioliasis	+	+	Hepatobiliary	Eggs in stool, serology
Fasciolopsiasis	+		GI	Eggs in stool
Filarial infections				
Lymphatic Filariasis				
Brugia, Wuchereria	+	+	Blood, lymphatics	Mf in blood, serology, CFA
Loa loa	+	+	Subcutaneous, eye	Mf in blood, worm extracted
Mansonella ozzardi	+	+	Blood	Mf in blood
Mansonella perstans	+	+	Blood, body cavities	Mf in blood, adult in tissue
Mansonella streptocerca	+	+	Skin, subcutaneous tissue	Mf in skin snips
Onchocerca volvulus	+	+	Skin, eye, subcutaneous tissue	Mf in skin snips, adults in nodules
Tropical pulmonary eosinophilia	+	+	Lung	Serology
Gnathostomiasis	+	+	Soft tissue	Serology, worm in specimen
Hookworm	+	+	GI, lung (acutely)	Eggs in stool
Opisthorchiasis	+	+	Hepatobiliary	Eggs in stool
Paragonimiasis	+	+	Lung, CNS, subcutaneous	Eggs in sputum, BAL, stool
Schistosomiasis	+			Serology
Schistosoma haematobium	+		Urinary tract	Eggs in urine
Schistosoma intercalatum	+		Hepatic, GI	Eggs in stool
Schistosoma japonicum	+		Hepatic, GI	Eggs in stool
Schistosoma mansoni	+		Hepatic, GI	Eggs in stool
Schistosoma mekongi	+		Hepatic, GI	Eggs in stool
Strongyloidiasis	+	+	GI, lung, skin	Larvae in stool, serology
Trichinosis	+	+	GI, muscle	Serology, muscle biopsy
Visceral larva migrans				
Toxocara canis; T catis	+	+	Liver, eye, lung	Serology, larvae in tissue
Baylisacaris procyois	+	+	CNS, eye	Larvae in specimen

Abbreviations: BAL, bronchoalveolar lavage; CFA, circulating filarial antigen; CNS, central nervous system; CSF, cerebrospinal fluid; GI, gastrointestinal; Mf, microfilariae.

Infections with protozoa rarely result in peripheral eosinophilia. However, the intestinal coccidian *Isospora belli* can be associated with eosinophilia [15,16]. Less commonly, eosinophilia can result from infection with the protozoan *Dientamoeba fragilis*. Rarely, infection with *Sarcocystis hominis*, a cause of eosinophilic myositis, has been accompanied by marked peripheral eosinophilia [17–19].

Ectoparasites, particularly scabies, are also associated with peripheral blood eosinophilia [20]. While eosinophilia can be associated with myiasis, this association occurs rarely [21]. Although uncommon in HIV infection, modest eosinophilia can be seen [22–25]. Marked hypereosinophilia has developed in some HIV-infected patients particularly in those with a pustular, exfoliative dermatitis [22,25–27]. Two fungal diseases have been also been associated with hypereosinophilia: coccidiomyocosis and aspergillosis (when presenting as ABPA). Although the eosinophilia is typically mild in coccidial infections, marked eosinophilia may develop with disseminated coccidiomycosis [28–30].

Atopic/allergic diseases

Blood eosinophilia rarely exceeds 1500/μL in allergic rhinitis, nonallergic rhinitis with eosinophilia syndrome (NARES), or even in asthma (both allergic and nonallergic) despite respiratory tract eosinophil infiltration.

Because so many medications (as well as nutritional supplements and alternative therapies) have been associated with eosinophilia, a detailed history of current and past medications should be obtained from all patients with eosinophilia. Although the mechanisms underlying the drug-associated rise in eosinophil levels have not been determined (apart perhaps from some of the cytokines used therapeutically [eg, IL-2, GM-CSF]) [31–33], medication-related drug reactions are likely the most common cause of persistently elevated eosinophil levels in areas where exposure to parasites is uncommon [11]. Medication-associated peripheral blood eosinophilia may present without accompanying symptoms or may be associated with specific signs and symptoms. Asymptomatic eosinophilia has been associated most often with quinine, penicillins, cephalosporins, or quinolones. Pulmonary infiltrates with peripheral eosinophilia have been particularly associated with nonsteroidal anti-inflammatory drugs (NSAIDs), sulfas, and nitrofurantoin. Drug-induced hepatitis with eosinophilia is most often induced by the tetracyclines or the semisynthetic penicillins, although, more recently this has been seen by some of the newer selective serotonin reuptake inhibitors (SSRIs) [34]. Interstitial nephritis with eosinophilia has been associated with cephalosporins (cefotaxime is most commonly reported but others such as cefoxitin, cefoperazone, and cefotriaxone have also been described) and semisynthetic penicillins. Drug reaction with eosinophilia and systemic symptoms (DRESS) can occur with sulfasalazine, hydantoin, carbamazepine, d-penicillamine, allopurinol, hydrochlorothiazide, and cyclosporine, associated with viral infection (human herpesvirus-6, Epstein-Barr virus, cytomegalovirus) [12,35,36]. Patients with DRESS present with fever, rash, systemic involvement, and an appropriate medication history. Various drug-associated eosinophilic disorders are listed in Table 2 and a more exhaustive list can be found in reference [12].

Hematologic/neoplastic disorders

Lymphoid malignancies

Apart from situations where eosinophils or their precursors are malignantly transformed [37–39], eosinophilia can be driven by the production of eosinophilopoetic cytokines. For example, eosinophilia is often associated with Hodgkin's disease, and the generation of IL-5 by Reed-Sternberg cells has been demonstrated [40,41]. In primary cutaneous T-cell lymphoma and Sezary syndrome, blood and dermal eosinophilia are also frequently observed [42]. Other types of lymphoid malignancies (acute lymphoblastic leukemia [43] and B-cell ALL [44]) have been associated with eosinophilia.

Solid tumors

In addition to lymphomas, other neoplasms may occasionally be associated with blood eosinophilia. Tumor-associated eosinophilia [45] occurs with large-cell nonkeratinizing cervical tumors, large-cell undifferentiated lung carcinomas [46]; squamous carcinomas of the lung, vagina, penis, skin, and nasopharynx [47,48]; adenocarcinomas of the stomach, large bowel, and uterine body; and transitional cell carcinoma of the bladder [49].

Mastocytosis

Systemic mast cell disease is accompanied by peripheral eosinophilia in about 25% of cases [50] and rarely by features and organ involvement

Table 2
Types of drug reactions associated with eosinophilia

Manifestations	Commonly associated drugs
Asymptomatic	Penicillins, cephalosporins
Soft tissue swelling	GM-CSF, IL-2
Pulmonary infiltrates	Nonsteroidal anti-inflammatory agents
Interstitial nephritis	Semisynthetic penicillins, cephalosporins
Myocarditis	Ranitidine
Hepatitis	Semisynthetic penicillins, tetracyclines
Hypersensitivity vasculitis	Allopurinol, phenytoin
Gastroenterocolitis	Nonsteroidal anti-inflammtory agents
Asthma, nasal polyps	Aspirin
Eosinophilia-myalgia syndrome	L-tryptophan contaminant
DRESS	Sulfasalazine, hydantoin, carbamazepine, allopurinol, hydrochlorothiazide, cyclosporine, nevirapine

typical of HES [51]. Recently, methods for distinguishing between HES (with mast cell involvement) and systemic mastocytosis with eosinophilia have been proposed [52].

Immunologic disorders

Immunodeficiency disorders
Among the many primary immunodeficiency disorders only a few are associated with high-grade eosinophilia, those being Omenn syndrome [53] and the HyperIgE syndrome [54,55].

Graft-versus-host disease
Chronic graft-versus-host disease (GVHD), particularly that which develops following allogeneic stem cell transplantation, most commonly affects the skin, liver, and gastrointestinal (GI) tract [56,57]. Marked eosinophilia has also been seen occasionally with acute GVHD [58].

Endocrine disorders

The loss of endogenous adrenoglucocorticosteroids in Addison's disease, adrenal hemorrhage, or hypopituitarism can cause cause increased blood eosinophilia. Eosinophilia may be a clue to adrenal insufficiency in some patients, including those whose illnesses require intensive care [59].

Other

Cholesterol embolization, typically after a vascular or intravascular procedure, can lead to eosinophilia [60]. Radiation therapy has also been linked to eosinophilia, although high-grade eosinophilia is rare in this setting [61]. Sarcoidosis, inflammatory bowel disease, and other disorders associated with immunodysregulation, can also be associated with marked eosinophilia [62].

Hypereosinophilia with organ-restricted involvement

It is most important to be able to distinguish between HES and those conditions with overlapping clinical presentations. Because, historically, HES has required organ dysfunction associated with high-grade eosinophilia, known disorders of specific organ systems accompanied by eosinophilia are those most often confused with HES (Box 2).

Skin and subcutaneous tissues

Atopic and blistering diseases
Eosinophils participate in the inflammatory infiltrate in numerous dermatologic conditions. Blood and tissue eosinophilia are common in atopic dermatitis [63]. Tissue eosinophils are seen in blistering diseases, such as bullous

Box 2. Diseases with organ-restricted involvement and marked peripheral eosinophilia

Skin and subcutaneous diseases
  Episodic angioedema with eosinophilia
  Eosinophilic cellulitis (Well's syndrome)
  Eosinophilic panniculitis
  Angiolymphoid hyperplasia with eosinophilia (and Kimura's
    Disease)
  Eosinophilic pustular dermatitis
  Cutaneous necrotizing eosinophilic vasculitis

Pulmonary diseases
  Drug- and toxin-induced eosinophilic lung diseases
  Helminth associated (Loeffler's syndrome; tropical pulmonary
    eosinophilia)
  Chronic eosinophilic pneumonia
  Acute eosinophilic pneumonia
  Churg-Strauss syndrome
  Other vasculitides

Gastrointestinal diseases
  Eosinophilic gastrointestinal disorders (EGIDs)
    Eosinophilic esophagitis (EE)
    Eosinophilic gastroenteritis (EG)
  Primary biliary cirrhosis
  Sclerosing cholangitis
  Eosinophilic cholangitis
  Eosinophilic cholecystitis

Neurologic diseases
  Eosinophilic meningitis
  Ventriculoperitoneal shunts
  Leukemia or lymphoma with central nervous system
    involvement (Hodgkin's)
  Nonsteroidal anti-inflammatory drugs
  Antibiotics
  Contrast agents

Rheumatologic diseases
  Churg-Strauss syndrome
  Other vasculitides
  Eosinophilia-myalgia syndrome

> Cardiac diseases
>   Hypersensitivity myocarditis
>   Churg-Strauss syndrome
>
> Genitourinary disease
>   Drug-induced interstitial nephritis
>   Eosinophilic cystitis

pemphigoid, pemphigus vulgaris, dermatitis herpetiformis, and herpes gestationis, and can be prominent in drug-induced lesions. An uncommon disorder, characterized by the association of nodules, eosinophilia, rheumatism, dermatitis, and swelling (NERDS), includes prominent para-articular nodules, recurrent urticaria with angioedema, and tissue and blood eosinophilia [64].

Eosinophilic panniculitis

Eosinophilic panniculitis is characterized by a prominent eosinophil infiltration of subcutaneous fat [65]. Lesions often are nodular and less frequently present as plaques or vesicles. Eosinophilic panniculitis is commonly associated with gnathostomiasis, leukocytoclastic vasculitis, and erythema nodosum [65]. Other disorders associated with eosinophilic panniculitis include atopic and contact dermatitis, eosinophilic cellulitis, arthropod bites, toxocariasis, polyarteritis nodosa, injection granuloma, lupus panniculitis, malignancy, diabetes, and chronic recurrent parotitis [65,66].

Episodic angioedema with eosinophilia

Although blood eosinophilia does not usually accompany angioedema, a distinct entity, episodic angioedema with eosinophilia, is characterized by recurrent episodes of angioedema, urticaria, pruritus, fever, weight gain with oliguria, elevated serum immunoglobulin (Ig)M, and leukocytosis with Imarked blood eosinophilia [67]. The level of blood eosinophilia parallels disease activity. This disease is associated with cyclic alterations in serum IL-5 or GM-CSF levels [68–70]. The clinical course of this disease with its periodic recurrences of angioedema and eosinophilia and its lack of association with cardiac damage distinguishes it from HES, although some consider it an overlapping syndrome with HES [4]. Indeed, some patients will develop clonal T-cell populations and progress to HES.

Kimura's disease and angiolymphoid hyperplasia with eosinophilia

Kimura's disease presents as large subcutaneous masses on the head or neck of Asian men, whereas angiolymphoid hyperplasia with eosinophilia occurs in all races and is characterized by generally smaller and more superficial lesions. Eosinophilia is common to both [71–73].

Eosinophilic fasciitis

Eosinophilic fasciitis (Shulman's syndrome) has an acute onset of erythema, swelling, and induration of the extremities, often with a history of antecedent exercise [74,75]. Skin lesions are accompanied by elevated blood eosinophil counts. Histologically, unlike scleroderma, the epidermis and dermis are normal with most pathology located in the subcutaneous tissue, fascia, and muscle.

Wells' syndrome (eosinophilic cellulitis)

Eosinophilic cellulitis is marked by recurrent swellings on the extremities [76,77]. Although involved skin appears cellulitic, minimal tenderness, absence of warmth, and failure to respond to antibiotics distinguish it from bacterial cellulitis. It resolves spontaneously leaving a granulomatous infiltration. Blood eosinophilia is present in 50% of cases.

Eosinophilic pustular folliculitis

Mixed eosinophilic and neutrophilic infiltrates occur in affected follicles, and blood eosinophilia may be present [78]. Although described in healthy individuals, it also occurs in those infected with HIV and less commonly in HIV-negative patients being treated for hematologic malignancies or following bone marrow transplantation [79,80].

Pulmonary

Eosinophilic lung diseases are a heterogeneous group of disorders unified by the presence of large numbers of eosinophils in the inflammatory cellular infiltrates in the airways or parenchyma of the lungs with a clinical presentation that usually consists of symptoms referable to the respiratory system accompanied by abnormal chest radiograph/CT and peripheral blood eosinophilia. These eosinophilic lung diseases are reviewed extensively by Wechsler elsewhere in this issue, and the major categories of pulmonary disorders associated with high-grade eosinophilia are listed in Box 2.

Besides the medication- and toxin-induced eosinophilic pulmonary diseases and allergic bronchopulmonary aspergillosis (discussed previously in this article), Churg-Strauss syndrome and helminth infections (particularly in the migratory phase early in the infection) have been associated with transient pulmonary infiltrates and marked eosinophilia (Loeffler's syndrome) [81]. Moreover, a very rare manifestation of *Wuchereria bancrofti*, termed tropical pulmonary eosinophilia, is a systemic disorder defined by pulmonary infiltrates, nocturnal wheezing, IgE elevations, and marked peripheral eosinophilia [82].

Chronic eosinophilic pneumonia

This is a disease of unknown etiology that typically present with cough, fever, dyspnea, and significant weight loss [83]. Laboratory findings include blood eosinophilia in almost 90% of patients [83]. Chronic eosinophilic pneumonia [84] is characterized radiographically by peripheral infiltrates. Mediastinal lymphadenopathy may be present as well [84].

Histologically, the lung biopsies show a predominantly eosinophilic infiltrate in the alveoli and interstitium [85]. Response to corticosteroid administration is dramatic, occurring within 24 hours. Blood eosinophilia can decline within 24 hours [83], and complete resolution of symptoms occurs within 2 weeks in two thirds of patients [83]. Radiographic improvement may be as early as 60 to 72 hours, and clearance can be expected to occur within 2 weeks in one half of patients [86]. Recurrences of clinical and radiographic changes were seen in 58% of patients after discontinuation of corticosteroids [83].

Acute eosinophilic pneumonia

Acute eosinophilic pneumonia is a clinical entity distinct from other eosinophilic pneumonias [87–89]. Patients commonly present with acute onset of cough, dyspnea, and fever. Diagnostic criteria for acute eosinophilic pneumonia have been defined and require both exclusion of other causes and the presence of a febrile illness of short duration, hypoxemic respiratory failure, diffuse alveolar or mixed alveolar-interstitial infiltrates on radiography, either bronchoalveolar lavage eosinophils greater than 25% (or biopsy confirmation of lung tissue eosinophilia) [87,90], and rapid response to corticosteroids.

Gastrointestinal

Blood eosinophilia can develop with a number of gastrointestinal and hepatobiliary disorders, but tissue eosinophilia is more characteristic. The eosinophilic gastrointestinal diseases (EGID) are discussed in full by Rothenberg and Zuo elsewhere in this issue. In brief, there are a number of GI diseases that have eosinophil-mediated pathology and marked peripheral blood eosinophilia.

Eosinophilic gastrointestinal diseases
Eosinophilic esophagitis. Characterized by eosinophilic infiltration of the esophagus, eosinophilic esophagitis (EE) is a disorder felt to have an allergic etiology. Adults typically present with dysphagia and/or food impaction while children have a more variable clinical presentation. Peripheral eosinophilia is common. Strictures may be seen on endoscopy; histopathology reveals mucosal infiltration with eosinophils [91,92].

Eosinophilic gastroenteritis. Eosinophilic gastroenteritis is an uncommon disorder characterized by gastrointestinal symptoms, blood eosinophilia, and eosinophilic infiltration of the gastrointestinal wall [93–96]. The peak age of onset is in the third decade. Although allergies to foods, including milk, contribute in some children, in adults, allergic etiologies are uncommon. Different layers of the GI tract may be involved, and as a consequence, different types of symptoms may occur. Mucosal involvement can result in abdominal pain, nausea, vomiting, diarrhea, weight loss, anemia, protein-losing enteropathy, and intestinal perforation. Patients with muscular layer involvement have symptoms of pyloric or intestinal obstruction and early satiety. Subserosal eosinophilic infiltration may result in development of eosinophilic ascites [94,96].

Hepatobiliary diseases

Eosinophilic hepatitis develops in response to some medications [97–100] and to helminth parasites (see Table 1). Marked peripheral eosinophilia has been seen in primary biliary cirrhosis [101], sclerosing cholangitis [102], eosinophilic cholangitis [103], and eosinophilic cholecystitis [104].

Neurologic

Marked tissue eosinophilia occurs within organizing chronic subdural hematomas [105]. Other eosinophil-associated neurologic diseases are uncommon and include the disorders that cause eosinophilic meningitis [106]. Cerebrospinal fluid eosinophilia can be a significant clue to central nervous system infections with coccidioidomycosis or *Angiostrongylus cantonensis* as well as to adverse drug reactions to NSAIDs or antibiotics.

Rheumatologic

Marked peripheral blood eosinophilia is not common in connective tissue diseases [107], although it has been described associated with dermatomyositis [107], rheumatoid arthritis [108], systemic sclerosis [109], and Sjögren's syndrome [110]. It should be remembered that many of the drugs used to treat these disorders can cause hypersensitivity reactions with eosinophilia (eg, NSAIDS).

Eosinophilia-myalgia syndrome and toxic oil syndrome

The eosinophilia-myalgia syndrome arose from ingestion of contaminated L-tryptophan [111] and toxic oil syndrome was caused by ingestion of cooking oil adulterated with denatured rapeseed oil [112–115]. Both are chronic, persisting multisystem diseases in which marked eosinophilia developed [116].

Vasculitis

Churg-Strauss syndrome (CSS), among the vasculitides, is the disorder that is associated with high-grade, persistent eosinophilia (see Wechsler and colleagues for fuller treatise). Although mild eosinophilia is common, marked eosinophilia is uncommon in many of the other vasculitides but has been seen in patients with cutaneous necrotizing vasculitis [117–119], thromboangiitis obliterans with eosinophilia of the temporal arteritis [120], and unusual cases of Wegener's granulomatosis [121,122].

Cardiac

The principal cardiac sequela of eosinophilic diseases is damage to the endomyocardium (see the article by Ogbogu and colleagues elsewhere in this issue). This can occur with hypersensitivity myocarditis [123] and with eosinophilias associated with eosinophilic leukemia, sarcomas, carcinomas, and lymphomas [124]; with GM-CSF [31] or IL-2 administration [125,126]; with prolonged drug-induced eosinophilia; and with parasitic infections [127–129].

Genitourinary

Interstitial nephritis with eosinophilia is typically drug-induced. Agents known to induce nephritis include semisynthetic penicillins, cephalosporins, NSAIDs, allopurinol, rifampin, and ciprofloxacin, among others.

Eosinophilic cystitis is a rare clinicopathological condition characterized by transmural inflammation of the bladder predominantly with eosinophils. It has been associated with bladder tumors, bladder trauma, parasitic infections, and some medications. The most common symptom complex consists of urinary frequency, hematuria, dysuria, and suprapubic pain [130].

Approach to the evaluation of a patient with high-grade eosinophilia

The approach to identifying the cause of marked, persistent eosinophilia is a challenging problem. Nevertheless, the prevention of morbidity by identifying the cause of the eosinophilia and intervening therapeutically is an important task that should be approached systematically. Although this article assumes that the presence of marked eosinophilia has been established, it should be borne in mind that some of the earlier automated methods used to assess leukocyte populations resulted in inaccuracies in establishing the presence of eosinophilia.

To evaluate a patient with persistent and marked eosinophilia, the approach suggested in Box 3 is recommended. A careful history should be taken directed specifically at the nature of the symptoms (if present) with an emphasis placed on disorders known to be associated with eosinophilia, previous eosinophil counts (if available), travel, and occupational and dietary history. A complete medication history should be taken that includes over-the-counter medications, supplements, herbal preparations, and vitamins; any medication known to induce eosinophilia should be discontinued. Patients should be asked about diseases commonly found in their family; previous allergies to medications or to environmental allergens must also be addressed.

Box 3. Approach to evaluation of marked eosinophilia

1. Eosinophil Determinations—Verify eosinophil count; estimate or get absolute eosinophil count
2. Medical History
   - Obtain history of previous eosinophil counts
   - Medical History
     - review medical history with emphasis placed on disorders know to be associated with eosinophilia including atopic disease
   - Medication History
     - review recent and current medication history
     - discontinue any drugs known to be associated with eosinophilia
     - make a detailed list of all medications (including nutritional supplements, vitamins, herbal preparations)
     - Note any history of allergy to medications
   - Travel/Geographic History
     - Review past history of travel to or residence in other countries
     - Review travel within indigenous country with emphasis on regions where particular eosinophilia-associated infections may be common
   - Occupational/Recreational History
     - Review occupational and recreational exposures
   - Dietary History
     - Review carefully; query dietary indiscretions, nutritional supplements
   - Family History
     - Review whether others in family have eosinophilia suggesting a common exposure or familial nature of disease

Physical examination
- Do a careful physical examination
- Close attention paid to skin, soft tissues, masses, lymphadenopathy

Initial laboratory evaluation
- Routine studies to assess general hematologic status (complete blood count, platelet count)
- Studies to assess organ function (liver function tests, renal function tests, urinalysis, chest radiograph), inflammation (C reactive protein/erythocyte sedimentation rate), immune status (immunoglobulins, IgE)

> *Further diagnostic evaluations (based on initial laboratory findings or localizing symptoms) that can help identify underlying cause*
> - Tissue examination (biopsies) if necessary
> - Specimen collection (cerebrospinal fluid, sputum, bronchoalveolar lavage, stool, urine) that can identify the
> - CT and MRI to define better focal lesions.
> - Bone marrow aspirates and biopsies to assess fully the nature of the process underlying the eosinophilia.
> - Additional disease-defining tests to exclude particular diagnoses (eg, serum tryptase/cKIT mutations for systemic mastocytosis, antineutrophil cytoplasmic antibodies (ANCA) for CSS and other vasculitides, serologies for helminths

Physical examination with special attention to skin, soft tissues, lungs, liver, and spleen as well as an additional directed examination based on the patient's specific symptoms or chief complaint is obviously important.

Initially, the approach to the evaluation of marked eosinophilia must be to assess general health status and to assess whether there is underlying organ dysfunction. The eosinophilia must be confirmed, and an estimation of the absolute eosinophil count (if not measured directly) must be made. Routine studies to assess hematologic status (CBC, platelet count, pro-thrombin time [PT]/partial thromboplastin time [PTT]), studies to assess organ function (liver function tests, renal function tests, urinalysis, chest radiograph, electrocardiogram), markers of inflammation (CRP/ESR), and immunologic status (quantitative immunoglobulins and IgE) should also be performed routinely. The presence of particular symptoms or physical findings may direct other laboratory studies.

Further diagnostic evaluation based on the initial studies is usually required to distinguish among the myriad disorders underlying hypereosinophilia. When a parasitic infection is suspected, the laboratory evaluation should be based on information gleaned from the history and physical examination, to avoid going on a "fishing expedition" by ordering needless laboratory tests; however, a minimum set of diagnostic tests directed toward establishing the presence of a particular parasite should be obtained (see Table 1). The localizing clinical findings in symptomatic patients as well as laboratory evidence of organ involvement must guide the subsequent evaluation. Access to tissue (biopsies) or material (eg, CSF, sputum, bronchoalveolar lavage, stool, urine) that can identify the underlying problem is often necessary. CT and MRI to define better focal lesions should be employed. Bone marrow aspirates and biopsies will often be necessary to assess fully the nature of the process underlying the high-grade eosinophilia. Additional disease-defining tests may be necessary to exclude particular diagnoses (eg, serum tryptase/assessment of cKIT mutations for systemic mastocytosis, antineutrophil cytoplasmic antibodies [ANCA] for CSS and other vasculitides, serologies for helminths).

Summary

The approach to the identifying the cause of marked, persistent eosinophilia is a challenging problem. Excluding many of these non-HES causes of marked peripheral blood eosinophilia is required for making the diagnosis of HES. Moreover, the prevention of morbidity by identifying the cause of the eosinophilia and intervening therapeutically is an important task that must be approached systematically.

Acknowledgments

This study was supported in part by the Division of Intramural Research (DIR) of the National Institute of Allergy and Infectious Diseases.

References

[1] Rothenberg ME. Eosinophilia. N Engl J Med 1998;338:1592–600.
[2] Simon D, Simon HU. Eosinophilic disorders. J Allergy Clin Immunol 2007;119:1291–300.
[3] Wilson ME, Weller PF, editors. Eosinophilia. Philadelphia: Churchill Livingstone; 1999.
[4] Klion AD, Bochner BS, Gleich GJ, et al. Approaches to the treatment of hypereosinophilic syndromes: a workshop summary report. J Allergy Clin Immunol 2006;117:1292–302.
[5] Weller PF. The immunobiology of eosinophils. N Engl J Med 1991;324:1110–8.
[6] Uhrbrand H. The number of circulating eosinophils: normal figures and spontaneous variations. Acta Med Scand 1958;160:99–104.
[7] Bass DA. Behavior of eosinophil leukocytes in acute inflammation. I. Lack of dependence on adrenal function. J Clin Invest 1975;55:1229–69.
[8] Beeson PB, Bass DA. The eosinophil. Major Probl Intern Med 1977;14:1.
[9] Mawhorter SD, Stephany DA, Ottesen EA, et al. Identification of surface molecules associated with physiologic activation of eosinophils: application of whole blood flow cytometry to eosinophils. J Immunol 1996;156:4851–8.
[10] Dvorak AM, Weller PF. Ultrastructural analysis of human eosinophils. Chem Immunol 2000;76:1–28.
[11] Moore TA, Nutman TB. Eosinophilia in the returning traveler. Infect Dis Clin North Am 1998;12:503–21.
[12] Weller PF. Eosinophilia and eosinophil-related disorders. In: Adkinson NF, Yunginger JW, Busse Wwea, editors. Allergy: principles and practices. 6th edition. St. Louis (MO): Mosby-Year Book; 2003. p. 1105–555.
[13] Weller PF. Eosinophilia in travelers. Med Clin North Am 1992;76:1413–32.
[14] Wilson ME. Eosinophilia. In: A world guide to infections: diseases, distributions, diagnosis. New York: Oxford University Press; 1991. p. 164–256.
[15] Brandborg LL, Goldberg SB, Briedenbach WC. Human coccidiosis—a possible cause of malabsorption: the life cycle in small-bowel biopsies as a diagnostic feature. N Engl J Med 1970;283:1306–13.

[16] Trier JS, Moxey PC, Schimmel EM, et al. Chronic intestinal coccidiosis in man: intestinal morphology and response to treatment. Gastroenterology 1974;66:923–35.

[17] Arness MK, Brown JD, Dubey JP, et al. An outbreak of acute eosinophilic myositis attributed to human Sarcocystis parasitism. Am J Trop Med Hyg 1999;61:548–53.

[18] Chen X, Zuo Y, Zuo W. [Observation on the clinical symptoms and sporocyst excretion in human volunteers experimentally infected with *Sarcocystis hominis*]. Zhongguo Ji Sheng Chong Xue Yu Ji Sheng Chong Bing Za Zhi 1999;17:25–7 [in Chinese].

[19] van den Enden E, Praet M, Joos R, et al. Eosinophilic myositis resulting from sarcocystosis: a review and report of five cases. J Trop Med Hyg 1995;28:819.

[20] Deshpande AD. Eosinophilia associated with scabies. Practitioner 1987;231:455.

[21] Starr J, Pruett JH, Yunginger JW, et al. Myiasis due to *Hypoderma lineatum* infection mimicking the hypereosinophilic syndrome. Mayo Clin Proc 2000;75:755–9.

[22] Drabick JJ, Magill AJ, Smith KJ, et al. Hypereosinophilic syndrome associated with HIV infection. Military Medical Consortium for Applied Retroviral Research. South Med J 1994;87:525–9.

[23] Simpson-Dent SL, Fearfield LA, Staughton RCD. HIV-associated eosinophilic folliculitis—diagnosis and management. Sex Transm Infect 1999;75:291–3.

[24] Skiest DJ, Keiser P. Clinical significance of eosinophilia in HIV-infected individuals. Am J Med 1997;102:449–53.

[25] Tietz A, Sponagel L, Erb P, et al. Eosinophilia in patients infected with the human immunodeficiency virus. Eur J Clin Microbiol Infect Dis 1997;16:675–7.

[26] Kaplan MH, Hall WW, Susin M, et al. Syndrome of severe skin disease, eosinophilia, and dermatopathic lymphadenopathy in patients with HTLV-II complicating human immunodeficiency virus infection. Am J Med 1991;91:300–9.

[27] May LP, Kelly J, Sanchez M. Hypereosinophilic syndrome with unusual cutaneous manifestations in two men with HIV infection. J Am Acad Dermatol 1990;23:202–4.

[28] Echols RM, Palmer DL, Long GW. Tissue eosinophilia in human coccidiomycosis. Rev Infect Dis 1982;4:656–64.

[29] Harley WB, Blaser MJ. Disseminated coccidioidomycosis associated with extreme eosinophilia. Clin Infect Dis 1994;18:627–9.

[30] Schermoly MJ, Hinthorn DR. Eosinophilia in coccidioidomycosis. Arch Intern Med 1988; 148:895–6.

[31] Donhuijsen K, Haedicke C, Hattenberger S, et al. Granulocyte-macrophage colony-stimulating factor-related eosinophilia and Loeffler's endocarditis. Blood 1992;79:2798.

[32] Ishimitsu T, Torisu M. The role of eosinophils in interleukin-2/lymphokine-activated killer cell therapy. Surgery 1993;113:192–9.

[33] Rodgers S, Rees RC, Hancock BW. Changes in the phenotypic characteristics of eosinophils from patients receiving recombinant human interleukin-2 (rhIL-2) therapy. Br J Haematol 1994;86:746–53.

[34] Dumortier G, Cabaret W, Stamatiadis L, et al. [Hepatic tolerance of atypical antipsychotic drugs]. Encephale 2002;28:542–51.

[35] Kim YJ, Nutman TB. Eosinophilia: causes and pathobiology in persons with prior exposures in tropical areas with an emphasis on parasitic infections. Curr Infect Dis Rep 2006;8:43–50.

[36] Wolf R, Davidovici B, Matz H, et al. Drug rash with eosinophilia and systemic symptoms versus Stevens-Johnson Syndrome—a case that indicates a stumbling block in the current classification. Int Arch Allergy Immunol 2006;141:308–10.

[37] Bain B. Eosinophilic leukemia and idiopathic hypereosinophilic syndrome are mutually exclusive diagnoses. Blood 2004;104:3836.

[38] Bain B. Hypereosinophilia. Curr Opin Hematol 2000;7:21–5.

[39] Bain BJ. Eosinophilic leukaemias and the idiopathic hypereosinophilic syndrome. Br J Haematol 1996;95:2–9.

[40] Gruss HJ, Brach MA, Drexler HG, et al. Expression of cytokine genes, cytokine receptor genes, and transcription factors in cultured Hodgkin and Reed-Sternberg cells. Cancer Res 1992;52:3353–60.

[41] Samoszuk M, Nansen L. Detection of interleukin-5 messenger RNA in Reed-Sternberg cells of Hodgkin's disease with eosinophilia. Blood 1990;75:13–6.

[42] Borish L, Dishuck J, Cox L, et al. Sezary syndrome with elevated serum IgE and hypereosinophilia: role of dysregulated cytokine production. J Allergy Clin Immunol 1993;92: 123–31.

[43] Hogan TF, Koss W, Murgo AJ, et al. Acute lymphoblastic leukemia with chromosomal 5;14 translocation and hypereosinophilia: case report and literature review. J Clin Oncol 1987;5:382–90.

[44] Robyn J, Noel P, Wlodarska I, et al. Imatinib-responsive hypereosinophilia in a patient with B cell ALL. Leuk Lymphoma 2004;45:2497–501.

[45] Lowe D, Jorizzo J, Hutt MS. Tumour-associated eosinophilia: a review. J Clin Pathol 1981; 34:1343–8.

[46] Knox AJ, Johnson CE, Page RL. Eosinophilia associated with thoracic malignancy. Br J Dis Chest 1986;80:92–5.

[47] Berkompas RJ. Isolated eosinophilia associated with a squamous cell lung cancer. J Tenn Med Assoc 1989;82:241–2.

[48] Lowe D, Fletcher CD. Eosinophilia in squamous cell carcinoma of the oral cavity, external genitalia and anus—clinical correlations. Histopathology 1984;8:627–32.

[49] Lowe D, Fletcher CD, Gower RL. Tumour-associated eosinophilia in the bladder. J Clin Pathol 1984;37:500–2.

[50] Parker RI. Hematologic aspects of systemic mastocytosis. Hematol Oncol Clin North Am 2000;14:557–68.

[51] Miranda RN, Esparza AR, Sambandam S, et al. Systemic mast cell disease presenting with peripheral blood eosinophilia. Hum Pathol 1994;25:727–30.

[52] Maric I, Robyn J, Metcalfe DD, et al. KIT D816V-associated systemic mastocytosis with eosinophilia and FIP1L1/PDGFRA-associated chronic eosinophilic leukemia are distinct entities. J Allergy Clin Immunol 2007 [epub ahead of print].

[53] Aleman K, Noordzij JG, de Groot R, et al. Reviewing Omenn syndrome. Eur J Pediatr 2001;160:718–25.

[54] Grimbacher B, Holland SM, Gallin JI, et al. Hyper-IgE syndrome with recurrent infections—an autosomal dominant multisystem disorder. N Engl J Med 1999;340:692–702.

[55] Grimbacher B, Holland SM, Puck JM. Hyper-IgE syndromes. Immunol Rev 2005;203: 244–50.

[56] Jacobsohn DA, Schechter T, Seshadri R, et al. Eosinophilia correlates with the presence or development of chronic graft-versus-host disease in children. Transplantation 2004;77: 1096–100.

[57] McNeel D, Rubio MT, Damaj G, et al. Hypereosinophilia as a presenting sign of acute graft-versus-host disease after allogeneic bone marrow transplantation. Transplantation 2002;74:1797–800.

[58] Basara N, Kiehl MG, Fauser AA. Eosinophilia indicates the evolution to acute graft-versus-host disease. Blood 2002;100:3055.

[59] Beishuizen A, Vermes I, Hylkema BS, et al. Relative eosinophilia and functional adrenal insufficiency in critically ill patients. Lancet 1999;353:1675–6.

[60] Wilson DM, Salazer TL, Farkouh ME. Eosinophiluria in atheroembolic renal disease. Am J Med 1991;91:186–9.

[61] Chabasse D, Oriot M, Larra F. [Blood eosinophilia in Hodgkin's disease and radiation therapy (author's transl)]. Sem Hop 1981;57:373–8.

[62] Renston JP, Goldman ES, Hsu RM, et al. Peripheral blood eosinophilia in association with sarcoidosis. Mayo Clin Proc 2000;75:586–90.

[63] Leiferman KM. Eosinophils in atopic dermatitis. J Allergy Clin Immunol 1994;94: 1310–7.

[64] Butterfield JH, Leiferman KM, Gleich GJ. Nodules, eosinophilia, rheumatism, dermatitis and swelling (NERDS): a novel eosinophilic disorder. Clin Exp Allergy 1993;23:571–80.

[65] Adame J, Cohen PR. Eosinophilic panniculitis: diagnostic considerations and evaluation. J Am Acad Dermatol 1996;34:229–34.

[66] Kato N. Eosinophilic panniculitis. J Dermatol 1993;20:185–7.

[67] Gleich GJ, Schroeter AL, Marcoux JP, et al. Episodic angioedema associated with eosinophilia. N Engl J Med 1984;310:1621–6.

[68] Banerji A, Weller PF, Sheikh J. Cytokine-associated angioedema syndromes including episodic angioedema with eosinophilia (Gleich's Syndrome). Immunol Allergy Clin North Am 2006;26:769–81.

[69] Bochner BS, Friedman B, Krishnaswami G, et al. Episodic eosinophilia-myalgia-like syndrome in a patient without L-tryptophan use: association with eosinophil activation and increased serum levels of granulocyte-macrophage colony-stimulating factor. J Allergy Clin Immunol 1991;88:629–36.

[70] Butterfield JH, Leiferman KM, Abrams J, et al. Elevated serum levels of interleukin-5 in patients with the syndrome of episodic angioedema and eosinophilia. Blood 1992;79: 688–92.

[71] Abuel-Haija M, Hurford MT. Kimura disease. Arch Pathol Lab Med 2007;131:650–1.

[72] Don DM, Ishiyama A, Johnstone AK, et al. Angiolymphoid hyperplasia with eosinophilia and vascular tumors of the head and neck. Am J Otolaryngol 1996;17:240–5.

[73] Helander SD, Peters MS, Kuo TT, et al. Kimura's disease and angiolymphoid hyperplasia with eosinophilia: new observations from immunohistochemical studies of lymphocyte markers, endothelial antigens, and granulocyte proteins. J Cutan Pathol 1995;22:319–26.

[74] Doyle JA, Ginsburg WW. Eosinophilic fasciitis. Med Clin North Am 1989;73:1157–66.

[75] Shulman LE. Diffuse fasciitis with eosinophilia: a new syndrome? Trans Assoc Am Physicians 1975;88:70–86.

[76] Aberer W, Konrad K, Wolff K. Wells' syndrome is a distinctive disease entity and not a histologic diagnosis. J Am Acad Dermatol 1988;18:105–14.

[77] Espana A, Sanz ML, Sola J, et al. Wells' syndrome (eosinophilic cellulitis): correlation between clinical activity, eosinophil levels, eosinophil cation protein and interleukin-5. Br J Dermatol 1999;140:127–30.

[78] McCalmont TH, Altemus D, Maurer T, et al. Eosinophilic folliculitis. The histologic spectrum. Am J Dermatopathol 1995;17:439–46.

[79] Basarab T. HIV-associated eosinophilic pustular folliculitis. J Am Acad Dermatol 1997;37: 670–1.

[80] Bull RH, Harland CA, Fallowfield ME, et al. Eosinophilic folliculitis: a self-limiting illness in patients being treated for haematological malignancy. Br J Dermatol 1993;129:178–82.

[81] Loeffler W. Transient lung infiltrations with blood eosinophilia. Int Arch Allergy Appl Immunol 1956;8:54.

[82] Ottesen EA, Nutman TB. Tropical pulmonary eosinophilia. Annu Rev Med 1992;43: 417–24.

[83] Jederlinic PJ, Sicilian L, Gaensler EA. Chronic eosinophilic pneumonia. A report of 19 cases and a review of the literature. Medicine 1988;67:154–62.

[84] Carrington CB, Addington WW, Goff AM, et al. Chronic eosinophilic pneumonia. N Engl J Med 1969;280:787–98.

[85] Olopade CO, Crotty TB, Douglas WW, et al. Chronic eosinophilic pneumonia and idiopathic bronchiolitis obliterans organizing pneumonia: comparison of eosinophil number and degranulation by immunofluorescence staining for eosinophil-derived major basic protein. Mayo Clin Proc 1995;70:137–42.

[86] Mayo JR, Muller NL, Road J, et al. Chronic eosinophilic pneumonia: CT findings in six cases. AJR Am J Roentgenol 1989;153:727–30.

[87] Allen JA, Pacht ER, Gadek JE, et al. Acute eosinophilic pneumonia as a reversible cause of noninfectious respiratory failure. N Engl J Med 1989;321:569–74.

[88] Hayakawa H, Sato A, Toyoshima M, et al. A clinical study of idiopathic eosinophilic pneumonia. Chest 1994;105:1462–6.

[89] Pope-Harman AL, Davis WB, Allen ED, et al. Acute eosinophilic pneumonia. A summary of 15 cases and review of the literature. Medicine 1996;75:334–42.

[90] Tazelaar HD, Linz LJ, Colby TV, et al. Acute eosinophilic pneumonia: histopathologic findings in nine patients. Am J Respir Crit Care Med 1997;155:296–302.

[91] Blanchard C, Wang N, Rothenberg ME. Eosinophilic esophagitis: pathogenesis, genetics, and therapy. J Allergy Clin Immunol 2006;118:1054–9.

[92] Walsh SV, Antonioli DA, Goldman H, et al. Allergic esophagitis in children: a clinicopathological entity. Am J Surg Pathol 1999;23:390–6.

[93] Khan S, Orenstein SR. Eosinophilic gastroenteritis: epidemiology, diagnosis and management. Paediatr Drugs 2002;4:563–70.

[94] Lee M, Hodges WG, Huggins TL, et al. Eosinophilic gastroenteritis. South Med J 1996;89:189–94.

[95] Rothenberg ME. Eosinophilic gastrointestinal disorders (EGID). J Allergy Clin Immunol 2004;113:11.

[96] Talley NJ, Shorter RG, Phillips SF, et al. Eosinophilic gastroenteritis: a clinicopathological study of patients with disease of the mucosa, muscle layer, and subserosal tissues. Gut 1990;31:54–8.

[97] Cleau D, Jobard JM, Alves T, et al. Cholestatic hepatitis induced by the amoxicillin-clavulanic acid combination. A case and review of the literature]. Gastroenterol Clin Biol 1990;14:1007–9.

[98] Fix OK, Peters MG, Davern TJ. Eosinophilic hepatitis caused by lamotrigine. Clin Gastroenterol Hepatol 2006;4:xxvi.

[99] Owens RC Jr, Ambrose PG. Antimicrobial safety: focus on fluoroquinolones. Clin Infect Dis 2005;41(Suppl 2):S144–57.

[100] Pompili M, Basso M, Grieco A, et al. Recurrent acute hepatitis associated with use of cetirizine. Ann Pharmacother 2004;38:1844–7.

[101] Terasaki S, Nakanuma Y, Yamazaki M, et al. Eosinophilic infiltration of the liver in primary biliary cirrhosis: a morphological study. Hepatology 1993;17:206–12.

[102] Grauer L, Padilla VM 3rd, Bouza L, et al. Eosinophilic sclerosing cholangitis associated with hypereosinophilic syndrome. Am J Gastroenterol 1993;88:1764–9.

[103] Rosengart TK, Rotterdam H, Ranson JH. Eosinophilic cholangitis: a self-limited cause of extrahepatic biliary obstruction. Am J Gastroenterol 1990;85:582–5.

[104] Dabbs DJ. Eosinophilic and lymphoeosinophilic cholecystitis. Am J Surg Pathol 1993;17:497–501.

[105] Golden J, Frim DM, Chapman PH, et al. Marked tissue eosinophilia within organizing chronic subdural hematoma membranes. Clin Neuropathol 1994;13:12–6.

[106] Weller PF, Liu LX. Eosinophilic meningitis. Semin Neurol 1993;13:161–8.

[107] Kargili A, Bavbek N, Kaya A, et al. Eosinophilia in rheumatologic diseases: a prospective study of 1000 cases. Rheumatol Int 2004;24:321–4.

[108] Winchester RJ, Koffler D, Litwin SD, et al. Observations on the eosinophilia of certain patients with rheumatoid arthritis. Arthritis Rheum 1971;14:650–65.

[109] Falanga V, Medsger TA Jr. Frequency, levels, and significance of blood eosinophilia in systemic sclerosis, localized scleroderma, and eosinophilic fasciitis. J Am Acad Dermatol 1987;17:648–56.

[110] Bavbek N, Kargili A, Cipil H, et al. Rheumatologic disease with peripheral eosinophilia. Rheumatol Int 2004;24:317–20.

[111] Belongia EA, Hedberg CW, Gleich GJ, et al. An investigation of the cause of the eosinophilia-myalgia syndrome associated with tryptophan use. N Engl J Med 1990;323:357–65.

[112] Kilbourne EM, Rigau-Perez JG, Heath CW Jr, et al. Clinical epidemiology of toxic-oil syndrome. Manifestations of a New Illness. N Engl J Med 1983;309:1408–14.

[113] Mayeno AN, Gleich GJ. Eosinophilia-myalgia syndrome and tryptophan production: a cautionary tale. Trends Biotechnol 1994;12:346–52.

[114] Posada de la Paz M, Philen RM, Borda AI. Toxic oil syndrome: the perspective after 20 years. Epidemiol Rev 2001;23:231–47.

[115] Tabuenca JM. Toxic-allergic syndrome caused by ingestion of rapeseed oil denatured with aniline. Lancet 1981;2:567–8.

[116] Kaufman LD, Gleich GJ. The expanding clinical spectrum of multisystem disease associated with eosinophilia. Arch Dermatol 1997;133:225–7.

[117] Chen KR, Pittelkow MR, Su D, et al. Recurrent cutaneous necrotizing eosinophilic vasculitis. A novel eosinophil-mediated syndrome. Arch Dermatol 1994;130:1159–66.

[118] Chen KR, Su WP, Pittelkow MR, et al. Eosinophilic vasculitis in connective tissue disease. J Am Acad Dermatol 1996;35:173–82.

[119] Chen KR, Su WP, Pittelkow MR, et al. Eosinophilic vasculitis syndrome: recurrent cutaneous eosinophilic necrotizing vasculitis. Semin Dermatol 1995;14:106–10.

[120] Lie JT, Michet CJ Jr. Thromboangiitis obliterans with eosinophilia (Buerger's disease) of the temporal arteries. Hum Pathol 1988;19:598–602.

[121] Krupsky M, Landau Z, Lifschitz-Mercer B, et al. Wegener's granulomatosis with peripheral eosinophilia. Atypical variant of a classic disease. Chest 1993;104:1290–2.

[122] Yousem SA, Lombard CM. The eosinophilic variant of Wegener's granulomatosis. Hum Pathol 1988;19:682–8.

[123] Kendell KR, Day JD, Hruban RH, et al. Intimate association of eosinophils to collagen bundles in eosinophilic myocarditis and ranitidine-induced hypersensitivity myocarditis. Arch Pathol Lab Med 1995;119:1154–60.

[124] Monsuez JJ, de Kerviler E, Barboteu M, et al. Non-Hodgkin's lymphoma related eosinophilic endomyocardial disease. Eur Heart J 1994;15:1423–7.

[125] Junghans RP, Manning W, Safar M, et al. Biventricular cardiac thrombosis during interleukin-2 infusion. N Engl J Med 2001;344:859–60.

[126] Schuchter LM, Hendricks CB, Holland KH, et al. Eosinophilic myocarditis associated with high-dose interleukin-2 therapy. Am J Med 1990;88:439–40.

[127] Andy JJ, Bishara FF, Soyinka OO, et al. Loiasis as a possible trigger of African endomyocardial fibrosis: a case report from Nigeria. Acta Trop 1981;38:179–86.

[128] Brockington IF, Olsen EGJ, Goodwin JF. Endomyocardial fibrosis in Europeans resident in tropical Africa. Lancet 1967;1:583–8.

[129] Ive FA, Willis AJP, Ikeme AC, et al. Endomyocardial fibrosis and filariasis. Quart J Med 1967;36:495–516.

[130] van den Ouden D. Diagnosis and management of eosinophilic cystitis. Eur Urol 2000;37: 386–94.

ELSEVIER
SAUNDERS

Immunol Allergy Clin N Am
27 (2007) 551–560

IMMUNOLOGY
AND ALLERGY
CLINICS
OF NORTH AMERICA

Approach to the Therapy
of Hypereosinophilic Syndromes

Amy D. Klion, MD

*Laboratory of Parasitic Diseases, National Institute of Allergy and Infectious Diseases,
National Institutes of Health, Bldg 4, Rm. 126, 4 Center Drive, Bethesda, MD 20892, USA*

With the introduction of new diagnostic methods and treatment modalities, it has become increasingly clear that hypereosinophilic syndromes (HES) are a heterogeneous group of disorders for which a single approach to treatment is insufficient. This situation is best exemplified by the group of patients now recognized as having chronic eosinophilic leukemia (CEL) on the basis of an interstitial deletion in chromosome 4 leading to the formation of the fusion tyrosine kinase FIP1L1/PDGFRA (F/P) [1]. Typically, this subgroup of patients is refractory to corticosteroid therapy, and before the availability of the tyrosine kinase inhibitor, imatinib, had extremely high morbidity and mortality [2]. Although corticosteroid therapy remains the first-line therapy for patients fulfilling the diagnostic criteria of HES who do not have F/P-positive CEL, the choice of a second-line agent depends on a number of factors, including the type of HES, the patient's concomitant therapies and medical history, cost, and patient preference. Sequential trials of several agents alone or in combination may be necessary to optimize treatment for an individual patient. Unfortunately, some patients who have HES are unresponsive to or intolerant of all currently available agents. With the development of new therapies specifically targeting eosinophils, including monoclonal antibodies directed at interleukin-5 (IL-5), the treatment algorithm is likely to change dramatically in the next several years.

General principles of treatment

Establishing the correct diagnosis is necessarily the first step in determining appropriate treatment for patients assumed to have HES. For this

This work was supported by intramural research funding from NIH/NIAID.
E-mail address: aklion@nih.gov

0889-8561/07/$ - see front matter. Published by Elsevier Inc.
doi:10.1016/j.iac.2007.07.006

purpose, the original diagnostic criteria of Chusid [3] continue to be useful with minor modifications. First, the patient should have a peripheral eosinophil count higher than 1500/μL. Although most would agree that this count should be documented on more than one occasion, a delay in treatment for the 6 months required to make the diagnosis using Chusid's criteria could prove fatal in patients who have aggressive disease, particularly those who have F/P-positive CEL. Next, secondary causes of eosinophilia, such as parasitic infection and drug hypersensitivity, should be excluded. Finally, signs and symptoms of organ involvement by eosinophilic infiltration should be demonstrated. This last criterion deserves special mention, because there are individuals who have marked eosinophilia with counts higher than 1500/μL sustained over many years who do not develop end-organ involvement. These individuals do not require specific therapy but should be followed closely, particularly in the first 5 years following the identification of marked eosinophilia, because the onset of signs or symptoms could herald the development of true HES. The initial evaluation of all patients who have sustained unexplained eosinophilia with counts higher than 1500/μL, regardless of the presence of symptoms or an abnormal physical examination, should include a bone marrow examination with cytogenetics, molecular or fluorescent in situ hybridization (FISH) testing for F/P, and assessment of lymphocyte clonality to identify occult CEL, lymphoma, or lymphocytic-variant HES (L-HES).

Regardless of the etiology of HES, the primary goal of treatment is to reduce tissue eosinophilia and eosinophil-mediated tissue damage. Although peripheral eosinophilia provides an inexpensive and accessible measure of treatment response in HES, the absolute eosinophil count does not predict reliably the extent of tissue involvement. Furthermore, some patients progress despite eosinophil counts below the 1500/μL threshold. A number of other potential markers of disease progression have been proposed, including serum levels of eosinophil granule proteins and surface expression of eosinophil activation markers; however, none have been validated to date. Consequently, patients need to be followed closely for clinical evidence of disease activity on therapy. In addition, because cardiac involvement may be relatively asymptomatic until irreversible damage has occurred, serial echocardiograms should be performed every 6 to 12 months in all patients. The need for and frequency of other testing, including assessment of pulmonary function and CT of the chest and/or abdomen, should be tailored to the clinical manifestations of the individual patient.

Myeloproliferative hypereosinophilic syndrome

Once the diagnosis of HES has been confirmed, it is important to identify patients who have evidence of myeloproliferative HES, because treatment for this subset of patients is markedly different from that for patients who have other types of HES (Fig. 1). For the purposes of treatment, patients

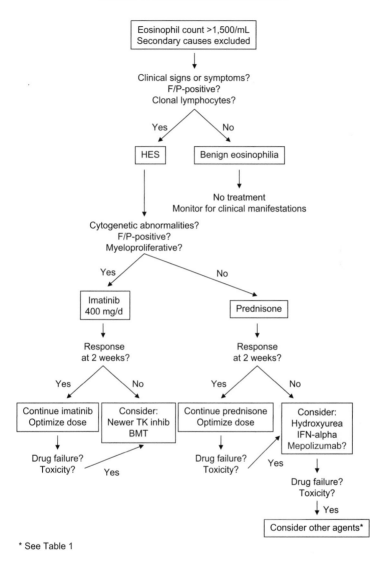

Fig. 1. Treatment algorithm for HES. BMT, bone marrow transplantation; F/P, FIP1L1/PDGFRA; IFN, interferon; TK inhib, tyrosine kinase inhibitors.

who have myeloproliferative HES can be divided into two categories: (1) patients who have cytogenetic or molecular evidence of *PDGFRA*-associated CEL and (2) patients who have features of myeloproliferative disease of unknown etiology. Features of myeloproliferative HES include the presence of dysplastic eosinophils or eosinophil precursors on peripheral blood smear, elevated serum B_{12} levels, anemia and/or thrombocytopenia, hepatosplenomegaly, bone marrow biopsy with increased cellularity, myelofibrosis and/or the presence of increased numbers of spindle-shaped mast cells, and elevated serum tryptase levels [2].

Imatinib is first-line treatment for F/P-positive disease and should be considered for all HES with myeloproliferative features, because successful therapy has been reported in patients lacking the F/P mutation [1,4]. Early treatment is essential, because structural damage from endomyocardial fibrosis is irreversible [2]. Mild side effects of imatinib therapy are common but rarely lead to discontinuation of therapy. These side effects include myelosuppression, elevated transaminase levels, nausea, vomiting, edema, muscle cramps, arthralgias, diarrhea, and skin rashes. Acute eosinophilic myocarditis has been reported following initiation of imatinib therapy in three patients who had HES [4,5]. In view of this finding, it has been suggested that a screening serum troponin level be obtained before imatinib therapy in patients who have eosinophilia and that corticosteroid therapy be initiated if the serum troponin level is elevated [5]. Congestive heart failure, possibly caused by a toxic effect of imatinib on heart muscle cells, has been reported in 0.7% of 1100 patients who had chronic myeloid leukemia (CML) treated with imatinib in an international phase III study (compared with 0.9% of those taking interferon and cytarabine) [6]. This side effect seems to be most common in patients who have other cardiac risk factors, such as advanced age or a prior history of cardiac disease. Because imatinib therapy is likely to be prolonged (possibly lifelong), oligospermia has been reported in a patient receiving imatinib for HES [7], and the majority of patients who have imatinib-responsive HES are young men, male patients should be counseled to consider storing sperm before the initiation of therapy.

Because the initial response to imatinib is rapid, a failure of response to 400 mg daily after 1 to 2 weeks is indicative of drug failure. Although many patients, especially those who have the F/P mutation, ultimately respond to doses of imatinib as low as 100 mg weekly, some patients do not achieve molecular remission on low-dose therapy [8]. Furthermore, data from CML suggest that the magnitude of the molecular response is a predictor of relapse and disease progression [9]. Thus, it seems prudent to use high-dose therapy (400 mg daily) initially to achieve molecular remission and then to decrease the dose slowly while following closely for evidence of molecular relapse by reverse transcriptase polymerase chain reaction or FISH. In the author's experience, patients who are F/P negative but have features of myeloproliferative disease have a less dramatic response to imatinib and often require higher doses to maintain hematologic and clinical remission (Klion AD, unpublished data). Once the eosinophil count has decreased, repeat bone marrow examination should be performed to exclude occult leukemia in all F/P-negative patients [10].

Imatinib resistance has been reported in F/P-positive CEL [1,11]. All cases reported to date have been caused by a T6741 mutation in *PDGFRA* similar to the most common imatinib-resistance mutation in CML. Thus, alternative tyrosine kinase inhibitors with activity against imatinib-resistant CML, including dasatinib, nilotinib, and sorafenib, are likely to be effective in F/P-positive patients and should be considered in patients who develop imatinib resistance or side effects necessitating discontinuation of imatinib therapy. The side-effect profiles of these agents are, in general, less favorable than that of imatinib and preclude their use as first-line agents. Nonmyeloablative allogeneic bone marrow transplantation has been used successfully in patients who have HES [12] and is the only curative therapy for this disease. Despite improvements in recent years, however, morbidity and mortality of the procedure itself remain a problem. Consequently, bone marrow transplantation should be reserved for patients who have progressive disease despite chemotherapy.

Idiopathic hypereosinophilic syndrome

Although corticosteroids have been used as therapy for HES for many decades and remain the first-line treatment for most patients who do not have F/P-associated disease, little is known about the most appropriate dosing regimen. An initial dose of 1 mg/kg or 40 mg/d or higher has been recommended and would seem most appropriate for patients who have evidence of severe symptoms or life-threatening complications [13]. In corticosteroid-responsive patients, symptomatic improvement and resolution of eosinophilia are extremely rapid, often occurring within 24 hours of initiation of therapy. Once a response is obtained, the dose can be decreased gradually to minimize side effects. Some patients, including those who have episodic eosinophilia and angioedema (Gleich's syndrome), can be managed with intermittent short courses of steroids.

Because corticosteroid-induced bone loss occurs early (even within the first 6 months) and can be observed in patients receiving doses as low as 5 mg/d, a baseline measurement of bone mineral density and supplementation with calcium and vitamin D is recommended for all patients for whom the duration of glucocorticoid treatment is anticipated to be 3 months or longer [14]. A bisphosphonate should be added unless contraindicated, because its efficacy in preventing and treating steroid-induced osteoporosis has been demonstrated in several large randomized, controlled clinical trials [14]. Prophylaxis against *Pneumocystis* pneumonia should be instituted for patients requiring long-term, high-dose corticosteroid therapy.

Despite a dramatic initial response to corticosteroids in the majority of patients with HES, most patients ultimately experience significant drug-related toxicities, and alternative therapies must be considered. Although a wide variety of therapies have been used to treat steroid-refractory and steroid-intolerant HES (Table 1), hydroxyurea and interferon-alpha are the most commonly used agents available for second-line therapy (for a detailed discussion, see the article by Butterfield in this issue). Of note, both hydroxyurea and interferon-alpha have a slow onset of action (1–2 weeks)

Table 1
Summary of treatment options for hypereosinophilic syndromes

Treatment	Indications	Dose	Comments
Corticosteroids	First-line therapy unless *PDGFRA*-associated	Varied	Initial dose $\geq$ 40 mg daily with slow taper to lowest effective dose
Hydroxyurea	Second-line therapy	1–3 g/d	Slow onset of action (1–2 weeks)
Vincristine	Consider for counts > 100,000/mm³	1–2 mg intravenously	For rapid reduction of eosinophilia; not for chronic therapy
Other cytotoxic agents (including cyclophosphamide, 6-thioguanine, methotrexate, cytarabine, 2-CDA)	Consider for refractory HES unresponsive to corticosteroids, hydroxyurea, IFN-α	NA	Myeleran and 6-mercaptopurine have been consistently ineffective in published studies
IFN-α	Second-line therapy	1–2 MU/d subcutaneously	Slow onset of action (1–2 weeks); pegylated IFN-α seems to have comparable efficacy
Anti-IL-5 antibody	Research indication to date	NA	Currently unavailable except in clinical trials or for compassionate use (mepolizumab, GlaxoSmithKline [Philadelphia, PA])
Other immuno-modulatory therapy (including alemtuzumab, cyclosporine, IVIG)	Consider for refractory disease	NA	Little published data
Imatinib mesylate	First-line therapy for *PDGFRA*-associated and myeloproliferative variant; consider for other refractory disease	100–400 mg/d	With corticosteroids if cardiac involvement; not useful in lymphocytic variant
Bone marrow transplantation	*PDGFRA*-associated and imatinib-resistant F/P-negative patients who have disease progression despite aggressive therapy	NA	Nonmyeloablative

Abbreviations: HES, hypereosinophilia syndrome; IFN-α, interferon-alpha; IL-5, interleukin 5; IVIG, intravenous immunoglobulin; MU, million units; NA, not applicable.

Adapted from Klion AD, Bochner BS, Gleich GJ, et al. Approaches to the treatment of hypereosinophilic syndromes: a workshop summary report. J Allergy Clin Immunol 2006;117:1295.

and should not be used as single agents for severe, progressive disease. Monoclonal anti-IL-5 antibody therapy seems to be a promising alternative, particularly for steroid-responsive patients experiencing drug toxicity [15–17]; however, it is currently available only for research use.

A number of factors should be considered in the choice of second-line therapy, including cost, ease of administration, the toxicity profile, and patient preference. Hydroxyurea is an alkylating agent with cytotoxic activity on developing cells in the bone marrow. Doses used to treat HES typically range from 1 to 3 g/d. Advantages of hydroxyurea include its low cost and oral route of administration. The most common dose-limiting toxicities are hematologic (anemia, thrombocytopenia, and neutropenia) and gastrointestinal. Idiosyncratic fever reactions necessitating drug discontinuation also have been reported [18]. The major disadvantage of hydroxyurea is that monotherapy rarely achieves a complete response [19].

The utility of interferon-alpha in the treatment of HES has been documented in numerous case series beginning in the early 1990s [20], and sustained remissions following discontinuation of therapy have been reported [21]. A wide variety of doses and regimens have been used, with efficacy demonstrated in some cases at doses as low as 0.5 million units every other day. The major disadvantages of interferon therapy are cost, the need for subcutaneous administration, and its side effect profile, which leads to drug discontinuation in a majority of patients. The most common side effects are flulike symptoms, gastrointestinal complaints, myalgias, cytopenias, and depression. Less commonly, development or exacerbation of autoimmune phenomena, including autoimmune thyroiditis and retinopathy, can occur. Administration of hydroxyurea at low doses (500–1000 mg/d) in combination with interferon seems to potentiate the therapeutic effect and can be used in situations of dose-limiting toxicity [22]. Interferon should be avoided in patients who have a significant history of depression because it can markedly exacerbate symptoms despite antidepressant therapy.

Numerous other treatment options exist for patients who do not respond to therapy with corticosteroids (see Table 1), although which treatment, if any, is likely to be effective in a given patient is unpredictable. In general, agents with the least toxicity should be tried first. Care should be taken to start agents one at a time and to evaluate the response to one agent completely before moving on to the next. Given the favorable side-effect profile and dramatic clinical improvement in patients who respond, a short (1- to 2-week) trial of imatinib is an attractive choice for patients who have steroid-unresponsive idiopathic HES, although the likelihood of response in patients who do not have myeloproliferative features is likely to be low. Because imatinib therapy is quite expensive (approximately $2400/mo at a dose of 400 mg/d) and is not without toxicity, therapy should be discontinued if a response is not evident within 2 weeks.

Clearly, new approaches to the therapy of HES are needed. Although a number of agents targeting cytokine and chemokine receptors on eosinophils are in preclinical development, only monoclonal anti-IL-5 anti-body has been tested in patients who have HES. Two different antibodies, mepolizumab and reslizumab, were developed independently by GlaxoSmithKline (Philadelphia, Pennsylvania) and Schering-Plough Research Institute (Kenilworth, New Jersey), respectively. Both were shown in early small clinical trials to be safe and effective in lowering blood eosinophil counts in patients who had HES [15,23]. More recently, a multicenter, randomized, double-blind, placebo-controlled trial of mepolizumab was conducted to assess the steroid-sparing effects of mepolizumab in 85 patients who had F/P-negative HES. Consistent with the results of the prior studies, mepolizumab was effective in reducing corticosteroid requirements in more than 80% of patients who had steroid-responsive, F/P-negative HES [17]. An open-label extension study is underway currently to assess long-term effects of mepolizumab in this group of patients.

Lymphocytic-variant hypereosinophilic syndrome

Although steroids are the initial treatment of choice for patients who have L-HES, there are some notable differences in the choice of a second-line agent and the approach to the monitoring of therapy in these patients as compared with patients who have true idiopathic HES. First, because clonal T cells are the primary cause of the eosinophilia in L-HES, therapies targeting eosinophils or eosinophil precursors, such as hydroxyurea and imatinib, would be expected to have little effect on the underlying cause of the disease. In fact, imatinib has been administered to several patients who had L-HES without response [24,25]. Interferon-alpha, on the other hand, has been shown to inhibit in vitro proliferation and IL-5 production by clonal T cells from such patients [26] and has shown clinical efficacy in this subgroup of patients. Because interferon also was found to prolong survival of CD3−/CD4+ clonal T cells in these studies, the authors suggest that interferon not be used as monotherapy in patients who have L-HES but be used in association with a proapoptotic agent, such as corticosteroids. Other agents that target T cells and/or IL-5, including cyclosporine A, alemtuzumab (anti-CD52 antibody), mepolizumab, and reslizumab (anti-IL5 antibodies) would be logical choices for therapy in patients who have L-HES refractory to corticosteroids.

Additional monitoring of therapy in L-HES should include periodic assessment for lymphadenopathy and/or increasing lymphocytosis (every 3–4 months), quantification of aberrant T cells (twice yearly), and karyotyping (yearly), because these patients can progress to lymphoma [27].

Summary

Although recent advances in the understanding of the pathogenesis of HES have altered the approach to therapy in some groups of patients, most notably those who have myeloproliferative disease, a standardized approach to treatment is lacking for most patients who have HES, largely because HES is extremely uncommon, and patients do not present to a single subspecialty for care. As new therapies become available, well-designed, multicenter trials to address the safety and efficacy of these agents in this heterogeneous group of patients will become increasingly important.

References

[1] Cools J, DeAngelo DJ, Gotlib J, et al. A tyrosine kinase created by the fusion of the PDGFRA and FIP1L1 genes as a therapeutic target of imatinib in idiopathic hypereosinophilic syndrome. N Engl J Med 2003;348:1201–14.

[2] Klion AD, Noel P, Akin C, et al. Elevated serum tryptase levels identify a subset of patients with a myeloproliferative variant of idiopathic hypereosinophilic syndrome associated with tissue fibrosis, poor prognosis, and imatinib responsiveness. Blood 2003;101:4660–6.

[3] Chusid MJ, Dale DC, West BC, et al. The hypereosinophilic syndrome: analysis of fourteen cases with review of the literature. Medicine (Baltimore) 1975;54:1–27.

[4] Pardanani A, Brockman SR, Paternoster SF, et al. FIP1L1-PDGFRA fusion: prevalence and clinicopathologic correlates in 89 consecutive patients with moderate to severe eosinophilia. Blood 2004;104:3038–45.

[5] Pitini V, Arrigo C, Azzarello D, et al. Serum concentration of cardiac troponin T in patients with hypereosinophilic syndrome treated with imatinib is predictive of adverse outcomes. Blood 2003;102:3456–7.

[6] Novartis. Gleevec. Available at: http://www.pharma.us.novartis.com/product/pi/pdf/gleevec_tabs.pdf. Accessed August 13, 2007.

[7] Seshadri T, Seymour JF, McArthur GA. Oligospermia in a patient receiving imatinib therapy for the hypereosinophilic syndrome. N Engl J Med 2004;351:2134–5.

[8] Klion AD, Robyn J, Akin C, et al. Molecular remission and reversal of myelofibrosis in response to imatinib mesylate treatment in patients with the myeloproliferative variant of hypereosinophilic syndrome. Blood 2004;103:473–8.

[9] Druker BJ, Guilhot F, O'Brien SG, et al. Five-year follow-up of patients receiving imatinib for chronic myeloid leukemia. N Engl J Med 2006;355:2408–17.

[10] Robyn J, Noel P, Wlodarska I, et al. Imatinib-responsive hypereosinophilia in a patient with B cell ALL. Leuk Lymphoma 2004;45:2497–501.

[11] von Bubnoff N, Sandherr M, Schlimok G, et al. Myeloid blast crisis evolving during imatinib treatment of an FIP1L1-PDGFR alpha-positive chronic myeloproliferative disease with prominent eosinophilia. Leukemia 2005;286–7.

[12] Ueno NT, Anagnostopoulos A, Rondon G, et al. Successful non-myeloablative allogeneic transplantation for treatment of idiopathic hypereosinophilic syndrome. Br J Haematol 2002;119:131–4.

[13] Klion AD, Bochner BS, Gleich GJ, et al. Approaches to the treatment of hypereosinophilic syndromes: a workshop summary report. J Allergy Clin Immunol 2006;117:1292–302.

[14] Recommendations for the prevention and treatment of glucocorticoid-induced osteoporosis: 2001 update. American College of Rheumatology Ad Hoc Committee on Glucocorticoid-Induced Osteoporosis. Arthritis Rheum 2001;44:1496–503.

[15] Klion AD, Law MA, Noel P, et al. Safety and efficacy of the monoclonal anti-interleukin 5 antibody, SCH55700, in the treatment of patients with the hypereosinophilic syndrome. Blood 2004;103:2939–41.

[16] Plötz SG, Simon HU, Darsow U, et al. Use of an anti-interleukin-5 antibody in the hypereosinophilic syndrome with eosinophilic dermatitis. N Engl J Med 2003;349:2334–9.

[17] Rothenberg M, Klion A, Roufosse F, et al. Corticosteroid reduction and clinical control in patients with hypereosinophilic syndrome treated with mepolizumab, an anti-interleukin-5 monoclonal antibody. Submitted for publication.

[18] Lossos IS, Matzner Y. Hydroxyurea-induced fever: case report and review of the literature. Ann Pharmacother 1995;29:132–3.

[19] Parrillo JE, Fauci AS, Wolff SM. Therapy of the hypereosinophilic syndrome. Ann Intern Med 1978;89:167–72.

[20] Butterfield JH, Gleich GJ. Interferon-α treatment of six patients with the idiopathic hypereosinophilic syndrome. Ann Intern Med 1994;121:648–53.

[21] Yoon TY, Ahn G-B, Chang S-H. Complete remission of hypereosinophilic syndrome after interferon-α therapy: report of a case and literature review. J Dermatol 2000;27:110–5.

[22] Demiroglu H, Dundar S. Combination of interferon-alpha and hydroxyurea in the treatment of idiopathic hypereosinophilic syndrome. Br J Haematol 1997;97:927–40.

[23] Garrett JK, Jameson SC, Thomson B, et al. Anti-interleukin-5 (mepolizumab) therapy for hypereosinophilic syndromes. J Allergy Clin Immunol 2003;113:115–9.

[24] Pardanani A, Reeder T, Porrata LF, et al. Imatinib therapy for hypereosinophilic syndrome and other eosinophilic disorders. Blood 2003;101:3391–7.

[25] Pitini V, Teti D, Arrigo C, et al. Alemtuzumab therapy for refractory idiopathic hypereosinophilic syndrome with abnormal T cells: a case report. Br J Haematol 2004;207:477.

[26] Schandene L, Roufosse F, de Lavareille A, et al. Interferon α prevents spontaneous apoptosis of clonal T2 cells associated wit chronic hypereosinophilia. Blood 2000;13:4285–92.

[27] Roufosse F, Cogan E, Goldman M. Recent advances in the pathogenesis and management of hypereosinophilic syndromes. Allergy 2004;59:673–89.

**ELSEVIER
SAUNDERS**

Immunol Allergy Clin N Am
27 (2007) 561–570

IMMUNOLOGY
AND ALLERGY
CLINICS
OF NORTH AMERICA

Index

Note: Page numbers of article titles are in **boldface** type.

0889-8561/07/$ - see front matter © 2007 Elsevier Inc. All rights reserved.
doi:10.1016/S0889-8561(07)00074-4   *immunology.theclinics.com*

Moving?

Make sure your subscription moves with you!

To notify us of your new address, find your **Clinics Account Number** (located on your mailing label above your name), and contact customer service at:

E-mail: elspcs@elsevier.com

800-654-2452 (subscribers in the U.S. & Canada)
407-345-4000 (subscribers outside of the U.S. & Canada)

Fax number: 407-363-9661

Elsevier Periodicals Customer Service
6277 Sea Harbor Drive
Orlando, FL 32887-4800

*To ensure uninterrupted delivery of your subscription, please notify us at least 4 weeks in advance of move.